Mathematical Methods for DNA Sequences

Editor
Michael S. Waterman, Ph.D.
Professor of Mathematics and Molecular Biology
University of Southern California
Los Angeles, California

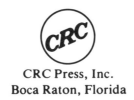

CRC Press, Inc.
Boca Raton, Florida

LIBRARY OF CONGRESS
Library of Congress Cataloging-in-Publication Data
Mathematical methods for DNA sequences / editor, Michael S. Waterman.
   p.   cm.
   Includes bibliographies and index.
   ISBN 0-8493-6664-X
   1. Nucleotide sequence—Mathematical models. 2. Nucleotide sequence—
Statistical methods. 3. Nucleotide sequence—Data processing. I. Waterman, Michael S.
QP624.M37   1989
574.87'322—dc 19   88-6336
CIP

Direct all inquires to CRC Press, Inc., 2000 Corporate Blvd., N.W., Boca Raton, Florida, 33431.

©1989 by CRC Press, Inc.

International Standard Book Number 0-8493-6664-X

Library of Congress Card Number 88-6336
Printed in the United States

PREFACE

The modern era of molecular biology began with the celebrated discovery in 1953 by Watson and Crick of the double helical structure of DNA. This revolution in biology has created a large body of fundamental data by directly reading DNA sequences. These data are taken from various regions of a large variety of genomes and include the complete sequences of several viruses and mitochondria. Rapid sequencing began about 10 years ago and the rate of DNA sequencing, measured in nucleotides per year, continues to accelerate. Currently over 2×10^7 nucleotides are entered into databases in approximately 1.7×10^3 entries, and sequencing is proceeding at more than 7×10^6 nucleotides per year. Partly as a consequence of reading the genetic material DNA, molecular biologists have made an astounding number of fundamental discoveries about biology. These discoveries include introns which interrupt protein coding regions, self-splicing RNAs, reverse transcription and pseudogenes, and identification of oncogenes and their mutant forms which cause cancer in humans. The molecular details of regulation, growth, and development are beginning to be understood. The entire AIDS virus sequence was known shortly after it was discovered. Ten years ago this would have been impossible. Biologists are now looking ahead to projects to map and sequence entire genomes.

While the field of molecular biology is primarily experimental and advances are based on observations of specific biological systems, there is an associated development of mathematical, statistical, and computer methods. This new branch of applied mathematics is rapidly gaining importance. As soon as DNA began to be sequenced, many individuals began to collect various subsets of the data and to design algorithms and software to analyze the new sequences. The computer revolution and the revolution in biology occurred at about the same time, much to the good fortune of those who have become involved with DNA sequence data. Computer sequence analysis seems to be everywhere today; in most biology centers there is someone, usually referred to as "the computer person", who performs tasks from making restriction maps of known sequences to the prediction of structure of proteins. Some of these analyses, often the most essential for the working molecular biologist, are mathematically elementary and involve straightforward algorithms. Others, such as reliable prediction of protein structure from amino acid sequences, are beyond current methods of mathematics and computer science.

The theme of this book is the new area of mathematical methods for DNA sequences. While molecular evolution could be included under this title since it has mathematical content and relates to sequences, it is a thriving field and has been treated elsewhere. The subjects of these chapters are in their infancy; it is even true that the mathematical content is not always deep, but I feel that in every case the work is motivated by real biological data and problems.

Since DNA sequence data motivate the mathematical work, the completeness, accuracy, organization, flexibility, and annotation of the data bases are essential to the research described in this book. The two major data bases were begun quite recently. In 1982, both the European Molecular Biology Laboratory (EMBL) at Heidelburg and the National Institutes of Health (NIH) in the U.S. established nucleic acids sequence databases. Japan has now joined this international effort. There are over 2×10^7 nucleotides in the databases and perhaps 10^7 sequenced nucleotides not yet entered. In simple terms of volume of nucleotides, what is the prospect for the near future? Currently, a skilled worker can sequence perhaps 1000 nucleotides per day at a cost of approximately $1 per nucleotide. Automated machines are already available which can increase the rate to about 5000 nucleotides per day. Under development are machines which might sequence 3×10^5 nucleotides per day with a goal of 10^6 nucleotides per day at a cost of 10¢ per nucleotide. Other promising approaches such as multiplex sequencing are also being tested. The data explosion in molecular biology has just begun!

Consider the massive task of organizing this important data into a useful database. First of all, the data must be entered into a computer. Alas, even in these days of the ubiquitous personal computer, the sequences do not always come to GenBank or EMBL on tape or floppy disks. Instead, some sequences still must be found in the literature and transcribed. In addition, many important decisions must be made about which biological features to describe in the database. The descriptions and their accuracy are essential to an informed use of the sequences. Of course, the importance of various features changes as the science matures, and features unheard of today will be essential tomorrow. One natural way to organize the sequences is by taxonomy or evolutionary relationships. We are learning that evolution is much more complex than previously imagined so that taxonomic classifications are also subject to change and to become more complicated.

We are fortunate to have Fickett and Burks, two GenBank workers, to discuss these issues in depth in Chapter 1. This is by no means a closed subject! One difficulty that does not seem solved is the vital one of software to allow easy access to the data. It is essential for a user to address the data in a language based on the biological features. Until the data are accessible in this natural way, users will be forced to write awkward interfaces between their analysis programs and the databases. In the near future we expect to have one international DNA data base with a database management system.

At the heart of the techniques of genetic engineering is a class of proteins known as restriction enzymes. They are essential to our ability to map, sequence, and manipulate DNA. These enzymes were evolved by bacteria to protect themselves against invading DNA, such as viruses. The restriction enzymes of interest here (known as type II enzymes) cut the invading DNA at the positions of short specific patterns called restriction sites; the enzymes do not cut the host DNA where these patterns occur due to modification (methylation) of the DNA. Several hundred restriction enzymes have been isolated and most are routinely available. The importance to biology of these enzymes cannot be overemphasized.

Chapter 2 by Lander treats several interesting mathematical problems arising from the biologist's use of restriction enzymes. First, he considers the statistical distribution of restriction sites along a long DNA molecule. Even if we assume the nucleotides are independent and identically distributed, the intuition of geometric waiting times between occurrences of a given site is not always valid. This is because some restriction sites can have overlapping occurrences, such as the four-letter site GCGC. The enzyme will cut GCGCGC which has two occurrences only once; therefore, the waiting time between cuts is increased. When combinations of enzymes are used, the problem becomes more complex. The nucleotides are statistically dependent, also complicating the distribution theory. Still, satisfactory answers have been given.

Lander next considers mapping the location of restriction sites on a sample of unsequencing DNA. Such a map is referred to as a physical map. The data are approximate fragment lengths of digested DNA. In the simplest problem, two enzymes are used alone and then together to obtain a total of three length sets from the three digests. Using these sets of lengths, the problem is to order the sites on a map which is consistent with the digest data. This is computationally a very difficult problem, known in computer science as an NP-complete problem. In addition, there are an exponentially increasing number of solutions as DNA length increases, only one of which is correct. Biologists routinely solve this problem, simply by changing enzymes or problem size when they are not certain of their answer. Most are unaware that they are working near such mathematically dangerous ground.

Very large genome sized samples of DNa can be mapped by first making a partial digest of the DNA, cutting each copy of the DNA at some, but not all, sites. Then the fragments within a certain size range can be cloned into what is called a DNA library. A ntural requisiste for a complete map is the inclusion in the library of all segments of genomic DNA. The statistical properties of sampling the clones from the library is important to the map construction. Lander describes what is known about this distribution.

Identification of genes which are associated with certain human diseases is of great interest in both the popular and scientific press. Some mutations in genomic DNA cause restriction fragment length polymorphisms (RFLPs) and these mutations are used as tools to trace inheritance of genetic traits. More generally, RFLPs can be used to make what is called a genetic linkage map of large regions of DNA. The human genome is being mapped at increasingly fine scale by these methods. Any advance in this area is big news; Lander reports on the methods and includes some recent results. This area will continue to attract our attention as more of the genes involved in well-known diseases are mapped.

Sequence comparison is a popular computer activity and many papers have been written about mathematical and algorithmic aspects. Sequence comparisons are needed for the detection of common structure and function as well as for studies of evolutionary relationships. I have written Chapters 3 and 4 on sequence alignment and consensus patterns.

The sequence alignments considered here are based on an explicit optimization function which rewards matches and penalizes mismatches, insertions, and deletions. Such alignments are known as similarity alignments. (Sequence alignments based on metric distance are not always as general as similarity alignments.) The two major problems are (1) alignment of full sequences and (2) finding segments of sequence that can be well aligned. While full sequence alignment is a problem of interest when protein evolution is being studied as, for example, cytochrome-c sequences.Current studies view the genome as a mosaic of variously sized blocks of DNA. Therefore, to detect evolutionary relationships and important homologies, it is essential to search for well-matched sequence segments. Both these problems can be approached with dynamic programming algorithms. If a great many comparisons are to be made or if more than two sequences are to be compared, then dynamic programming is usually too expensive in terms of time. Hashing techniques have been used, especially for database searches where they have been responsible for the discovery of unexpected homologies. Some lack of precision in hashing methods arises from difficulties with including insertions and deletions. A new algorithm based on consensus sequence analysis solves the problem of aligning several sequences. Consensus methods are discussed below, but a dynamic programming algorithm is coupled with the basic consensus pattern calculation to achieve a multiple alignment.

No matter how a sequence alignment is obtained, the question of statistical significance comes up. The idea is to study how unlikely a certain alignment is. If explicit alignment criteria are given and the sequences are assumed to be generated from a statistical model, this is a very well-posed problem. Some recent elegant results in probability theory relate this problem to the extreme value distribution and shed new light on these problems. Karlin et al. in Chapter 6 further treat this approach in depth, enlarging the scope of pattern considered. In the alignment and consensus chapters (3 and 4), significance of alignments is also considered.

Consensus sequence analysis is based on the idea that functionally important sequence features are conserved in the sequence while other portions of the sequence are free to evolve. An important example of consensus patterns occurs in promoter sequences where the consensus patterns are protein binding sites. These patterns are not precise in sequence location or in sequence pattern. The basic mathematical problem is to find unknown patterns that occur imperfectly in a set of several sequences. Neither dynamic programming nor hashing techniques work for this problem. Frequently, a large number of sequences must be examined before the consensus pattern can be determined. Even though the number of alignments is huge, a new technique has been derived to rapidly find consensus patterns of up to ten letters. The limitation on pattern size is due to limited computer storage, not time. Sometimes protein binding patterns are approximately palindromic in nature, so that the pattern is made up of an inverted, complimentary repeat. Knowing more about the pattern's nature gives us the added power to find weaker patterns. These analyses can be extended to find imperfect repeats along a single sequence. When the patterns of interest are too long for these methods, the set of possible consensus patterns must be reduced and a new, less elegant algorithm employed. Many statistical and algorithm issues remain to be resolved in this important area.

Many papers have been written about the statistical properties of DNA and protein sequences. Motivation comes in part from a desire to characterize functional domains by statistical properties. Some of the studies have been weak statistically, and moreover, the initial hopes for characterization of important domains seems to have been overly optimistic. Still, the studies continue and very interesting features are sometimes revealed. Tavaré and Giddings discuss statistical techniques for DNA sequences in Chapter 5. They give a new approach to modeling DNA sequences by Markov chain models. Earlier approaches were not able to test for higher order dependence due to the relatively short sequence lengths. They also present the first DNA sequence analysis that uses Walsh transforms to discover periodicities.

The useful Chapter 6 of Karlin, Ost, and Blaisdell gives a broad treatment of the statistical properties of a variety of patterns in sequences. Theoretical significance measures are given for the length of long patterns common to two or more sequences. These results relate to the sequence alignments discussed above. In addition, long repeats with two or more occurrences in a single sequence are treated as well as long dyad symmetries and other long runs. An approach to alignment can be based on significant repeated patterns between sequences. Extensions to first order Markov dependence are outlined. What is especially nice about the presentation is the variety of biological examples, the variety of patterns, and the variety of statistical models.

The three-dimensional form of biological molecules is an important determinant of their function. Single-stranded RNAs fold onto themselves making various helices which we refer to as secondary structure. If free energies are assigned to the base pairs, end loops, bulges, interior loops, and multibranch loops, then the analytical problem is to find the minimum free energy secondary structure of an RNA with known sequence. The problem often comes up and the program of choice is by Zuker, who has written Chapter 7 about the dynamic programming method of prediction. The graphs associated with secondary structures are very pretty, and Zuker also discusses those. The algorithms are a nice modification of those used in sequence alignment, although they are quite a bit more complex. Zuker's approach, using special assumptions about the energy functions, implements an algorithm which runs in time proportional to n^3 where n is sequence length. Recently, a fairly general version of a problem was shown to have a polynomial time algorithm; until then, the best general result had exponential time.

Frequently these algorithms do not find the correct structure, that is, the one used by the cell. This can happen because of the more complex environment of biological systems, as well as our incomplete knowledge of the energy functions. Still, the biologically correct structure is likely to have a (model) free energy close to the minimum, so it is an appealing idea to search the structure neighborhood of the minimum. It was only recently that it became practical to produce all solutions in a neighborhood of the minimum for a dynamic programming algorithm. The drawback for secondary structure is that a huge number of structures are in a small neighborhood, many with only slight differences. Zuker gives us a way to approach this problem.

In multiple sequence alignment, the sequence set can be aligned by matching words. Sets of RNAs can have a common secondary structure and the structure can be deduced by matching helices rather than by base pairs. I give in Chapter 8 the first description of RNA folding on a computer by a consensus method. The consensus patterns here are helices and the search becomes quadratic in time due to the choice of the two helix locations along the sequence. Initially, the sequences are aligned by their ends or by other sequence features. As the folding proceeds, the sequence set can be realigned on the helices that are formed. The basic ideas motivating the analytical work are due to Woese and Noller, who, essentially by hand, found consensus foldings of large rRNA molecules. The new computer method is successful, folding the entire set of *E. coli* tRNA molecules into the correct cloverleaf shape. As in any of these sequence analyses, it is important only to accept statistically significant results.

Much of this volume deals with nucleic acids as words over a four-letter alphabet. In reality, DNA exists as a complex, three-dimensional structure. In Chapter 9, White treats the geometry and topology of closed, circular DNA. His famous formula relates the linking number (Lk) to twist (Tw) and writhing (Wr) by Lk = Tw + Wr. Lk is a topological property that is invariant (unchanged) under continuous deformation of the DNA. Both Tw and Wr are geometric quantities.

While biologists sometimes treat the quantities in White's formula in an elementary way, the concepts are actually much more subtle. White gives us a guided tour of the subject, with several perspectives on the fundamental quantities. First, linking numbers are defined by crossing numbers, then by surface intersection, and finally by the Gauss map and its associated integral. Then the writhing number is defined by crossing numbers as well as the Gauss map and its integral. After taking us through his basic formula, White then applies the mathematical results to study structural aspects of DNA. Twist and writhing numbers are computed for several situations, including DNA wound around a nucleosome. The analysis of enzymatic action is very nice, especially that concerning the actions of types I and II topoisomerases.

Recent applications of knot theory allow the analysis of catenated DNA but are not treated here. The results from knot theory have attracted a great deal of attention and seem to have begun a new era of applications of mathematics to DNA.

With Benham's Chapter 10, we turn from the geometry and topology to the mechanics of superhelical DNA. This author's approach is to analyze conformational equilibria. Here we see the local conformations of superhelical DNA changing between the B-form, A-form, and the left-handed Z-form. Many regulatory events depend on DNA conformation so that these structural transitions are very important.

This is a realm of classical applied mathematics. DNA is modeled as a symmetric, linearly elastic rod. It is possible in this context to bring the effects of individual base pairs into play. Z-form DNA, for example, is frequently composed of alternating purine-pyrimidines. Benham constructs partition functions and uses statistical mechanics to study equilibria of superhelical DNA, of secondary structure, and of tertiary structure. An important future direction for this research is to include kinetics. How do the transitions occur and how rapidly are the equilibria reached?

The future of this subject is dependent on progress in molecular biology and on the cooperation between the mathematical sciences and biology. Computational methods become more important to biology as the amount of data increases. There has recently been much talk of sequencing the human genome of about 3×10^9 nucleotides. There are already projects underway to make both genetic and physical maps of various chromosomes. *E. coli* has recently been physically mapped and other bacterial genomes will soon follow. *E. coli* will probably be sequenced in a few years. In the near future, the sequencing rate will increase by one or two orders of magnitude because of improved sequencing technology, including multiplex sequencing and robotics. Sequence and map information at the genomic level will become commonplace. Precisely what analytical questions will be posed by the new data is not yet clear. Certainly it will be a serious and exciting challenge to organize and analyze this explosion of information.

THE EDITOR

Michael S. Waterman, Ph.D. is Professor of Mathematics and Molecular Biology, University of Southern California, Los Angeles. Dr. Waterman earned his B.S. and M.S. in Mathematics at Oregon State University in 1964 and 1966 and an M.A. and a Ph.D. in Statistics at Michigan State University in 1968 and 1969. He was both Assistant and Associate Professor at Idaho State University from 1969 to 1975. He left in July 1975 to serve as a staff member and eventually Project Leader at Los Alamos National Laboratory. In 1982, Dr. Waterman accepted his current position at USC. In addition to these duties, he has also worked as a consultant to Energy Incorporated, visiting professor at the University of Hawaii, and visiting research professor of structural biology at UC San Francisco.

Dr. Waterman has received the following awards and grants: National Science Foundation (NSF) trainee, Michigan State University; AWU Faculty Participant, Los Alamos National Laboratory; Outstanding Educator of America Award (1971 and 1972); NSF research grants (1971, 1972, 1975); New Research Initiatives Award from Director's Office, Los Alamos National Laboratory (1976 and 1981); Outstanding Presentations Award of the SPES section of the American Statistical Association (1977); National Institutes of Health Research Grants (1980, 1981, 1986—1988); and System Development Foundation Grants (1982—1987).

His other professional activities include Collaborator, Center for Prokaryotic Gene Analysis, University of Illinois (1987 to present); Advisory Board, Center for Mathematics and Molecular Biology at UC Berkeley (1987 to present); International Advisory Committee for Nucleotide Databases, NIH (1988 to present); Advisory Board, Protein Identification Resource, Georgetown University (1988 to present); and NIH Special Review Committee (1988 to present).

He has worked in an editorial capacity on the journals *Bulletin of Mathematical Biology, Journal of Molecular Biology and Evolution, Advances in Applied Mathematics*, and *Genomics* and has authored or coauthored over 100 articles, book chapters, and reports.

Dr. Waterman is a member of the Institute of Mathematical Statistics, the American Association for the Advancement of Science, the American Statistics Association, the Society for Mathematical Biology, and the Society for Industrial and Applied Mathematics.

CONTRIBUTORS

Craig Benham, Ph.D.
Biomath Sci
Mount Sinai School of Medicine
New York, New York

B. Edwin Blaisdell, Ph.D.
Linus Pauling Institute of Science and
Medicine
Palo Alto, California

Christian Burks, Ph.D.
Theoretical Biology and Biophysics
Los Alamos National Laboratory
Los Alamos, New Mexico

James W. Fickett, Ph.D.
Theoretical Biology and Biophysics
Los Alamos National Laboratory
Los Alamos, New Mexico

Barton W. Giddings, Ph.D.
Department of Biology
Massachusetts Institute of Technology
Cambridge, Massachusetts

Samuel Karlin, Ph.D.
Department of Mathematics
Stanford University
Stanford, California

Eric S. Lander, Ph.D.
Whitehead Institute for Biomedical
  Research
Cambridge, Massachusetts

Friedemann Ost, Ph.D.
Technische Universtität
München, BRD

Simon Tavaré, Ph.D.
Department of Mathematics
University of Utah
Salt Lake City, Utah

Michael S. Waterman, Ph.D.
Department of Mathematics
University of Southern California
Los Angeles, California

James White, Ph.D.
Professor
Department of Mathematics
University of California
Los Angeles, California

Michael Zuker, Ph.D.
Research Officer
Division of Biological Sciences
National Research Council
Ottawa, Ontario, Canada

TABLE OF CONTENTS

Chapter 1

DEVELOPMENT OF A DATABASE FOR NUCLEOTIDE SEQUENCES

James W. Fickett and Christian Burks

TABLE OF CONTENTS

I. INTRODUCTION

The appearance of DNA sequence data is nothing less than revolutionary. For the first time we are gaining a look at the most fundamental determinant of biological reality. Furthermore, our knowledge is increasing at a dizzying rate: only 10 years after the appearance of efficient DNA-sequencing methods[1,2] it is common to see yet another report of the complete sequence of a viral genome (see Table 1). The first complete bacterial genomic sequence may be done over the next few years, and there is serious talk of a concentrated effort to sequence all 24 human chromosomes.

What will we have when these sequences are determined? What do we have now in the 10 million nucleotide of sequence data determined to date? We are in the position of Johann Kepler when he first began looking for patterns in the volumes of data that Tycho Brahe had spent his life accumulating. We have the program that runs the cellular machinery, but we know very little about how to read it. Bench biologists, by experiment and by close association with the data, have found meaningful patterns. Theoreticians, by careful reasoning and use of collections of data, have found others, but we still understand frustratingly little.

Computer analysis can greatly aid our understanding of these data. The sequences are often meaningless to the human eye; there is abundant evidence that humans cannot even copy over a DNA sequence without making frequent errors. Patterns that seem significant

Table 1
COMPLETELY SEQUENCED GENOMES

Organism[a]	Genome type[b]	Sequence length[c]	Accession no.[d]
Organelles			
Mouse mitochondrion	ds-DNA, circular	16295	J01420
Bovine mitochondrion	ds-DNA, circular	16338	J01394
Human mitochondrion	ds-DNA, circular	16569	J01415
X. laevis mitochondrion	ds-DNA, circular	17553	M10217
Eukaryotic plasmids			
S. cerevisiae 2 μm plasmid	ds-DNA, circular	6318	J01347
K. lactis K1 plasmid	ds-DNA, circular	8874	X00762
Prokaryotic plasmids			
pSN2	ds-DNA, circular	1288	J01763
pC194	ds-DNA, circular	2910	J01754
pBR327	ds-DNA, circular	3273	J02549
pE194	ds-DNA, circular	3728	J01755
pVH51	ds-DNA, circular	3847	K03114
pBR329	ds-DNA, circular	4150	J01753
pJD1	ds-DNA, circular	4207	M10316
pBR322	ds-DNA, circular	4363	J01749
pT181	ds-DNA, circular	4437	J01764
ColE1	ds-DNA, circular	6646	J01566
RSC13	ds-DNA, circular	7894	J01783
Animal viruses			
Duck hepatitis B virus	ms-DNA, circular	3021	K01834
Human hepatitis B virus (ayw)	ms-DNA, circular	3182	J02203
Human hepatitis B virus (adr)	ms-DNA, circular	3188	V00867
Human hepatitis B virus (adw)	ms-DNA, circular	3200	V00866
Woodchuck hepatitis virus (WHV1)	ms-DNA, circular	3308	J02442
Woodchuck hepatitis virus (WHV2)	ms-DNA, circular	3320	M11082
Ground squirrel hepatitis virus	ms-DNA, circular	3311	K02715
Avian sarcoma virus Y73	ss-RNA, linear	3718	J02027
FBR murine osteosarcoma virus	ss-RNA, linear	3791[e]	K02712
FBJ murine osteosarcoma virus	ss-RNA, linear	4026[e]	J02084
Black beetle virus	ss-RNA, 2 linear segments	4504	K02560
Adeno-associated virus 2	ss-DNA, linear	4675	J01901
Fujinami sarcoma virus	ss-RNA, linear	4788[e]	J02194
Human polyomavirus BK (MM)	ds-DNA, circular	4963	J02039
Minute virus of mice	ss-DNA, linear	5081	J02275
Human polyomavirus JC	ds-DNA, circular	5130	J02226
Human polyomavirus BK (Dunlop)	ds-DNA, circular	5153	J02038
Parvovirus H1	ss-DNA, linear	5176	J02198
Simian virus 40	ds-DNA, circular	5243	J02400
Lymphotropic papovavirus	ds-DNA, circular	5270	K02562
Polyoma virus (a3)	ds-DNA, circular	5296	J02289
Polyoma virus (a2)	ds-DNA, circular	5297	J02288
Simian sarcoma virus	ss-RNA, linear	5319[e]	J02394
Crawford small-plaque polyomavirus	ds-DNA, circular	5350	K02737
Abelson murine leukemia virus	ss-RNA, linear	5659[e]	J02009
Moloney murine sarcoma virus (1)	ss-RNA, linear	5828[e]	J02266
Moloney murine sarcoma virus (124)	ss-RNA, linear	5833[e]	J02263
Spleen focus-forming virus	ss-RNA, linear	6296[e]	K00021
Human rhinovirus type 14	ss-RNA, linear	7212	K02121
Poliovirus type 3	ss-RNA, linear	7431	K01392
Poliovirus type 3 attenuated	ss-RNA, linear	7432	K00043

Table 1 (continued)
COMPLETELY SEQUENCED GENOMES

Organism[a]	Genome type[b]	Sequence length[c]	Accession no.[d]
Poliovirus type 1	ss-RNA, linear	7440	J02281
Poliovirus type 1 attenuated	ss-RNA, linear	7441	V01150
Human hepatitis A virus	ss-RNA, linear	7478	K02990
Human papillomavirus 1A	ds-DNA, circular	7811	V01116
Cottontail rabbit papillomavirus	ds-DNA, circular	7868	K02708
Human papillomavirus 6b	ds-DNA, circular	7902	X00203
Human papillomavirus type 16	ds-DNA, circular	7904	K02718
Bovine papillomavirus type 1	ds-DNA, circular	7945	J02044
Maloney murine leukemia virus	ss-RNA, linear	8332	J02255
AKV murine leukemia virus	ss-RNA, linear	8371	J01998
Bovine leukemia virus	ss-RNA, linear	8714	K02120
Human T-cell leukemia virus type II	ss-RNA, linear	8952[e]	M10060
Human T-cell leukemia virus type I	ss-RNA, linear	9032[e]	J02029
Lymphadenopathy-associated virus[f]	ss-RNA, linear	9193	K02013
Visna lentivirus	ss-RNA, linear	9202	M10608
Rous sarcoma virus	ss-RNA, linear	9625[e]	J02342
AIDS-associated virus-2[f]	ss-RNA, linear	9737[e]	K02007
Human T-cell leukemia virus type III[f]	ss-RNA, linear	9751[e]	K02083
Yellow fever virus	ss-RNA, linear	10862	K02749
Vesicular stomatitis virus	ss-RNA, linear	11162	J02428
Sindbis virus	ss-RNA, linear	11703	J02363
Influenza type A	ss-RNA, 8 linear segments	13588	J02143
Adenovirus 2	ds-DNA, linear	35937	J01917
Epstein-Barr virus	ds-DNA, linear	172282	V01555
Plant viruses			
Coconut cadang-cadang viroid (fast)	ss-RNA, circular	246	J02050
Avocado sunblotch viroid	ss-RNA, circular	247	J02020
Coconut cadang-cadang viroid (slow)	ss-RNA, circular	287	J02051
Hop stunt viroid	ss-RNA, circular	297	X00009
Cucumber pale fruit viroid	ss-RNA, circular	303	X00524
Chrysanthemum stunt viroid (CSV2)	ss-RNA, circular	354	M19506
Chrysanthemum stunt viroid (CSV1)	ss-RNA, circular	356	M19505
Potato spindle tuber viroid	ss-RNA, circular	359	J02287
Tomato apical stunt viroid	ss-RNA, circular	360	K00818
Tomato planta macho viroid	ss-RNA, circular	360	K00817
Citrus exocortis viroid (C)	ss-RNA, circular	371	J02053
Citrus exocortis viroid (DE25)	ss-RNA, circular	371	K00964
Citrus exocortis viroid (DE26)	ss-RNA, circular	371	K00965
Satellite tobacco necrosis virus	ss-RNA, linear	1239	J02399
Maize streak virus	ss-DNA, circular	2687	K02026
Tomato golden mosaic virus	ss-DNA, 2 circular segments	5096	K02030
Bean golden mosaic virus	ss-DNA, 2 circular segments	5233	M10070
Cassava latent virus	ss-DNA, 2 circular segments	5503	J02057
Tobacco mosaic virus (vulgare)	ss-RNA, linear	6395	J02415
Cauliflower mosaic virus (D/H Hungary)	ds-DNA, circular	8016	J02047
Cauliflower mosaic virus (Strasbourg)	ds-DNA, circular	8024	J02048
Cauliflower mosaic virus (CM1841)	ds-DNA, circular	8031	J02046
Brome mosaic virus	ss-RNA, 3 linear segments	8213	K02706
Alfalfa mosaic virus	ss-RNA, 3 linear segments	8274	J02000
Cowpea mosaic virus	ss-RNA, 2 linear segments	9370	X00206
Bacteriophage			
MS2	ss-RNA, linear	3569	J02467
φX174	ss-DNA, circular	5386	J02482

Table 1 (continued)
COMPLETELY SEQUENCED GENOMES

Organism[a]	Genome type[b]	Sequence length[c]	Accession no.[d]
G4	ss-DNA, circular	5577	J02454
f1	ss-DNA, circular	6407	J02448
M13	ss-DNA, circular	6407	J02461
fd	ss-DNA, circular	6408	J02451
IKe	ss-DNA, circular	6883	K02750
T7	ds-DNA, linear	39936	J02518
λ	ds-DNA, circular	48502	J02459

[a] Based on the May 1986 release (#42.0) of the database. The strains are indicated (in parentheses) only when more than one complete strain is known.
[b] ds, double-stranded; ms, mixed single- and double-stranded; ss, single-stranded.
[c] Length given in units of nucleotides.
[d] The number given is the primary GenBank/EMBL accession number; for genomes spread over several entries, only one entry's number is given.
[e] This length represents the cellular proviral form of the virus, which is slightly longer than the virion form.
[f] There is evidence that these viruses, though named differently, are actually variant strains of the same virus.

when one person looks at five or ten genes often turn out to be the result of random variation when a larger scale analysis is carried out.

To make these data available for significant analysis, one must first gather and organize them into a comprehensive database. Although several specialized computer collections of nucleic acid sequence data are mentioned briefly, our primary focus in this chapter is on general applications of the data and on comprehensive collections. We know of only two data banks currently attempting comprehensive coverage of nucleotide sequence data: the GenBank* *gen*etic sequence data *bank* in the U.S., and the data bank at EMBL (European Molecular Biology Laboratory at Heidelberg, West Germany). We will describe one approach, undertaken by the GenBank staff at LANL (Los Alamos National Laboratory), to the development of a database that does justice to the natural structure of the data, facilitates current applications, and allows expansion for the foreseeable future. Of course, this development has benefited considerably from close collaboration and many discussions both with our colleagues on the GenBank project at BBN (BBN Laboratories, Inc.) and with our colleagues at EMBL.

II. HISTORICAL BACKGROUND

A. A New Kind of Data

Only 10 years ago, our knowledge of genomic structure at the molecular level was limited to the order of a few genes relative to one another. Today sequencing of nucleic acids, the determination of genetic information at the most fundamental level, is a major tool of biological research. In fact, since all biological processes are believed to have determinants encoded in nucleotide sequences, there are few areas of the biological sciences where investigators are not addressing major problems by isolating and sequencing nucleic acids (*Science,* for example, has published several issues with collections of articles illustrating this point[3-6]).

In 1978, when sequencing was a new tool, about 200 articles appeared reporting nucleotide sequences. Now that sequencing is routine, dedicated laboratories can generate up to 1000 nucleotides per day per skilled technician and about 2500 articles per year, and report roughly 2 million nucleotides of new sequence data. The nucleic acids being sequenced span the range of known functions: protein coding, structural RNA coding, and regulatory regions of DNA, as well as messenger RNA and several species of structural RNA. Furthermore, regions whose functions are as yet unknown are increasingly being sequenced.

B. Need for Computer Storage and Analysis

It was already clear in the late 1970s that nucleic acid sequencing would become a major tool of biological research. As the volume of data rapidly mounted (the number of papers publishing nucleotide sequences almost doubled between 1978 and 1979, and again from 1979 to 1980; see Appendix I), many people observed that a computer-based data bank would be needed to fully exploit it.

The great advantage of a centralized repository is that information fragmented in the literature can be assembled for easier access and comprehension. For example, the GenBank entry HUMHBB (GenBank/EMBL accession number J00179) is a synthesis of information from 74 articles, spanning a region of 73,360 nucleotides. It gives an overview of the entire human locus for β-like globin genes and pseudogenes, and probably for all of their proximal control elements. A centralized repository can present the most correct view of the data by keeping track of published and unpublished corrections and by communicating with the authors when the acts of gathering, comparing, and distributing the data uncover inconsistencies.

Computers offer a natural and highly effective means for making sequence comparisons and for searching sequences for meaningful patterns; moreover, by far the most facile means of transmitting sequence data at a tolerable error rate is on electronic data processing media. Thus it was clear from the beginning that the centralized repository should be computer based. A well-designed computer database also allows the data to be reorganized and displayed in various ways for different purposes. Printed copy adapted to visual scanning is just as easily produced as derived amino acid sequences, based on the genes specified in the nucleic acid data.

In the long run, computer networks will allow significant interactions among widely separated databases, and supercomputers will allow large scale analyses (e.g., database-wide complex pattern searches) and simulations (e.g., of the simultaneous regulation of thousands of genes in a changing environment).

C. From Pilot Projects to the Current Scene

Needs and opportunities were first explored in a 1979 meeting at Rockefeller University sponsored by the National Science Foundation and, subsequently, at workshops organized by EMBL in Europe, and by the NIH (National Institutes of Health) in the U.S. A number of groups in the U.S., Europe, Israel, and Japan were active in developing and applying computer methods for handling and analyzing sequence data, and several of these were actively collecting and organizing the data. Most of the pilot projects (several of which continue as independent databases) covered specialized domains; a well-known example is the tRNA sequence database,[7] published annually in a supplement to *Nucleic Acids Research*.

These efforts, in conjunction with much work and discussion within the molecular biology community, and the support of both the NIH in the U.S. and EMBL in Europe, have led to an international effort to collect, organize, and make available all nucleotide sequence data in computer-readable form.

In the spring of 1982, the EMBL Nucleotide Sequence Data Library issued its first collection. In July 1982, the National Institute of General Medical Sciences and several co-sponsors established the GenBank database, with LANL collecting and organizing the data, and BBN making it available to the public. GenBank began making monthly releases in

October 1982. Current co-sponsors of GenBank are the National Institute of General Medical Sciences, the National Cancer Institute, the National Institute of Allergy and Infectious Diseases, the National Institute of Arthritis, Diabetes, Digestive and Kidney Diseases, the Division of Research Resources of NIH, the National Library of Medicine, the National Science Foundation, the Department of Energy, and the Department of Defense. For recent announcements of the databases, see the articles by Hamm and Cameron[8] and Bilofsky et al.[9]

Throughout this period, the spirit of various national groups collecting sequence data has been one of friendly cooperation. The EMBL-GenBank collaboration is discussed in detail in several places below.

III. CONCEPTUAL VIEW OF THE DATABASE

This section deals with the abstract design of a comprehensive nucleotide sequence database (at the conceptual level, the GenBank and EMBL databases are essentially identical, and this section makes no distinction between them). We discuss the selection of information for the database and how the information is most naturally arranged in entries and fields, but not the methods for physically storing, transmitting, or retrieving the data. In standard database terminology,[10] this section is concerned with the external and conceptual views of the database. Section IV deals with the physical organization of the data.

A. Data Covered
1. Sources of the Data

The information in GenBank is drawn primarily from articles reporting original sequence data in biological journals. Journals publishing at least 12 sequence papers per year are covered systematically; sequences published in other journals, books, symposium proceedings, and theses are generally included only if brought to our attention by a citation in an article we do cover, or by an author. Unpublished data that are contributed directly by the authors are also included (and clearly marked as unpublished). Papers which report facts about sequences, but do not report new sequence data per se, are sometimes included, but are not covered systematically.

The GenBank charter is to collect all published nucleotide sequences greater than 50 nucleotides in length. The size restriction is used, with discretion, to eliminate fragmentary data such as RNAase-generated oligonucleotides that have not been combined into a longer sequence or groups of variants formed by site-directed mutagenesis.

Not all the information in the entries is from the articles that report sequences. When original articles are unavailable, secondary sources (e.g., published collections) are sometimes used. Data in the published articles are often supplemented by information taken from standard reference works on taxonomy, genetic maps, biochemical nomenclature, and the like.

2. What to Include

The primary data are, of course, the nucleotide sequences. Next, each sequence needs to be accompanied by identifying information of both a biological and bibliographical nature. The biological definition is comprised of the biological setting — the source organism, the location in the genome, the means of isolation — and the biological function, if known. The bibliographical definition is the citation information necessary to locate the sources of the data. For the database to be a serious analytical tool, it also needs to present enough of the biological context to make the sequence meaningful. Thus, it must include full information on the products encoded by the nucleotide sequences as well as all known information on the biological function of regions of the sequence. Henceforth we shall use the term "annotation'' to mean all the information accompanying the sequence other than the sequence itself.

Since the database is intended to portray biological reality, we ordinarily try to include all the data associated with the sequence that is of proven biological relevance, but we do not ordinarily include conjectural or evaluative information. The sites along the sequence that most journal articles present provide a good example of the practical difficulties involved in deciding what and what not to include. Some of these sites are identified as a result of a great deal of direct experimental evidence; some are identified merely as the result of visual or computer-aided pattern recognition; most fall somewhere between these two extremes. In this situation, our guidelines for what to include are first, to limit selections to those sites that have been experimentally verified; second, to exclude sites that can be identified purely by pattern recognition, as these can be reconstructed without the aid of the annotation; and finally, to try to anticipate and emphasize those sites that appear to be ubiquitously emphasized in the sequence literature.

The resources necessary to gather all these data, enter it into a computer database, organize it, and check its consistency were unfortunately underestimated at the outset of the project. (To get some idea of the quantity of data, see Section VI and Appendix I.) Thus, it has been impossible to enter the sequences with full annotation as quickly as we would like, and priorities have had to be set on completion of various phases of data entry. GenBank is used by different people in many ways: for some, only those sequence entries that have been fully annotated with all known facts are useful; for others, all that matters is that the sequence itself is quickly entered. Currently, we enter the sequences as rapidly as possible and make them available immediately in unannotated form; the entries are then fully annotated in a later release.

B. Nature of the Database

The database is organized biologically rather than bibliographically; the fundamental unit of database is therefore a contiguous sequence, derived from one paper or many, rather than a citation and the one or more sequences are derived from the corresponding paper. (Each database entry contains both the citations and the information necessary to reconstruct exactly the sequence(s) contributed by each paper.) In general, a database entry consists of a sequence, its biological definition, and a table of intervals and points on the sequence whose function is known. Just as a single sequence in the database may represent overlapping data from several papers, so one paper may contribute to several database entries.

To consistently implement this design philosophy requires that each time a paper is annotated for the database, the sequence reported must be checked for overlaps with any sequence already in the database; if there is an overlap, the new and old entries should be merged. Unfortunately, this is a very time consuming operation: we have had to make some tradeoffs between full and consistent merging, on the one hand, and timely entry of new data, on the other.

When fragments of a sequence are published, each contiguous fragment is put in its own entry. Thus, some entries include the statement that they are part of a larger group of entries, as well as a description of how they fit into that larger group.

The data organization is also designed for efficient computer maintenance and access. For example, any piece of sequence going into the database is assigned an arbitrary accession number that remains associated with those data forever. If the sequence is later renamed, merged into another entry, or has its definition corrected, it can still be found by means of the accession number (which is identical in the EMBL and GenBank databases). Cross references to related databases are also an important part of the database.

C. Data Items

In the next few paragraphs we will define the data items that are included in the GenBank database. After the list is complete, we will describe their organization. We group the data items (somewhat arbitrarily) as the sequence and its biological setting, bibliographical information, the biological annotation of regions within the sequence, and the items used for computer processing of the data. The list is essentially complete, but occasionally other information in included.

1. The Sequence and its Biological Setting

1. Sequence — the fundamental item is a contiguous stretch of sequence. The sequence in an entry must all be continuous as it occurs in nature but may have been reported a piece at a time in the literature. If more than one article is involved, the sequence is a mosaic, with the sequence in a region of overlap chosen arbitrarily from one article. (Any differences are annotated; see below.) When sequencing of a region is incomplete (e.g., an article presents the exon sequences of a gene but only restriction maps of the introns), each continuous sequence is put in a separate entry, and another data item specifies the connection between the pieces. The sequence is a text string, normally composed of a, c, g, and t. For the sake of uniformity, uridine is also represented as t when presenting RNAs. Ambiguities in the sequence data are represented using the standard IUPAC code.[11] Modified nucleotides (e.g., in tRNAs) are represented as the underlying unmodified nucleotide, and the modification is given in the sites (see below).

2. Length — the number of nucleotides in the sequence, listed separately for convenience.

3. Nucleic acid species — the nucleic acid species that was isolated for sequencing (DNA, genomic RNA, mRNA, rRNA, tRNA, or uRNA) and its strandedness.

4. Topology — sequences are presented as a single linear string; this data item determines whether they should be interpreted as a single linear string, as a circular string, or as a complete single element of a tandem repeat.

5. Location — specifies the location of the 5′ end of the sequence on a restriction map, genetic map, or physical map.

6. Segment — specifies the connection between neighboring, but not overlapping, pieces of sequence. When the distance(s) between two (or more) sequences is (are) known, each entry has a data item containing the notation "segment i of n", meaning that this sequence is the ith in a series of n.

7. Source — specifies the organism, developmental stage, tissue type, cell line, clone number, and molecule type used in determining the sequence.

8. Definition — a concise, biological definition of the sequence, mentioning at least the source organism and the primary product or function.

2. Bibliographical Information

1. References — the bibliographic source(s) of the data. Each reference is really a composite data item that gives the span of sequence contributed by a particular article, the authors of the article, the title, and the citation.

2. Sites of bibliographical interest — notations, associated with particular points on the sequence, that enable the reconstruction of the sequence as reported in any particular reference. When two articles differ in the reported version of a particular location on the sequence, the difference is noted and the nature of difference classified as revision (the difference is due to experimental error in one of the articles; which article it is has been resolved), or variation (the difference exists in nature), or conflict (source of difference undetermined). The numbering scheme used in each reference is included as a site. A site consists of a key which gives the type of site, a location and span, and a prose description.

3. Biological Annotation

1. Products — any cellular products coded for by the nucleic acid molecule. Each product is specified by a type (e.g., tRNA or protein), the span(s) of the coding region, a specification of the coding strand, and a prose description of the product.
2. Sites of biological interest — notations of points of known biological function on the sequence. These include endpoints of the products mentioned above, points of product processing (e.g., the boundary between signal peptide and mature peptide), mutations, recombination sites, protein-binding regions, and control sequences. Modified nucleotides are noted here. A site of biological interest has the same component parts as a site of bibliographical interest (see above).
3. Comment — normally this contains background information on the biology, mention of patterns that do not fit in the framework of sites, references to other sources of information, etc.

4. Items for Computer Processing

1. Entry name — a short name (one to nine alphanumeric characters) for the entry. These are made so that when alphabetized in a short directory, groups of related entries sort together: sequences from one organism sort together; within an organism, sequences with related function usually sort together; and entries within a segment group also sort together.
2. Accession number(s) — each sequence is assigned an accession number on entry into the database. When entries are renamed or merged, the accession number remains associated with the sequence to which it was originally assigned. This is a data item by which any sequence can always be tracked.
3. Taxonomy — a full taxonomy is listed for each entry, primarily for purposes of retrieval.
4. Keywords — keywords from a standard list, again for retrieval.
5. Footnote — notes for database staff (not distributed).
6. Base count — how many of each base appear in the sequence, primarily for a rudimentary error check on transmission.
7. Status — primarily indicates the degree of annotation.
8. Date — date of last change to the entry.

D. Organizing Data Items in Records and Fields

The distributed database is made up of records, in turn made up of fields. Each record consists of a sequence and its annotation; with a few exceptions, a record contains one field for each of the data items mentioned above. The reference-related fields may occur more than once in one entry.

- The LOCUS contains the entry name, the length of the sequence, the nucleic acid species, the topology, the status, and the date. It functions as a summary or header.
- The DEFINITION field contains the definition.
- The ACCESSION field contains the accession number list.
- The KEYWORDS field contains the keywords.
- The SEGMENT field contains the segment information.
- The SOURCE field contains the source.
- The ORGANISM field contains the taxonomy (including the formal species name).
- A REFERENCE field contains a number for a reference and information on how much of the sequence in the current entry was contributed by the given reference.
- A TITLE field contains a title for a reference.

- An AUTHORS field contains a list of authors for a reference.
- A JOURNAL field contains a citation (which can be to a book or other source as well as to a journal).
- The COMMENT field contains the comment.
- The FEATURES field is a table containing the products.
- The SITES field is a table containing the sites, both those of a bibliographical nature and those of a biological nature.
- The BASE COUNT field contains the base count.
- The ORIGIN field contains the location and the sequence.

Internally, GenBank is moving toward a more standard relational structure.[10] There are many reasons for spreading the data among several types of records; perhaps the most pressing one is to control data redundancy. For example, consider the taxonomy field: if the taxonomy is maintained in the primary entries, and the taxonomy of, say, mouse needs revision, then that same revision must be made in each of several hundred entries. It is better to maintain a separate file of the organism-to-taxonomy mapping and to maintain the taxonomies there. Then the master taxonomy for mouse would be called into each mouse entry at the time of distribution or application. GenBank currently has separate data files for the taxonomies, special genetic codes, and references. The reference data file includes references not only for entries in GenBank but also for all references currently in the data entry process. It also includes status information for all references, mailing addresses for authors, and other information that is not included in the public releases.

IV. PHYSICAL STRUCTURE OF GenBank

In the last section, we discussed the conceptual view of the database. This section is concerned with the physical arrangement of the data. GenBank is unusual in that the stored database itself is distributed, and there is no one DBMS (database management system) common to even a majority of users. BBN, the primary distributor under the GenBank contract, has an on-line version, with one DBMS. They also distribute the database on tape (in one format, identical to the stored form) and on floppy diskette (in another format). Secondary distributors put the data in other arrangements and provide different software for access.

This section is about the form in which the data is maintained at LANL and distributed on tape. This form embodies our conceptual view of the database and is the form most commonly available to users. The distribution format of EMBL is close enough to that of GenBank that the file formats themselves provide no barrier to completely automatic machine interconvertability.

In the following section, we explain our reasons for using text files for data storage; then we describe the general storage method we use locally for most data files.

A. Portable Data Files

A DNA sequence of any length up to that of a full chromosome is really a single data item. We originally chose to develop our own data storage method because no DBMS available at that time supported a data type of character strings of variable and unlimited length. Since we deal primarily with textual data, we chose ordinary text files as our medium; this choice has turned out very well.

An advantage of ordinary text files is that they can be manipulated with a wide variety of existing utilities. As a relatively small project on a limited budget, we were able to start work right away with standard tools for text files — editors, pattern finders, file transfer programs, etc. As we grew, we added specialized database software that cooperated with, but did not replace, the standard tools. Most of our data entry is still done with an ordinary screen editor to which a few special functions have been added to handle the sequence itself a little more smoothly. End users of the database can similarly do many significant searches with just existing utilities or with simple programs written in a familiar language.

One of the greatest advantages of having the data in text files is portability. We commonly use many machines for different aspects of our work, and we maintain all or part of the database under six different operating systems (of course, the end users of the data work under many more operating systems). Text files are the easiest to move from one machine to another; furthermore, since a text file looks nearly the same to programs anywhere, programs which use data from text files are easier to move to another machine.

Of course, there are disadvantages in choosing not to store the data in some highly compressed and more structured format. We lose something in both space and speed. This database is still of a relatively modest size (about 20 megabytes), however, and fits easily in uncompressed form, even on a well-equipped personal computer. By constructing indexes (which are also text files) for entry name, accession number, article citation, author name, and keyword, and by using them with relatively simple access schemes, access time has been very good on minicomputers, and satisfactory on microcomputers. The amount of data is, of course, growing rapidly, but hardware capacity is growing even faster. Only a few years ago, 64 kbyte memories were standard on personal computers; now a megabyte of memory is common. Custom software is far more expensive than hardware; in the end, simple and portable software is more economical than more complex software that squeezes the ultimate performance out of just one piece of equipment.

B. GenBank's Line Type Format

One general format, called the line type format, is used both for the distributed database and for all of GenBank's internal record keeping. Not only GenBank data, but even system files and indexes, are kept in text files of this format. This allows for a great simplification in the maintenance of all of our software. The line type format is described precisely in Appendix II; here, we only describe it as it applies to the GenBank distribution files (see the sample GenBank entry in Figure 1).

The basic idea of the line type format is that a data field is stored as a line plus continuation lines: the first line of the field has an identifier at the left margin to give the field name, and continuation lines have blanks in the first few columns. In the GenBank format, any line beginning with at least three blanks is a continuation line.

A record is a successive group of fields defined by a beginning-of-record field (in GenBank, LOCUS) and an end-of-record field (in GenBank, //).

In line with the goals of fifth generation computer projects, this format makes life a little easier for humans, while still allowing efficient computer processing. The structure of the file is immediately apparent to humans, so that casual users and programmers can use the data without having to resort to unreadable manuals. The files can be printed and used as text without any special processing; those who are uncomfortable with computers can use the data, at least in simple ways, in printed form.

The conceptual differences between the EMBL and GenBank formats are covered in Appendix II.

The line type format description above does not specify the files in which various records occur. The primary GenBank database is currently distributed in 13 files, or divisions. These are nuclear DNA and mRNA from (1) primates, (2) rodents, (3) other mammalian vertebrates, (4) nonmammalian vertebrates, (5) invertebrates, and (6) plants; DNA and mRNA from (7) organelles and (8) bacteria; (9) structural RNA sequences; (10) eukaryotic virus and (11) bacteriophage sequences; (12) synthetic and recombinant sequences; and (13) unannotated (and therefore unclassified) sequences.

```
LOCUS        HUMACTCA1    232 bp ds-DNA              updated   06/17/86
DEFINITION   Human alpha-cardiac actin gene, 5' flank and exon 1.
ACCESSION    J00070
KEYWORDS     alpha-cardiac actin.
SEGMENT      1 of 4
SOURCE       Human: DNA, (beta-thalassemic library of Fritsch et al.), clone
             lambda-HA-25 [1]; cDNA to skeletal muscle mRNA, clone pHMCA-1[2].
  ORGANISM   Homo sapiens
             Eukaryota; Metazoa; Chordata; Vertebrata; Tetrapoda; Mammalia;
             Eutheria; Primates.
REFERENCE    1  (bases 1 to 232)
  AUTHORS    Hamada,H., Petrino,M.G. and Kakunaga,T.
  TITLE      Molecular structure and evolutionary origin of human cardiac muscle
             actin gene
  JOURNAL    Proc Nat Acad Sci USA 79, 5901-5905 (1982)
REFERENCE    2  (bases 104 to 158)
  AUTHORS    Gunning,P., Ponte,P., Blau,H. and Kedes,L.
  TITLE      alpha-skeletal and alpha-cardiac actin genes are coexpressed in
             adult human skeletal muscle and heart
  JOURNAL    Mol Cell Biol 3, 1985-1995 (1983)
COMMENT      [1] provides the following summary.  There appear to be six isoforms
             of actin in mammals: cytoplasmic beta- and gamma-actin,
             co-expressed in non-muscle cells; two smooth muscle actins,
             co-expressed in smooth muscle (in varying ratios from cell type to
             cell type), but not detected elsewhere; and alpha-cardiac and
             alpha-skeletal actin, co-expressed in human adult striated muscle
             cells (though in varying ratios -- alpha-cardiac actin predominates
             in cardiac muscle, alpha-skeletal actin predominates in skeletal
             muscle).

             The initial Met-Cys of the alpha-cardiac coding sequence is
             post-translationally removed.  The complete coding sequence consists
             of six exons; all intron boundaries obey the "gt" and "ag"
             consensus intron boundary rules.
FEATURES         from  to/span      description
    pept         30  +   158       alpha-cardiac actin propeptide, exon 1
    matp         36  +   158       alpha-cardiac actin mature peptide
  SITES
    refnumbr      1       1        sequence not numbered in [1]
    ->pept       30       1        actin cds propept start
    pept/pept    36       0        actin cds propept end/mature pept start
    refnumbr    104       1        numbered 1 in [2]
    unsure      140       1        n in [2]
    pept/IVS    159       0        actin cds exon 1 end/intron I start
    IVS/IVS     233       0        actin cds intron I sequenced/unsequenced
BASE COUNT       39 a     85 c      69 g       39 t
ORIGIN         5 bp upstream of PstI site.
        1 ctgcagaaac cccctgaagc tgtgccaaga tgtgtgacga cgaggagacc accgccctgg
       61 tgtgcgacaa cggctctggg ctggtgaagg ccggctttgc gggcgatgac gcgccccgcg
      121 ctgtcttccc gtccatcgtg ggccgcccgc ggcaccaggt aaacttcccg ccgagccccc
      181 cgtcccactc gggacccctt cagtccagcg atctaggaaa tggctctcac ct
//
```

FIGURE 1.   Sample entry from GenBank. This entry covers the first exon of the human α-cardiac actin gene. The format corresponds to that for the version of the GenBank database distributed on magnetic tape in June 1986 (release #43.0).

V. GATHERING THE DATA

A. International Collaboration

Even before the GenBank and EMBL nucleotide sequence databases were officially chartered, staff on both sides of the Atlantic were exchanging data and sharing ideas. Once the projects were in full swing, an informal agreement was made to split the work of incorporating data into what is essentially one database. The list of journals that are regularly covered

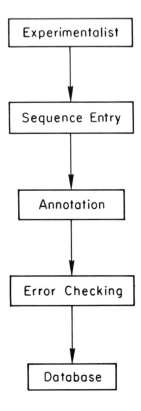

FIGURE 2.   The GenBank
data flow pipeline.

was divided such that each group locates and enters half of the data. The regular releases
of the database are then exchanged so that all data entered by each group finds its way into
the database of the other group. EMBL normally handles distribution to scientists in Europe,
while GenBank normally supplies the data to those in the Americas.

B. GenBank Data Entry

Just as the data are more useful if centrally gathered and organized, so they are more
useful if completed, corrected, and checked for consistency. We do much more than just
take data out of the papers and put it into the computer. During data entry, numerous checks
for consistency are made and problems are corrected by contacting the authors of the original
articles. We often add information that is missing in the articles (e.g., taxonomy), and we
enforce uniform terminology to enable efficient data retrieval.

As the sequence publication has increased, it has become increasingly difficult to have
the GenBank staff itself do all of this work. In this section, we discuss steps taken so far
to further involve the molecular biology community in the process of data entry and correction. Optimal models for community involvement are discussed in the final section.

The steps involved in the overall flow of data into the database are shown in Figure 2.
Though this view is greatly simplified, it does provide a good overview of the direction of
flow.

1. From the Experimentalist to the Database Staff

The data flow in Figure 2 begins with a research group which, having completed the
determination and study of a given sequence, either publishes it or distributes it as unpublished

data (the former alternative has predominated in the past, but journal restrictions on space for displaying sequence data are increasing the frequency of the latter alternative).

Half of the data flows from research groups to EMBL, half to GenBank. The flow to GenBank is treated in detail in the next few paragraphs; the point at which the EMBL data joins the GenBank stream is noted further on.

We discover most sequence data by scanning the literature, but there has been some progress toward eventually eliminating this step; more and more people are becoming aware of the value of the database and are submitting their data without being asked. *Nucleic Acids Research* and *The Journal of Biological Chemistry* now request or require the authors of accepted manuscripts to submit sequence data to the data bank.

When the project was young, we relied on hand entry of all sequence data from photocopied articles. With the explosive growth rate of sequence data, this approach quickly became impractical, so we have turned increasingly to a model involving direct submission (electronic, when possible) of data by the authors to the data bank. Now, when a sequence paper is identified, a data submission form (designed jointly with EMBL) is sent to the authors. This form requests both the sequence and the relevant biological annotation. An electronic version of the form is also posted on BIONET for use by authors we have not yet contacted. When there is no response to the request, we resort to the old model. The responses we do receive range from simply a reprint of the original article (least useful to us), to a clean hardcopy of the sequence data with hardcopy of the relevant annotation laid out in the format provided on the request form (more useful), to electronic responses (e.g., electronic mail, floppy disks, or magnetic tapes) containing both the sequence and the relevant annotation in the format suggested on the request form (most useful). When data are submitted electronically, one source of possible error — mistakes made in hand data entry — is eliminated. Currently, close to 1 million nucleotides per year of sequence data are being submitted on machine readable media.

When this first stage of data input is complete, we have a reprint or photocopy of the article and on our computer, the bare bones of a GenBank entry, with the sequence, citation, accession number, and a rough biological definition. If annotation has been submitted electronically by the author, it is stored at this stage in the COMMENT field of the entry.

2. Annotation of Entries

The information in each field of a GenBank entry answers one of a list of standard questions about the sequence. What is the biological definition of the sequence? What is the formal species name of the organism it came from? What mRNAs and proteins does it code for? The answers to these questions are ordinarily embedded in the article that originally reported the sequence. Developing this annotation involves abstracting it from the article and any additional direct information the authors have submitted to the database staff, and then adding it to the computer file containing the sequence. This is probably the most labor-intensive aspect of the database effort because it most often requires careful reading of what are quite often very complex articles. The time required for doing this has been reduced somewhat by the use of the GenBank/EMBL data submission forms, which ask explicitly for exactly the information we usually put into an entry. As authors become more cognizant of the kinds of information in database entries, and as direct contact between the authors and the database staff becomes more regular, we should be able to reduce the demands of this step on the data entry process.

An important part of the data bank work is what might be called deep annotation: the completion, interconnection, and unification of the annotation on a complicated entry or set of entries. In this regard, the cooperation of collectors of specialized databases has been invaluable, including that of Sprinzl et al. (tRNAs[7] and tRNA genes[12]), and Gold and co-workers (prokaryotic sequences[13]). In addition, we have benefitted immensely from the overview of specific genes or genome groups provided by investigators who specialize in those groups. For example, Blattner and co-workers assisted with developing the GenBank entry for bacteriophage lambda, as have Roberts with the adenovirus 2 entry, Kabat with immunoglobulin entries, Stormo with bacteriophage T4 entries, and Spritz with the human globin entries.

3. Error Checking

When the annotation has been added to an entry, and before the entry is inserted into the database, we seek to eliminate any errors that may have crept into the entry during the process of building it up. These errors (and the methods of detecting and correcting them) fall into two broad categories: semantic errors and syntactic errors.

The errors in the first category arise in the process of abstracting the meaning of an article. These are checked by having a second database staff member look at the article and make sure that the entry accurately and completely portrays the relevant information given in the article. Inter-line type consistency (e.g., that the composition given in BASE COUNT and the actual composition of the sequence are identical) is checked by computer.

The errors in the second category appear as divergences from the body of format rules that govern the information structure in the various line type fields. These errors can be detected by computer; we have several programs that check whether the entry format matches the specifications of format we have developed for the various line types.

4. Gathering Entries Into the Database

Approximately every 6 weeks, all new and modified entries that are in final form are gathered together and the primary database updated. Some final consistency checks are made; for example, a complete translation of all protein coding regions in the database is made and the correctness of the reading frames verified. The database is then transmitted to BBN for other checks and distribution.

The update process also includes making a log file of changes to the database, noting in the citation data file which papers have passed from the annotation stage into the database, etc.

5. It Is Not Quite So Simple

It should be pointed out that the flow of data is neither as simple as indicated in the above discussion nor as linear as indicated in Figure 2. The elaborated data flow diagram (which we will not detail here) could best be represented by imposing a number of circular paths on the diagram in Figure 2. For example, an entry that is inserted into the database is likely to be revised more than once as new papers appear reporting overlapping (and perhaps conflicting) data, or as corrections of earlier sequence or annotative information appear. Also, though we try to minimize it, our database format specifications are occasionally changed or augmented, requiring format revisions of some or all of the database entries.

VI. EXTENT OF THE DATA

We present here a characterization of the sequence data that are now available. The numbers given in the text and accompanying table are based on release 42.0 (May 1986) of the GenBank database. A detailed listing of several other database subsets has been prepared by Foley et al.[14]

We also include a brief list of a few other databases we are familiar with that contain either sequence or related data.

Table 2
NUMBER OF ENTRIES AND
NUCLEOTIDES IN EACH OF THE
GenBank SUBDIVISIONS

Division	No. of entries[a]	No. of nucleotides[a]
Primate	822	1036742
Rodent	1090	871093
Other mammal	217	194118
Nonmammalian vertebrate	409	297985
Invertebrate	525	342404
Plant	489	491971
Organelle	322	418336
Bacteria	680	870600
Structural RNA	563	61192
Virus	995	1372894
Bacteriophage	138	248342
Recombinant/synthetic	209	64041
Unannotated	957	495758
Total	7416	6765476

[a]   Based on the May 1986 release (#42.0) of the database.

A. The Quantity of Data
1. Overall Totals

The database contains 6,765,476 nucleotides in 7416 entries (an average of 912 nucleotides per entry). The amount of data for each database division is given in Table 2. There are now a number of individual entries in the database that contain quite long contiguous sequences. In Table 3, we list 27 entries that contain >10,000 nucleotides each; the longest such sequence corresponds to the complete genome of the Epstein-Barr virus (172,282 nucleotides).

An interesting characterization of the complexity of the available sequence data is that all 65,536 possible DNA octanucleotides (as well as, of course, all possible shorter oligomers) could be isolated in short restriction fragments from clones sequenced to date; for longer oligomers, the fraction that could be so isolated drops off rapidly.[15]

2. Totals by Sequence Taxonomy

Of course, with respect to understanding the complete "program" for any given organism, we are interested not simply in how many nucleotides are known, but in how big that number is with respect to the total genome size. In fact, the database now contains over 100 complete genomes, listed in Table 1. It will be seen that all of the complete genomes currently available correspond to extremely parasitic organisms that depend in large part on the genetic complement of the host organisms they prey upon (or exist symbiotically with). Though we expect that independent organisms will soon be completely sequenced, Table 4 indicates that we are still quite short of the complete sequences of these more elaborate genomes.

In a very few cases, we have many sequences corresponding to related variants of a single organism. For example, the database contains 211 entries, with a total of 138,340 nucleotides, for the influenza virus; all told, 78 different strains of this virus are represented.[14]

3. Totals by Sequence Function

What is the distribution of database sequences among product-coding regions, introns, and extra-genic regions? Table 5 shows that protein-coding regions have dominated the

Table 3
ENTRIES IN GenBank WITH GREATER THAN 10,000
NUCLEOTIDES OF CONTIGUOUS SEQUENCE

Sequence definition	Sequence length[a]	Accession no.
S. cerevisiae mitochondrial cytochrome oxidase gene	10168	J01481
Human fibrinogen γ-chain gene	10564	M10014
Yellow fever virus, complete genome	10862	K02749
E. coli gltA gene, sdhDCAB operon, and sucAB operon	10902	J01619
Adenovirus type 7, left end of genome	10948	V00032
Vesicular stomatitis virus, complete genome	11162	J02428
Adenovirus type 5, left end of genome	11570	V00025
Human β-nerve growth factor gene	11594	V01511
Chicken aldolase B gene	11651	M10946
Sindbis virus, complete genome	11703	J02363
Human α_1-antitrypsin gene	12222	K02212
E. coli rpl and rpo operons	12337	J01678
Human α-globin gene cluster	12847	J00153
Bacteriophage T4 fragment	12977	M10160
A. nidulans mitochondrial fragment	14440	J01390
Mouse mitochondrion, complete	16295	J01420
Bovine mitochondrion, complete	16338	J01394
Human mitochondrion, complete	16569	J01415
X. laevis mitochondrion, complete	17553	M10217
Ti plasmid *(A. tumefaciens)* fragment	24595	X00493
Adenovirus type 2, complete genome	35937	J01917
Human tissue plasminogen activator gene	36594	K03021
Human factor IX gene	38059	K02402
Bacteriophage T7, complete genome	39936	J02518
Bacteriophage λ, complete genome	48502	J02459
Human β-globin gene cluster	73360	J00179
Epstein-Barr virus, complete genome	172282	V01555

[a] Based on the May 1986 release (#42.0) of the database. Length given in units of nucleotides.
[b] Only the primary GenBank/EMBL accession number is given.

Table 4
AVAILABLE PERCENTAGE OF
SEVERAL LARGE GENOMES

Organism	No. of entries[a]	No. of nucleotides[a]	Total genome (%)[b]
E. coli	274	412750	12
S. cerevisiae	197	226142	1
D. melanogaster	235	166154	0.1
Mouse	750	559192	<0.02
Human	758	1004374	<0.03

[a] Based on the May 1986 release (#42.0) of the database.
[b] These numbers are only approximate and would be affected (in opposing directions) by taking into account the relatively small number of (1) overlapping but unmerged entries in the database and (2) entries in the unannotated division.

Table 5
FUNCTIONAL SUBSETS OF GenBank

Function	Total nucleotides[a]
Product coding	
Protein	48.04
Ribosomal RNA	2.32
Transfer RNA	1.36
Small nuclear RNA	0.11
Other structural RNA	0.08
Total	51.91
Introns	11.91
Noncoding[b]	36.18

[a] These numbers were generated by scanning the FEA-
TURES tables in the May 1986 release (#42.0) of
the database.
[b] Included in this category are open reading frames
and other potential product-coding regions that have
not been identified and experimentally verified.

interest of those determining sequences (due in part to the use of nucleic acid sequence
analysis as an indirect approach to determining amino acid sequences). Forty-eight percent
of the sequence data in the database correspond to known protein-coding spans; 3662 protein-
coding genes (2104 of them complete) coding for 872,143 amino acid residues are represented
in the database (recall that only experimentally confirmed coding regions are annotated in
the FEATURES table).

In some cases, particular products are represented across many gene copies and organisms.
For example, the database contains 275,252 nucleotides (in 401 entries) from human and
mouse immunoglobulin genes, 178,119 nucleotides (in 138 entries) from mouse and human
major histocompatibility complex regions, 194,600 nucleotides (in 119 entries) from globin-
coding regions, and 32,743 nucleotides (in 55 entries) from variant surface glycoprotein-
coding regions in *Trypanosoma*.

B. Related Collections

There are many specialized collections of nucleotide sequences that have annotations
particular to their special domains and are complementary to the GenBank and EMBL
collections. A few of these have had extensive interactions with GenBank and are mentioned
here; we make no attempt to be exhaustive. We also mention some other databases collecting
data that are closely related to nucleotide sequences. A few of the databases we mention
exist primarily in published form rather than as computer databases; it is very likely that
these will soon be available in computer-readable form.

1. Specialized Nucleotide Sequence Databases

In addition to the GenBank and EMBL collections, there are others that cover nucleotide
sequence data, although usually a smaller set of sequences defined by common function or
organism.

Several databases specialize in small structural RNAs: the tRNA collection,[7] which now
includes ~370 tRNAs; the tRNA gene collection,[12] which now includes ~465 tRNA genes;
the 5S, 5.8S, and 4.5S ribosomal RNA collection,[16] which now includes ~255 small
ribosomal RNAs; and the small nuclear RNA collection, [17] which now includes ~55 small
RNAs. The catalog of restriction enzyme recognition patterns[18] now lists the patterns cor-

responding to 515 enzymes. Schneider et al.[13] have collected a number of prokaryotic sequences centered about known transcription promoters as well as other sites of protein-DNA interaction.

There are many cases where individuals or small groups have maintained all the available sequence data (and in some cases, annotation) relative to a particular organism. A few examples include the 35,937 nucleotide adenovirus 2 genomic sequence,[19] the 48,502 nucleotide bacteriophage λ genomic sequence,[20,21] and the bacteriophage T4 collection,[22] which at ~43,000 nucleotides represents about 25% of that genome.

2. Related Databases

Computer databases of biological information are sprouting and growing quite rapidly. Here we list just a few of those that cover data most closely related to nucleotide sequence data.

Several databases provide collections of protein sequences (many of which are now derived indirectly from DNA and RNA sequences). The Protein Identification Resource is a national resource that contains all known protein sequences.[23] Other collections focus on narrower groups of proteins; an example is the collection of immunoglobulin (and immunoglobulin-related) sequences.[24] The Protein Data Bank, another national resource, contains the atomic coordinate files for known protein and nucleic acid crystal structures.[25]

Many of the clones that contain specific regions of particular genomes are also now being centrally stored and distributed. The American Type Culture Collection serves as a repository of such fragments; their staff is in the process of developing a computer directory of the available human DNA fragments.[26]

An effort focused on the human genetic map has been undertaken by the Human Gene Mapping Library,[27] which additionally includes data sets for known restriction fragment length polymorphisms, a directory of available probes and where to get them, and a related bibliography. McKusick[28] provides a database, MIM (mendelian inheritance in man), that catalogs human genetic diseases and related information. The large-scale organization of many other genomes is now known, including in some cases the location on the genome of many genes of basic and clinical interest. O'Brien[29] edits a collection of genetic maps for 100 organisms ranging from viruses to human.

VII. MAKING USE OF THE DATA

This section is about applications of the data. Access to the GenBank database has been discussed elsewhere.[9,30,31] In brief, the data are distributed on magnetic tape, floppy diskettes, and on-line by BBN and in hardcopy[32,33] as a supplement to *Nucleic Acids Research*. Essentially the same data, though provided in the format of their own database, are also distributed on magnetic tape by EMBL [contact G. Cameron at Postfach 10.2209, 6900 Heidelberg, West Germany (telephone 6221-387)]. There are also many secondary distributors.

A. Using GenBank on Different Machines

The following paragraphs broadly sketch what kinds of things can be done with GenBank in three sample computing environments. By a ''PC'' we mean something comparable to an IBM PC® XT, by ''minicomputer'' something comparable to a VAX 11/780, and by ''mainframe'' a machine on the scale of a Cray 1.

To use the database on a given machine, there must first of all be the capability to receive and store either the entire database or the portion which will be analyzed. The full database currently stands at about 20 megabytes, or 300,000 lines. This will fit on a well-equipped PC and on almost any minicomputer. Transmission by tape or floppies is reasonable, by computer network marginal, by telephone impractical. One division of the database is on the order of 2 megabytes, or 30,000 lines. This will easily fit on any machine with a hard disk and can reasonably be transferred over most networks, but it is still impractical to transfer over a telephone line. A single entry in the database ranges from a few tens to a few thousands of lines, from a few hundred bytes to a few hundreds of kbytes. A small set of entries can thus be handled on floppy disks and can reasonably be transferred over telephone lines.

A simple search for an entry of interest is practical on a PC if the database is indexed on the search key, but if a PC has to read through the whole database to find something, it is likely to take hours. A minicomputer can read through the whole database in a few minutes and can find indexed information with no noticeable delay. A search through the whole database on a mainframe takes on the order of 1 min. All these estimates assume an unloaded machine — an assumption that becomes progressively less likely the bigger the machine.

As for analysis, essentially anything that only involves a small set of entries can be done on a PC. An analysis that makes one pass over all the data, for example making a protein translation or searching for similarities between one sequence and all others, is practical, but not fast, on a minicomputer. A mainframe will do such an analysis in a few minutes. An analysis that has to deal with every entry in the entire database many times, such as making a catalog of all significant local similarities in all pairs of sequences, is currently at the limit of what can reasonably be done with supercomputers.

B. Writing Programs that Use GenBank

Many people are writing software to use GenBank (see the article by Lewitter and Rindone[34] as well as other reviews mentioned below). There is an implicit partnership between the architects of GenBank and those writing programs to use it: the architects must provide some continuity even while improving the design of the database, and programmers need to provide feedback to the architects as well as write programs that can be adapted as the database changes.

The basic line type format of the database (Section IV and Appendix II) is unlikely to change for quite some time. We think it is a good format, we know that a great deal of user software depends on it, and we ourselves have a heavy investment in software that assumes this general format. (We are happy to share our library of C language functions and utilities for handling details of input, output, and search in the line type format.)

Particular line types are less stable, although we try to maintain continuity. New line types may be added, old ones deleted, names of fields changed, and order of fields changed. The programmer should plan for this kind of change by putting all dependencies on individual line type identifiers in easily changed macros.

Stability of the format inside a given field is also subject to change. Any code that depends on the format of a particular field should be carefully isolated. The best procedure is to have a subroutine that translates the external format to an internal one that the rest of the program uses and that need not change, even if GenBank does.

A common mistake in writing programs for GenBank is in not allowing sufficient room for growth of the data. In only a few years, both the largest entry in the database, and also the database as a whole, have grown by a factor of 10. It is quite likely that future growth will be at least as fast. If repetitive analysis is being done, intermediate results should be saved, since recalculating them will be more expensive with a larger database. Code which might be run on a machine without virtual memory should never try to hold entire entries or full sequences in memory. Most search programs should be designed to use indexes on the search keys.

Although the difference between the GenBank and EMBL line type formats is not great, we feel that it is usually a mistake to try to make one program work on both. It is better to choose the preferred line type format and to write a program which converts the other.

C. Scientific Applications

Several recent reviews and dedicated volumes (including this book) have covered both individual analytical algorithms (and software implementing them) and integrated program packages for analyzing and manipulating sequence data.[34-46] As the database has matured, its usefulness in both facilitating and extending experimental work has grown. A few examples of current approaches taking advantage of the database follow.

The database can serve as an aid to experimentalists. One of the most common uses of the database is simply to see whether a particular region of interest has already been sequenced. Another is to compare a newly determined sequence to all or part of the database. (Waterman[47,48] provides surveys of alignment algorithms.) Such searches have at times uncovered unexpected and interesting similarities. A possible use of the database explored by Tung and Burks[15] is in connection with the synthesis of DNA molecules. They suggest the possibility of identifying relevant, naturally occurring oligomers by means of the database and then acquiring these cloned fragments, rather than synthesizing the final molecule one nucleotide at a time.

Amino acid sequences of proteins are now most often determined indirectly from nucleotide sequence data. Thus, it is very useful to maintain an up-to-date translation of all protein coding regions in GenBank. Another example of derived data that should be continually maintained as new sequence data accumulates is a database of all significant similarities between pairs of sequences. Codon usage tables and oligomer frequency tables would also be useful.

The importance of the protein coding region is such that we (1) have a number of special checks on the accuracy of their annotation and (2) make, at the time of each GenBank release, a derived database of the amino acid sequences coded for by genes in GenBank. Although other protein translations of GenBank are available (e.g., that of Claverie and Sauvaget[49]), the program that we use is the only one we know of that makes full and complete use of the information in the GenBank entries (Fickett[50] discusses the intricacies of protein translation from GenBank). The program is highly portable and publically available. We are exploring the possibility of making the derived protein database itself available either with regular GenBank releases or through other channels. A sample amino acid sequence entry resulting from translation of a protein-coding region is shown in Figure 3.

The most exciting use of the database is for exploratory data analysis. The data are still relatively new, and many important functional patterns lie near the surface, easy to discover. The TESTCODE algorithm[51] for discriminating protein-coding from noncoding DNA, depends primarily on simple periodicities in coding regions. The FEATURES tables allow the easy collection of, for example, all intron donor sequences currently known; this is a prerequisite for a search for regular patterns. Most analyses to date have treated nucleotide sequences as one-dimensional strings of characters. It is, of course, the three-dimensional structure of the nucleic acid polymer that is most relevant to the cell. Much work has been done on developing algorithms for predicting and characterizing the folding into secondary structure of nucleic acids.[52] Most recently, the dependence of the three-dimensional structure of DNA on nucleotide sequence has begun to be worked out,[53-55] and scientists have begun to analyze groups of sequences for similarity of structure rather than similarity of primary sequence.[56-59]

The database is a unique resource for evaluating the statistical significance of patterns found in exploratory data analysis. In developing the TESTCODE algorithm mentioned above, the usefulness of a large number of possible discriminants was tested by evaluating them on all coding and noncoding regions in the database. Although many putative tests for coding regions have been published, few have been evaluated in this way. (A notable exception is found in the work of Nakata et al.[60] on recognizing mRNA splice junctions.) A basic problem in evaluating the significance of almost any pattern is to assign probabilities

```
ID         HUMACTCA1
           alpha-cardiac actin propeptide (exon 1)
LOCUS      HUMACTCA1    232 bp    DNA              updated    07/02/84
ACCESSION  J00070
  ORGANISM Homo sapiens
           Eukaryota; Metazoa; Chordata; Vertebrata; Tetrapoda; Mammalia;
           Eutheria; Primates.
FEATURES       from  to/span      description
     pept      30  +   158    1 alpha-cardiac actin propeptide (exon 1)
LOCUS      HUMACTCA2   1846 bp    DNA              updated    07/02/84
ACCESSION  J00071
  ORGANISM Homo sapiens
           Eukaryota; Metazoa; Chordata; Vertebrata; Tetrapoda; Mammalia;
           Eutheria; Primates.
FEATURES       from  to/span      description
     pept    +  110     434    0 alpha-cardiac actin propeptide (exon 2)
              1105    1266    0 alpha-cardiac actin propeptide (exon 3)
              1393  +  1584    0 alpha-cardiac actin propeptide (exon 4)
LOCUS      HUMACTCA3    442 bp    DNA              updated    07/02/84
ACCESSION  J00072
  ORGANISM Homo sapiens
           Eukaryota; Metazoa; Chordata; Vertebrata; Tetrapoda; Mammalia;
           Eutheria; Primates.
FEATURES       from  to/span      description
     pept    +  173  +   354    0 cardiac actin propeptide (exon 5)
LOCUS      HUMACTCA4    749 bp    DNA              updated    07/02/84
ACCESSION  J00073
  ORGANISM Homo sapiens
           Eukaryota; Metazoa; Chordata; Vertebrata; Tetrapoda; Mammalia;
           Eutheria; Primates.
FEATURES       from  to/span      description
     pept    +  233     376    0 cardiac actin propeptide (exon 6)
COMPLETE   5':y  3':y
LENGTH     378
ORIGIN     Translated using phase 1
         1 mcddeettal vcdngsglvk agfagddapr avfpsivgrp rhqgvmvgmg qkdsyvgdea
        61 qskrgiltlk ypiehgiitn wddmekiwhh tfynelrvap eehptlltea plnpkanrek
       121 mtqimfetfn vpamyvaiqa vlslyasgrt tgivldsgdg vthnvpiyeg yalphaimrl
       181 dlagrdltdy lmkiltergy sfvttaerei vrdikeklcy valdfenema taasssslek
       241 syelpdgqvi tignerfrcp etlfqpsfig mesagihett ynsimkcdid irkdlyannv
       301 lsggttmypg iadrmqkeit alapstmkik iiapperkys vwiggsilas lstfqqmwis
       361 kqeydeagps ivhrkcf*
//
```

FIGURE 3. Sample translation of a protein-coding region in GenBank. This entry covers the complete coding region for a human α-cardiac actin and corresponds to GenBank entries HUMACTCA1, HUMACTCA2, HUMACTCA3, and HUMACTCA4 in the December 1985 release. The protein extraction and translation were done automatically with the program described by Fickett.[50]

to the occurrence of each possible sequence. Again, many people fail to use the data available and simply assume that all sequences are equally likely. It is much better to count oligomer frequencies in (a relevant subset of) the database and use a Markov chain model.[61] Similarity searches are widely used, and the assignment of a significance level to an alignment is a very important — and very difficult — problem. An empirical approach, based on aligning all pairs of sequences in a large subset of GenBank, is described by Smith et al.[62]

VIII. THE FUTURE

The explosive growth of sequence data is likely to continue. In fact, not only the amount of data, but the scope and interconnectedness of the data will grow at a pace hard to keep abreast of. As the age of biological hard data matures, one of the greatest challenges will be to organize the data in a connected way so that significant applications can access multiple related databases in meaningful ways. Another challenge, of primarily a social nature, will be to restructure the mechanics and the rewards of publishing so that the community will naturally be motivated to keep the databases complete and correct.

A. Growth of the Data

How much data will there be? Currently, the increase in publication rate seems to be slowing down a little; the total number of articles published per year seems to be increasing only linearly (Appendix I). However, journals are reluctant to publish data which do not bear on an issue of great current interest, and there are many indications that the volume of unpublished data is growing much faster than the volume of published data.

As the applications of sequence data grow, people become increasingly ambitious in sequencing projects. The complete sequence of simian virus 40 (5243 nucleotides) once was exciting news. Now, many complete viral genomes (Table 1) are known, including that of Epstein-Barr virus (172,282 nucleotides). Those involved most directly in sequencing say that the sequencing rate of 10^5 nucleotides per man-year will soon be 10 to 100 times what it is now.[63-65] Rumor has it that the complete *Escherichia coli* genome will be done in the next few years, and there is serious talk of a concerted effort to determine the sequence of the complete human genome in the next 10 to 20 years.[63,66-70] What kind of expansion of the database are we talking about here? The human sequences determined so far only constitute about 0.02% of the genome (Table 4). Thus, it is not at all hard to imagine that GenBank might grow to 1000 times its current size in only 10 to 20 years.

There are currently on the order of 400 species represented in GenBank. If, in the long run, all protein coding regions of, say, 1000 genomes were included, the database would contain on the order of 10^{12} nucleotides — 1 million times its current size.

Furthermore, though the database does contain a limited amount of sequence data corresponding to variation at specific loci within a population, these data are going to be expanding considerably due to a rapidly increasing interest in using large volumes of population data for distinguishing significant from less significant regions of a sequence (whether on the level of protein or DNA). The sequences of viral genomes are highly variable, and annotating the variations can require as much information as recording one version of the sequence. Though variation is not as great in, say, the coding regions of human β-globin genes, other regions of the human genome, such as repetitive elements and other "noncoding" DNA, vary considerably from individual to individual (in fact, some regions of the human genome are now being used with great success in "fingerprinting" individuals[71]). We will want to represent these data, which can be conceptually realized as variation along an axis orthogonal to the individual sequence, so that the relationships between the entries containing the data are preserved and can be used for automatically extracting and assembling the variational data.

Computer storage and data transmission capabilities are growing so rapidly that just storing and moving this amount of information is unlikely to be the main problem. Rather, the main problem will be one of organization, both of the data and of human resources.

B. Fuller Use of Biological Knowledge

The knowledge gained by science is expensive and valuable, but because of a lack of communication, it is very often not used by those who would most benefit from it. As the volume of information grows, the work required to organize that information and make it easily available becomes as valuable as the generation of the information in the first place.

It is steadily getting more difficult to keep up with published (let alone unpublished) information relevant to a given field. The result is not simply that some people fail to be current with their field; much worse, many never gain a unified view of the field they work in, and there is a great deal of unnecessary work done to get answers that could have been derived from known data.

Databases are coming of age and can usefully enter into a partnership with journals. Journals should answer the question, "what is new?" while databases should answer the question, "what is known?". Browsing in journals to find what is new makes sense, but retrieving cataloged facts from a database is far more efficient than looking them up in a library.

A recent report[72,73] emphasized the importance of developing a "matrix of biological knowledge". The two main aspects of this matrix are the interconnectedness of knowledge and the unifying principles which can be used to organize and comprehend knowledge. These ideas are very useful for database design.

The interconnections between mapping data, nucleotide sequence data, and protein sequence and structure data are great. So, although these data are maintained by different groups, it should be possible to easily move from one of the databases to another. The connections between these databases should allow queries like, "show sequences of all human genes on the short arm of chromosome 11", "retrieve available crystal structures for all proteins whose genes have more than three introns", and "display the -35 region for all genes of membrane proteins". Interconnecting the data is primarily a matter of deciding on standard nomenclature for the objects in the databases, so that each individual data bank can point to related information in all other databases. Implementing retrieval schemes will depend, in the near term, on adopting a standard format for portable data files and on exchanging data frequently. In the long run, highly sophisticated networking will make exchange of data unnecessary.

It should be noted that strong interconnectedness of the databases, at least of the mapping and the sequence databases, is a prerequisite for the sequencing of a mammalian chromosome or genome.

Room for expansion is important. There will always be new databases that need to be connected into the matrix. Additions to the above list might include two-dimensional gel data on proteins and expression data on mRNAs according to genomic location, developmental stage, and cell type.

GenBank has been planned with this cross-referencing in mind. When data are incorporated from specialized collections, the identifiers from the other collections are preserved. We include mapping data whenever we can. We have tried to incorporate standard nomenclature when it is available and applicable. We have also experimented in cross-referencing of different sequence databases.[74]

The second theme of the matrix of biological knowledge, that of unifying principles, might be implemented as follows. The application of a unifying principle is, in essence, the use of a parallel organization for two or more disparate data sets. Thus, taxonomic organization is useful in studying such widely different data as morphology, metabolic pathways, and strategies for gene control and expression. The application of unifying principles to databases is made possible by highly modular data structures and software which can easily reorganize large data sets according to the natural order within one field. For example, each GenBank entry contains a taxonomy field, and the whole database could be ordered and distributed as a (rather sparse) taxonomic tree. When GenBank is closely linked with the protein databases, it could easily be reorganized along the lines of protein superfamilies.

C. The Database as a Community Project

The value of the databases depends strongly on the degree to which they represent the true and complete knowledge of the community. Thus, a major goal of the data banks is to motivate all scientists to take an active part in organizing, correcting, and completing the data.

It is clear that as the volume of data grows, several steps of data entry must be totally automated. First, the community cannot afford to support a data bank staff sufficiently large to be solely responsible for finding, entering, and annotating new sequences. Rather, all published data should be submitted simultaneously to the journal and, accompanied by annotation, to the data banks, and unpublished data should, if made publicly available, be put in the databases for wider circulation. If the database is to reflect our current state of understanding, then additions and corrections to the data, which are often only circulated among friends, should also be submitted in a timely manner. In turn, the data bank staff must develop standardized and foolproof formats for data submission which can be automatically reformatted, checked for errors, and entered into the database with no human intervention. The database needs to be updated continuously so that there will be no significant delay between the submission of data and its availability.

Currently, the database staff, with the help of occasional visitors, provide all curatorial care of the database, that is, all review and reorganization of the data to clarify interconnections and unifying principles. However, the database staff can never replace the expertise of the community, and as the databases grow in size and importance, we envision the curatorial function being filled by a steady stream of scientists coming to review their areas of expertise.

It is true now and will probably be true for some time that many scientists do not take full advantage of computer analysis and simulation based on information in the databases. The data banks may serve as training centers for advanced use of computer tools, and one motive for curatorial work will be that scientists will have a chance to collaborate with the data bank staff, learning new techniques for use in their own work.

APPENDIX I
ESTIMATION OF SEQUENCE DATA PUBLICATION RATE

One of the divisions of labor between GenBank and EMBL is in routine scanning of the set of journals publishing sequence data. We made an independent audit of that process in August 1985. A set of journals, including all those cited in GenBank, was systematically sampled for the years 1978 through 1985, providing an overall picture of the publication of sequence data.

First, the June 1985 issues of the journal set were scanned to see which journals published a "significant" number of sequence papers, and the list was pared to 24 journals that can be expected to publish at least 12 papers per year. For each of the 24 and each of the years 1978 to 1985, the June issue(s) was scanned for papers with figures presenting what appeared to be a nucleotide sequence. Our experience indicates that 95% of such papers contain original data. For each journal, the number of expected sequences per annum is computed from the June sample. For a few journals not available to us, an estimate was based on titles from *Current Contents*.

From several checks on the method we conclude that (1) the journals not included in the main scan contribute less than 5% of all sequence data and (2) that the publication rates estimated from the June issues are probably about 15% higher; more sequence papers seem to be published in the summer.

Table 6 is a list of journals publishing at least 12 articles per year with sequence data. For each journal, the estimated number of sequence papers per year is given for the last 8 years. Overall, we estimate that 8180 papers were published in the period 1978 to 1985.

The rate at which sequence data are being published is still increasing significantly but no longer growing exponentially. This audit made no attempt to estimate the rate of accumulation of unpublished data.

Table 6
NUMBER OF SEQUENCE ARTICLES PUBLISHED,[a] BY JOURNAL AND YEAR

Journal	1985	1984	1983	1982	1981	1980	1979	1978
BBRC	36	0	0	0	0	0	0	0
Biochem. U.S.A.	39	13	13	13	39	0	13	0
Bioorg. Khim.	48	12	0	36	0	0	0	0
Cell	150	252	120	108	108	120	24	24
CSHSQB[b]	(20)	20	8	12	0	36	16	40
Curr. Gen.	48	72	60	(50)	(40)	(30)	(20)	(10)
DNA	43	48	48	48	0	0	0	0
EMBO J.	180	108	84	72	0	0	0	0
Eur. J. Biochem.	72	36	12	36	12	0	12	12
FEBS Lett.	52	28	28	28	28	28	0	14
Gene	105	72	24	52	40	40	16	8
J. Bacteriol.	108	(66)	24	24	12	0	0	0
J. Biol. Chem.	192	180	84	72	48	12	36	12
J. Gen. Virol.	24	(24)	(24)	12	0	0	0	0
J. Mol. Biol.	132	60	96	36	72	24	12	12
J. Mol. Evol.	16	(11)	6	5	0	0	0	0
J. Virol.	120	108	72	60	24	0	60	0
Mol. Cell. Biol.	192	60	24	0	12	0	0	0
Mol. Gen. Genet.	66	132	20	16	8	6	9	0
Nature (London)	117	117	65	91	65	78	52	26
NAR	408	372	276	276	228	108	48	36
PNASU	348	348	288	144	132	144	24	12
Science	91	65	39	26	13	0	0	0
Virology	32	32	0	48	0	16	0	0
Totals	2639	2236	1415	1265	881	642	342	206
Totals * 85%	2243	1901	1203	1072	749	546	291	175

[a] Where there are no data available to us, projections from other years are given in parentheses.
[b] For CSHQB (Cold Spring Harbor Symposia), the first $1/4$ of the proceedings were examined and the results multiplied by 4.

APPENDIX II
FORMAL DEFINITION OF LINE TYPE FORMAT

A. Line Type Format

An LT (line type) format is a way of interpreting the data in a text file. Formally, almost any text file may be considered an LT file and may be interpreted according to an LT format. Intuitively, an LT file is one in which a few of the leftmost columns are reserved for specifying the type of information on each line, a line of a given type may be continued with indented lines to form a field, and fields may be grouped in records.

GenBank uses a line type format as described here. The EMBL nucleotide sequence database uses a closely related format.

B. Line Type File

● *Definition.* An LTDF (line type data file) is an ASCII text file, all of whose lines are at most 255 characters long (excluding any end-of-line characters).

Long lines are allowed but are really intended only for temporary files. LT format was developed partly for ease of editing, printing, and scanning by eye; normally an LTDF will have lines no more than 79 characters long, so as to print well on most terminals.

C. LT Identifier and Type

If a line in an LT file has nonblank characters in the first few columns, it is explicitly identified as having a certain type of information in it. We say its "type" is given by the first word on the line. If the first few characters are blank, the line is regarded as a continuation of previous line(s); its type is implicitly identified as the same as that of the one(s) before it. To specify the LT format we are using, we must say how many columns we mean when we say "first few".

- *Definition.* An LTIL format is specified by an integer INDENT.
- *Definition.* An LTIL, LT identifier line, is a line with a nonblank character in one of the first INDENT columns (or first n columns if the line has fewer than INDENT characters).
- *Definition.* At LTID, LT identifier, is the initial segment of an LTIL, beginning at column 1 and ending with the first nonblank character followed by a blank or the end of the line.
- *Definition.* An LTCL, LT continuation line, is a line with blanks in the first INDENT columns (or the first n columns if the line has fewer than INDENT characters).

The difference between this scheme and that used by the EMBL data bank is that every line in the EMBL files has an identifier, and an LTCL is a line whose identifier is the same as that of the preceding line.

The LTIDs of GenBank are the familiar keywords "LOCUS", "DEFINITION", etc. The only difference between the formal definitions and the informal usage is the GenBank keyword "BASE COUNT". Here the LTID is "BASE".

LTIDs beginning "#" are reserved for programmers' use. It is safest to only use alphanumerics and underscore in LTIDs.

If a group of successive lines at the head of a file all lack characters in the first INDENT columns, then their type is undefined. The LT software will ignore such lines; this allows for a comment header on LT files. These lines will still be called LTCLs though a "continuation" is somewhat inappropriate.

D. Fields

A "field" is a line with an explicit identifier together with its following continuation lines.

- *Definition.* An LTF, LT field, is a maximal set of successive lines such that the first, and only the first, is an LTIL.

A consequence of the definitions is that every line in the file either belongs to the file header or to a field.

The grouping of lines into fields depends on INDENT. For example, with GenBank format, INDENT = 1 makes the FEATURES and SITES all one field, INDENT = 3 makes the FEATURES and SITES two separate fields, and INDENT = 20 makes each feature or site, with its continuation lines, a separate field.

E. Records

A record is a group of (usually successive) related fields, like the entries of the GenBank and EMBL databases. Whereas the fields of an LT file are completely determined by the number INDENT, and will usually be the same for all applications, a record is a very flexible construct that will often be different with different applications of the same file.

- *Definition.* An LTRD, LT record description, consists of a BOR (beginning-of-record) pattern, an EOR (end-of-record) pattern, and an IIR (include-in-record) pattern. Each of these is a possibly ambiguous pattern meant to match an initial portion of the first line of a field (normally the LTID).
- *Definition.* For any field F1 matching BOR, the LTR (LT record) with beginning boundary F1 is defined as follows: (1) the end of record boundary, F2, is the first field

following F1 which both matches EOR and is followed by either the end of the file or a field not matching EOR; (2) the record itself consists of all fields between F1 and F2 (inclusive) which match IIR and do not begin with "#".

Note that the boundaries F1 and F2 might not be included in the record itself.

● *Definition.* The KEY of the record with beginning boundary F1 is the field F1, with LTID removed, leading and trailing white space removed, and strings of internal white space replaced by single blanks.

The most common record associated with the sequence databases is one beginning with LOCUS (GenBank) or ID (EMBL) and ending with //. Another common one is that beginning with REFERENCE (GenBank) or RN (EMBL) and ending with JOURNAL (GenBank) or RL (EMBL).

The concept of record as defined here may be usefully applied to the EMBL database even though their definition of field is different.

Note that the concept of LTR depends strongly on the order of the fields in the file.

NOTE ADDED IN PROOF

GenBank is like the body of information it represents: it changes and expands rapidly. The following notes briefly update the information presented in the article above.

A New GenBank Contract. In September 1987, NIGMS awarded a new 5-year contract (NO1-GM-7-2110) for GenBank to IntelliGenetics, Inc. and Los Alamos National Laboratory.

Inquiries regarding submission of new or revised data to GenBank should be addressed to:

GenBank
T-10, MS K710
Los Alamos National Laboratory
Los Alamos, NM 87545
Telephone: 505-665-2177
e-mail: gb-sub%life@lanl.gov (new data submissions)
            genbank%life@lanl.gov (suggested revisions and general queries
               regarding data collection)

Inquiries regarding access to and distribution of GenBank should be addressed to:

GenBank
IntelliGenetics
700 El Camino Real East
Mountain View, CA 94040
Telephone: 415-962-7364
e-mail   genbank@bionet-20.arpa

Note that the most recent information on the size as well as the format of the GenBank database can be found in the release notes for any current release; additionally, related and more general information is presented in *News from GenBank* (contact IntelliGenetics for more information about both).

The Size of the GenBank Database. The most recent release (June 1988, #56.0) of the GenBank database contains over 18,000 entries with almost 21 million nucleotides. The distributed flat file version of the database amounts to about 60 megabytes.

Database Structure. There have been several changes to the distributed format over the past year. The SITES field was removed, with all the data items there being converted to data items in the FEATURES field (this was a preparative step in anticipation of eventually implementing a new FEATURES format that will be common to EMBL and GenBank). A new field, STANDARD, was added as part of the REFERENCE block; this field is used to provide information about the amount of annotation abstracted from a citation (previously provided in the LOCUS field) and the amount of in-house review this abstracting has received. Increasingly, we are moving data submitted by authors directly into entries without requiring in-house review of the entry by staff (though we still pass all submissions through any software-based checks that we have). Finally, the LOCUS field has been modified to include an explicit indication of the database division to which any given entry has been assigned.

As alluded to in the previous paragraph, the EMBL and GenBank have begun working on a new FEATURES syntax and descriptive keys that will be more flexible, richer, and identical in the formats distributed by the two databases.

A most important development — though one that will not be immediately evident to the user — has been the move away from maintaining the GenBank data in the same form as that in which it is distributed. We are in the process of developing a relational schema[75] for GenBank that will allow us to port the data into a relational database management system (RDBMS). This effort has forced us to modularize much of the data that was previously maintained in conglomerate form, and to formally specify the relationships (including that of redundancy) between the various data items in the database.

Collaborations. The EMBL Data Library and GenBank have been joined by a third collaborator, the DNA Data Bank of Japan (DDBJ). In the data collection split, they are currently covering journals published in Japan.

Both EMBL and GenBank have greatly expanded their interactions with journals that publish nucleotide sequence data; most of the journals publishing significant amounts of sequence data are now requesting authors to submit their data directly to GenBank or EMBL, and a few journals have begun to require authors to do so. In conjunction with this effort, EMBL and GenBank developed a common submission form; this has also recently been adopted by the Protein Identification Resource and its collaborators in Germany (MIPS) and Japan (JIPID).

The National Library of Medicine has also begun contributing to the data collection effort by providing GenBank with listings of articles (identified with MeSH headings that are developed for MEDLINE entries) that are likely to contain nucleotide sequences. This is quite useful for selectively scanning journals that one would otherwise not scan because sequences are so infrequently published there.

Related Databases. We discussed the report of Morowitz et al.[72] and the concept it introduced of a matrix of biological knowledge. In the summer of 1987, a workshop was held to discuss this topic, focusing on identifying new databases that were needed, developing links between existing and planned databases, and identifying computer science tools that could be brought to bear on these tasks.[76]

An important requirement for developing an overview of existing databases and future areas of research and development is an extensive listing and characterization of databases pertaining to molecular biology. Our group has developed such a listing, LiMB, a listing and description of databases relevant (but not limited) to molecular biology, and is now providing formal releases of this information.[77]

For purposes of cross-referencing, we have (in GenBank human nucleotide sequence entries) introduced pointers to corresponding mapped human genes listed in the Human Gene Mapping Library.[78]

Recent Publications. We have written several articles on various aspects of the database. Burks has discussed projected rates of appearance of new sequence data and the consequences for the database effort,[79] and also has presented a detailed account of publications in which sequence data have been published and the consequences of the increasing amount of unpublished data becoming available.[80] We have also discussed the challenges for the GenBank data management effort that will arise in the context of the proposed effort to completely map and sequence the human genome.[81] The 1988 issue of *Nucleic Acids Research* devoted to computer-related topics also contains an update on GenBank,[82] and the most recent — and perhaps last for some time to come — published version of the entire database appeared in 1987.[83]

ACKNOWLEDGMENTS

We recognize the many contributions to the database effort from our colleagues at LANL, BBN, and EMBL. We are grateful for enlightening conversations with W. Goad and M. Cinkosky; for a critical reading of the manuscript by M. Fickett and M. Waterman; for proofreading by P. Reitemeier; and for the graphical expertise of B. Atencio. The GenBank project is funded through a contract with the National Institutes of Health, National Institute of General Medical Sciences (N01-GM-2127); portions of this work were done under the auspices of the U.S. Department of Energy.

REFERENCES

1. **Maxam, A. M. and Gilbert, W.,** A new method for sequencing DNA, *Proc. Natl. Acad. Sci. U.S.A.,* 74, 560, 1977.
2. **Sanger, F., Nicklen, S., and Coulsen, A. R.,** DNA sequencing with chain-terminating inhibitors, *Proc. Natl. Acad. Sci. U.S.A.,* 74, 5463, 1977.
3. **Abelson, J. and Butz, E., Eds.,** Recombinant DNA, *Science,* 209, 1317, 1980.
4. **Abelson, P. H., Eds.,** Biotechnology, *Science,* 219, 611, 1983.
5. **Blattner, F. R., Eds.,** Biological frontiers, *Science,* 222, 719, 1983.
6. **Koshland, D. E., Jr., Eds.,** Biotechnology, *Science,* 229, 1193, 1985.
7. **Sprinzl, M., Moll, J., Meissner, F., and Gauss, D. H.,** Compilation of tRNA sequences, *Nucl. Acids Res.,* 13, r1, 1985.
8. **Hamm, G. and Cameron, G.,** The EMBL data library, *Nucl. Acids Res.,* 14, 5, 1986.
9. **Bilofsky, H. S., Burks, C., Fickett, J. W., Goad, W. B., Lewitter, F. I., Rindone, W. P., Swindell, C. D., and Tung, C.-S.,** The GenBank genetic sequence data bank, *Nucl. Acids Res.,* 14, 1, 1986.
10. **Date, C. J.,** *An Introduction to Database Systems,* Addison-Wesley, Reading, Mass., 1981.
11. **Cornish-Bowden, A.,** Nomenclature for incompletely specified bases in nucleic acid sequences: recommendations 1984, *Nucl. Acids Res.,* 13, 3021, 1985.
12. **Sprinzl, M., Vorderwülbecke, T., and Gauss, D. H.,** Compilation of sequences of tRNA genes, *Nucl. Acids Res.,* 13, r51, 1985.
13. **Schneider, T. D., Stormo, G. D., Haemer, J. S., and Gold, L.,** A design for computer nucleic-acid-sequence storage, retrieval, and manipulation, *Nucl. Acids Res.,* 10, 3013, 1982.
14. **Foley, B. T., Nelson, D., Smith, M. T., and Burks, C.,** Cross-sections of the GenBank database, *Trends Genet.,* 2, 233, 1986.
15. **Tung, C.-S. and Burks, C.,** Characterization of the distribution of potential short restriction fragments in nucleic acid sequence databases: implications for an alternative to chemical synthesis of oligonucleotides, *FEBS Lett.,* 205, 299, 1986.
16. **Erdmann, V. A., Wolters, J., Huysmans, E., and De Wachter, R.,** Collection of published 5S, 5.8S and 4.5S ribosomal RNA sequences, *Nucl. Acids Res.,* 13, r105, 1985.
17. **Reddy, R.,** Compilation of small RNA sequences, *Nucl. Acids Res.,* 13, r155, 1985.
18. **Roberts, R. J.,** Restriction and modification enzymes and their recognition sequences, *Nucl. Acids Res.,* 13, r165, 1985.
19. **Roberts, R. J., Akusjaervi, G., Alestroem, P., Gelinas, R. E., Gingeras, T. R., Sciaky, D., and Pettersson, U.,** A consensus sequence for the adenovirus-2 genome, in *Adenovirus DNA,* Doerfler, W., Ed., Martinus Nijhoff, Boston, 1986, 1.

20. **Daniels, D. L., Schroeder, J. L., Szybalski, W., Sanger, F., and Blattner, F. R.,** A molecular map of coliphage lambda, in *Lambda II,* Hendrix, R. W., Roberts, J. W., Stahl, F. W., and Weisberg, R. A., Eds., Cold Spring Harbor Laboratory, Cold Spring Harbor, N.Y., 1983, 469.

21. **Daniels, D. L., Schroeder, J. L., Szybalski, W., Sanger, F., Coulson, A. R., Hong, G. F., Hill, D. F., and Blattner, F. R.,** Complete annotated lambda sequence, in *Lambda II,* Hendrix, R. W., Roberts, J. W., Stahl, F. W., and Weisberg, R. A., Eds., Cold Spring Harbor Laboratory, Cold Spring Harbor, N.Y., 1983, 519.

22. **Stormo, G.,** T4 sequences collection effort, personal communication, 1986.

23. **George, D. G., Barker, W. C., and Hunt, L. T.,** The protein identification resource (PIR), *Nucl. Acids Res.,* 14, 11, 1986.

24. **Kabat, E. A., Wu, T. T., Bilofsky, H., Reid-Miller, M., and Perry, H.,** *Sequences of Proteins of Immunological Interest,* U.S. Department of Health and Human Resources, Bethesda, Md., 1983.

25. **Bernstein, F. C., Koetzle, T. F., Williams, G. J. B., Meyer, E. F., Brice, M. D., Rodgers, J. R., Kennard, O., Shimanouchi, T., and Tasumi, M.,** The protein data bank: a computer-based archival file for macromolecular structures, *J. Mol. Biol.,* 112, 535, 1977.

26. **Felix, J. S. and Badman, W. S.,** Human DNA repository, *Science,* 231, 203, 1986.

27. **Human Gene Mapping Library at New Haven,** unpublished manual, July 1986.

28. **McKusick, V.,** *Mendelian Inheritance in Man,* 8th ed., Johns Hopkins University Press, Baltimore, 1988.

29. **O'Brien, S. J., Ed.,** *Genetic Maps: A Compilation of Linkage and Restriction Maps of Genetically Studied Organisms,* Vol. 3, Cold Spring Harbor Laboratory, Cold Spring Harbor, N.Y., 1984.

30. **Bilofsky, H. S., Burks, C., Fickett, J. W., Goad, W. B., Lewitter, F. I., Rindone, W. P., Swindell, C. D., and Tung, C.-S.,** Data banks of nucleic acid sequences: GenBank, in *Introduction to Computing with Protein and Nucleic Acid Sequences,* Lesk, A., Ed., CODATA, 1988, in press.

31. **Burks, C., Fickett, J. W., Goad, W. B., Kanehisa, M., Lewitter, F. I., Rindone, W. P., Swindell, C. D., Tung, C.-S., and Bilofsky, H. S.,** The GenBank nucleic acid sequence database, *Computer Appl. Biosci.,* 1, 225, 1985.

32. **Andersen, J. S., Anderson, J., Atencio, E., Bergman, B. E., Bilofsky, H. S., Brown, L., Burks, C., Cameron, G. N., Channin, D. S., Elbe, U., England, C., Fickett, J. W., Goad, W., Hamm, G. H., Hayter, J. A., Kay, L., Kanehisa, M., Koile, K., Lennon, G., Linder, R., Lewitter, F. I., McLeod, M., Melone, D. L., Myers, G., Nelson, B., Nelson, D., Nial, J. L., Perry, H. M., Rindone, W. P., Rudloff, A., Simon, S., Smith, T. F., Stoesser, G., and Stueber, K.,** *Nucleotide Sequences 1984: A Compilation from the GenBank and EMBL Data Libraries,* Vols. 1 and 2, IRL Press, Oxford, 1984.

33. **Armstrong, J., Atencio, E. J., Bergman, B. E., Bilofsky, H. S., Brown, L. B., Burks, C., Cameron, G. N., Cinkosky, M. J., Elbe, U., England, C. E., Fickett, J. W., Foley, B. T., Goad, W. B., Hamm, G. H., Hayter, J. A., Hazledine, D., Kanehisa, M., Kay, L., Lennon, G. G., Lewitter, F. I., Linder, C. R., Leutzenkirchen, A., McCaldon, P., McLeod, M. J., Melone, D. L., Myers, G., Nelson, D., Nial, J. L., Perry, H. M., and Rindone, W. P., Sher, L. D., Smith, M. T., Stoesser, G., Swindell, C. D., and Tung, C.-S.,** *Nucleotide Sequences 1985: A Compilation from the GenBank and EMBL Data Libraries,* Vols. 1 to 4, IRL Press, Oxford, 1985.

34. **Lewitter, F. I. and Rindone, W. P.,** Computer programs for analyzing DNA and protein sequences, *Methods Enzymol.,* 151, 582, 1987.

35. **Söll, D. and Roberts, R. J., Eds.,** *The Applications of Computers to Research on Nucleic Acids,* IRL Press, Oxford, 1982 (originally published in *Nucl. Acids Res.,* 10, 1, 1982).

36. **Sankoff, D. J. and Kruskall, J. B., Eds.,** *Time Warps, String Edits, and Macromolecules: The Theory and Practice of String Comparison,* Addison-Wesley, Reading, Mass., 1983.

37. **Gingeras, T. R.,** Computers and DNA sequences: a natural combination, in *Statistical Analysis of DNA Sequence Data,* Weir, B. S., Ed., Marcel Dekker, New York, 1983, 15.

38. **Korn, L. J. and Queen, C.,** Analysis of biological sequences on small computers, *DNA,* 3, 421, 1984.

39. **Martinez, H. M., Ed.,** *Mathematical and Computational Problems in the Analysis of Molecular Sequences,* Pergamon Press, Oxford, 1984 (originally published in *Bull. Math. Biol.,* 46, 461, 1984).

40. **Söll, D. and Roberts, R. J., Eds.,** *The Application of Computers to Research in Nucleic Acids II,* Parts 1 and 2, IRL Press, Oxford, 1984 (originally published in *Nucl. Acids Res.,* 12, 1, 1984).

41. **Davison, D.,** Sequence similarity (''homology'') searching for molecular biologists, *Bull Math. Biol.,* 47, 437, 1985.

42. **Kneale, G. G. and Bishop, M. J.,** Nucleic acid and protein sequence databases, *Computer Appl. Biosci.,* 1, 11, 1985.

43. **Mount, D. W.,** Computer analysis of sequence, structure and function of biological macromolecules, *BioTechniques,* 3, 102, 1985.

44. **Smith, R. J.,** The analysis of nucleic acid sequences, in *Microcomputers in Biology: A Practical Approach,* Ireland, C. R. and Long, S. P., Eds., IRL Press, Oxford, 1985, 151.

45. **Goad, W. B.,** Computational analysis of genetic sequences, *Ann. Rev. Biophys. Biophys. Chem.,* 15, 79, 1986.

46. **Söll, D. and Roberts, R. J.,** Eds., *The Applications of Computers to Research on Nucleic Acids III,* IRL Press, Oxford, 1986 (originally published in *Nucl. Acids Res.,* 14, 1, 1986).

47. **Waterman, M. S.,** General methods of sequence comparison, *Bull. Math. Biol.,* 46, 473, 1984.

48. **Waterman, M. S.,** Sequence alignments, this volume (Chapter 3).

49. **Claverie, J.-M. and Sauvaget, I.,** A new protein sequence data bank, *Nature (London),* 318, 19, 1985.

50. **Fickett, J. W.,** Correct translation of protein-coding regions in GenBank, *Trends Biochem. Sci.,* 11, 190, 1986.

51. **Fickett, J.,** Recognition of protein-coding regions in DNA sequences, *Nucl. Acids Res.,* 10, 5303, 1982.

52. **Zuker, M.,** The use of dynamic programming algorithms in RNA secondary structure prediction, this volume (Chapter 7).

53. **Calladine, C. R.,** Mechanics of sequence-dependent stacking of bases in B-DNA, *J. Mol. Biol.,* 161, 343, 1982.

54. **Dickerson, R. E.,** Base sequence and helix structure variations in B and A DNA, *J. Mol. Biol.,* 166, 419, 1982.

55. **Tung, C.-S. and Harvey, S. C.,** Base sequence, local helix structure, and macroscopic curvature of A-DNA and B-DNA, *J. Biol. Chem.,* 261, 3700, 1986.

56. **Suyama, A. and Wada, A.,** Correlation between thermal stability maps and genetic maps of double-stranded DNAs, *J. Theor. Biol.,* 105, 133, 1983.

57. **Nussinov, R. and Lennon, G. G.,** Structural features are as important as sequence homologies in *Drosophila* heat shock gene upstream regions, *J. Mol. Evol.,* 20, 106, 1984.

58. **Konopka, A. K., Reiter, J., Jung, M., Zarling, D. A., and Jovin, T. M.,** Concordance of experimentally mapped or predicted Z-DNA sites with positions of selected alternating purine-pyrimidine tracts, *Nucl. Acids Res.,* 13, 1683, 1985.

59. **Tung, C.-S. and Burks, C.,** A quantitative measure of DNA curvature enabling the comparison of predicted structures, *J. Biomol. Struct. Dyn.,* 4, 553, 1987.

60. **Nakata, K., Kanehisa, M., and DeLisi, C.,** Prediction of splice junctions in mRNA sequences, *Nucl. Acids Res.,* 13, 5327, 1985.

61. **Waterman, M. S.,** Frequencies of restriction sites, *Nucl. Acids Res.,* 11, 8951, 1983.

62. **Smith, T. F., Waterman, M. S., and Burks, C.,** The statistical distribution of nucleic acid similarities, *Nucl. Acids Res.,* 13, 645, 1985.

63. **Bitensky, M. W.,** *Genome Sequencing Workshop Report,* Los Alamos National Laboratory, Los Alamos, N.M., 1986.

64. **Smith, L. M., Sanders, J. Z., Kaiser, R. J., Hughes, P., Dodd, C., Connell, C. R., Heiner, C., Kent, S. B. H., and Hood, L. E.,** Fluorescence detection in automated DNA sequence analysis, *Nature (London),* 321, 674, 1986.

65. **Lewin, R.,** DNA sequencing goes automatic, *Science,* 233, 24, 1986.

66. **Dulbecco, R.,** A turning point in cancer research: sequencing the human genome, *Science,* 231, 1055, 1986.

67. **Palca, P.,** Department of Energy on the map, *Nature (London),* 321, 371, 1986.

68. **Lewin, R.,** Proposal to sequence the human genome stirs debate, *Science,* 232, 1598, 1986.

69. **Robertson, M.,** The proper study of mankind, *Nature (London),* 322, 11, 1986.

70. **Noll, H.,** Sequencing the human genome, *Science,* 233, 143, 1986.

71. **Newmark, P.,** DNA fingerprints go commercial, *Nature (London),* 321, 104, 1986.

72. **Morowitz, H. J., Hastings, J. W., Bennett, M. V. L., Bischoff, K. B., Cristofalo, V. J., Flamm, W. G., Gilbert, L. I., Lederberg, J., Porter, K. R., Sato, G., Streisinger, G., and Ward, S.,** *Models for Biomedical Research: A New Perspective,* National Academy of Sciences, Washington, D.C., 1985.

73. **Holden, C.,** An omnifarious data bank for biology?, *Science,* 228, 1412, 1985.

74. **Kanehisa, M., Fickett, J. W., and Goad, W. B.,** A relational database system for the maintenance and verification of the Los Alamos sequence library, *Nucl. Acids Res.,* 12, 149, 1984.

75. **Nelson, D., Cinkosky, M., and Marr, T. G.,** Relational Schema for GenBank, unpublished, 1988.

76. **Morowitz, H. J. and Smith, T. F.,** *Report of the Matrix of Biological Knowledge Workshop,* Santa Fe Institute, Santa Fe, NM, 1987.

77. **Burks, C. and Lawton, J. R.** LiMB Database: Release 1.0, unpublished release notes, 1988.

78. **Schermer, C. R., Smith, M. T., Nelson, D., Miller, R. L., McLeod, M. J., Lewitter, F. I., Hayden, J. E.-D., Foley, B. T., Fickett, J. W., Esekogwu, V. I., Cohen, I. H., and Burks, C.,** Cross-referencing the GenBank and HGML databases, *Cytogenet. Cell Genet.,* in press.

79. **Burks, C.,** How much sequence data will the data banks be processing in the near future?, in *Proceedings of the First CODATA Workshop on Nucleic Acid and Protein Sequencing Data,* Schwarz, D., Ed., Oxford University Press, New York, in press, 1988.

80. **Burks, C.,** Sources of data in the GenBank database, in *Proceedings of the First CODATA Workshop on Nucleic Acid and Protein Sequencing Data,* Schwarz, D., Ed., Oxford University Press, New York, in press, 1988.

81. **Burks, C.,** The GenBank database and the flow of sequence data for the human genome, in *Proceedings of the Brookhaven National Laboratory Symposium on the Human Genome,* Woodhead, A., Ed., Brookhaven National Laboratory, Long Island, NY, in press, 1988.

82. **Bilofsky, H. S., Burks, C., Atencio, E. J., Bossinger, J., Cinkosky, M. J., Esekogwu, V. I., Fickett, J. W., Foeller, C., Foley, B. T., Goad, W. B., Hayden, J. E.-D., Lewitter, F. I., Lopez, N., MacInnes, K. A., Marr, T. G., Martinez, A. V., Martinez, F. A., McLeod, M. J., Mishra, S. K., Nelson, D., Rindone, W.P., Schermer, C. R., Smith, M. T., Swindell, C. D., Trujillo, B. L., and Tung, C.-S.,** The GenBank genetic sequence data bank, *Nucl. Acids Res.,* in press, 1988.

83. **Atencio, E. J., Bilofsky, H. S., Bossinger, J., Burks, C., Cameron, G. N., Cinkosky, M. J., England, C. E., Esekogwu, V. I., Fickett, J. W., Foley, B. T., Goad, W.B., Hamm, G. H., Hazledine, D J., Kahn, P., Kay, L., Lewitter, F. I., Lopez, N., MacInnes, K.A., McLeod, M.J., Melone, D. L., Myers, G., Nelson, D., Nial, J. L., Norman, J. K., Rasmussen, E. D., Revels, A. A., Rindone, W. P., Schermer, C. R., Smith, M. T., Stoesser, G., Swindell, C. D., Trujillo, B. L., and Tung, C.-S.,** *Nucleotide Sequences 1986/1987: A Compilation from the GenBank and EMBL Data Libraries,* Academic Press, Orlando, FL, 1987.

Chapter 2

ANALYSIS WITH RESTRICTION ENZYMES

Eric S. Lander

TABLE OF CONTENTS

I. INTRODUCTION

A cornerstone of the genetic engineering revolution was the discovery of restriction enzymes.[1] Restriction enzymes are endodeoxyribonucleases that recognize specific nucleotide sequences in double-stranded DNA and cleave both strands of the double helix. In the cells of origin, restriction enzymes act to destroy foreign DNA such as from a virus; the cell protects its own DNA by methylating the recognition site so as to render it unrecognizable by the enzyme.

The first restriction enzymes to be characterized, type I, had a specific recognition site but cleaved nonspecifically. Much more useful for genetic engineering are type II enzymes which produce a reproducible double-stranded break at the recognition site itself. Fragments can be ligated together in new combinations, producing recombinant DNA molecules. We shall restrict attention to type II enzymes.

The recognition sequences are almost always 4, 6, or 8 nucleotides in length and consist of reverse palindromes, such as CATG, which read the same on the complementary DNA strand.

A number of partly mathematical issues arise in the use of restriction enzymes. We shall consider four below:

1. The distribution of the distance between consecutive sites
2. Algorithms for constructing maps showing the location of restriction sites
3. Choices in constructing a partial digest DNA library
4. Ways to use restriction enzymes as probes for sequence differences between individuals in a population and, thereby, to study inheritance of genetic traits in natural populations such as humans

This chapter is meant to be illustrative; it is by no means a comprehensive survey. In a few instances, I have tried to indicate interesting open questions.

II. DISTRIBUTION OF RESTRICTION FRAGMENT LENGTHS

A rather fundamental question about a restriction enzyme is the average length of the fragments it produces. For simplicity, let us suppose that the four nucleotides occur independently and with equal frequency 1/4 in a genome. In this case, it is usually assumed that the average fragment size will be 4^6 on average. Contrary to intuition, this is not necessarily correct!

To explain this apparent paradox, we must be specific about how to handle overlapping occurrences of a restriction site, such as GCGC (HhaI) in TGCGCGCT. By cutting at one of these sites, the enzyme will destroy the other. For concreteness, we shall imagine the enzyme precessively scans the DNA from left to right, cutting at any site that does not overlap a site which has already been cut. (This arbitrary choice is made for the sake of concreteness as to which sites are cut when overlaps occur; we do not suggest that enzymes necessarily work in this manner.) In probability theory,[2] each site of this sort is then called a "renewal".

The mathematics of renewals was worked out by Feller[3] 40 years ago for the case of flipping a fair coin. Applying renewal theory, Waterman[2] showed that renewals of the DNA pattern GGGGGG are spaced farther apart than renewals of the pattern TTTGGG. An intuitive explanation is the following: the law of large numbers guarantees that runs of six G's will occur on the average every 4^6 bases. However, since two such runs can overlap, not all runs of six G's are renewals. Thus, renewals of the pattern GGGGGG occur less often than runs of six G's. By contrast, the pattern TTTGGG cannot overlap itself. Hence, the average distance between occurrences is 2^6.

In general, the mean distance between renewals of a six letter pattern is given by the formula:

$$4^6 + e_1 4^5 + e_2 4^4 + e_3 4^3 + e_4 4^2 + e_5 4^1$$

where $e_i = 1$ if the pattern can overlap itself when shifted i bases to the right and 0 otherwise. The mean fragment lengths for enzymes with the following recognition sites would be as follows:

Site	Mean distance
ATTAAT	4096
TAGCTA	4112
TTTTTT	5460

The most serious deviation from expectation occurs for an enzyme whose recognition site is a run of six letters. (As almost all enzymes recognize sites that are reverse palindromes, however, no such enzyme has yet been found.) In the other cases, the deviation from expectation is small enough that it can effectively be ignored.

The foregoing analysis can be generalized to include the fact that nucleotides do not occur equally often and do not occur independently. In particular, the $(A + T):(G + C)$ ratio varies between organisms and the dinucleotide frequencies (probabilities of a particular pair of nucleotides being adjacent) often differ significantly from the product of the frequencies of the two nucleotides in the pair. For example, the CG dinucleotide is underrepresented in mammalian DNA (perhaps because the cytosine in the CG pair is frequently methylated, in which case deamination gives rise to a T). In such a case, a better estimate of the frequency of a pattern is obtained by including the dinucleotide frequencies.

As an illustration, the frequency of EcoR1 (GAATTC) sites in mammalian DNA based on single base frequencies would be

$$\mu = (P_G P_A P_A P_T P_T P_C)^{-1}$$

while incorporating dinucleotide frequencies it would be

$$\mu' = (P_A P_{GA} P_{AA} P_{AT} P_{TT} P_{TC})^{-1}$$

where P_A is a single nucleotide frequency and P_{GA} is a dinucleotide frequency (viewing a DNA sequence as a Markov chain). Using the published frequencies,[4] Seed[5] computed that $\mu = 3.5$ kb while $\mu' = 2.7$ kb. In fact, the average distance between EcoR1 sites observed in single copy mammalian DNA[6] is about 2.5 kb, which agrees much more closely with μ'.

As in the case of equal frequency and independence, further slight corrections can be made according to renewal theory[2].

It is also possible to ask about the expected renewals of several patterns simultaneously.[7]

III. CONSTRUCTING RESTRICTION MAPS

The construction of a restriction map — a map indicating the positions in a DNA molecule of restriction sites for various restriction enzymes — is a prerequisite for almost all genetic engineering. Although restriction maps reveal only a portion of the information in the complete nucleotide sequence, they require much less laboratory work than sequencing while providing a rough-and-ready fingerprint suitable for most purposes. A variety of methods

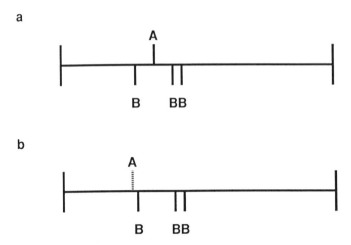

FIGURE 1. Measurement errors almost always occur in determining the lengths of restriction fragments. Even if the single digest fragments are ordered correctly, the computed lengths of the double digest fragments may not even lie in the same order as the actual lengths. An actual map is shown in a, with the inferred positions shown in b. Because of measurement errors, the order of the actual and inferred double digest fragments lengths does not correspond. This problem causes some algorithms for the double-digest problem not to be robust to measurement error.

have been used for restriction mapping. Simple and rapid methods for restriction mapping will likely acquire even greater importance when large-scale genome mapping projects are eventually undertaken.

A. Methods for Making Restriction Maps

Conceptually, the simplest method is via partial digestion. Cloned DNA molecules (i.e., a pure population) are first labeled at one end with a radioisotope. They are then incubated with a restriction enzyme under conditions (of time and concentration) that favor cleavage of about one restriction site per molecule. The partially digested mixture is then size-separated by electrophoresis through a gel which is then exposed to X-ray film. The bands on the film correspond to fragments stretching from the labeled end to one of the restriction sites. In this manner, the distance from the labeled end to the site can be simply read from the gel.

In practice, partial digestion is often not the method of first choice for several reasons: (1) determining appropriate conditions for partial digestion requires some care even under favorable circumstances; (2) for reasons that are poorly understood, different sites for an enzyme may have substantial heterogeneity in their rate of cleavage (thus, partial digest fragments terminating in sites with low cleave rates, but including a site with a high cutting rate, will be grossly underrepresented); (3) radiolabeling entails time and expense; and (4) the fragment sizes are relatively long, and the error in measurement of molecules by gel electrophoresis is roughly proportional to their length. Despite these problems, it is important to remember that one can resort to partial digestion when other approaches yield ambiguities.

A different approach is to use two different enzymes, for instance, A and B. Taking three aliquots of the DNA sample, one digests them (to completion) with (1) A alone, (2) B alone, and (3) both A and B. The three mixtures are then size-separated on a gel. All the fragments can be visualized by staining with ethidium bromide and their lengths recorded (Figure 1). So far, the laboratory work involved is minimal.

The trick is to determine which A-, B- and (A + B)-fragments overlap one another. It is easy to assemble the map once one knows which A- and B-fragments overlap. (Indeed, Griggs and Waterman[8] show that there is an algorithm with linear running for doing this.)

One can determine the overlaps either biochemically or mathematically. There are at least two biochemical approaches.

One approach is to purify the DNA from a band (the "probe" band), radioactively label it, and hybridize it to a second copy of the size-separated pattern of fragments (which has been transferred to a solid membrane via Southern blotting). After exposing the hybridized membrane to X-ray film, one can visualize exactly which other bands contain DNA from the probe band.

A related approach is to separately purify fragments obtained using the one enzyme and then redigest using the other enzyme. This shows the relationship between the single and double digest restriction fragments. Unfortunately both methods are quite time consuming.

The simplest approach, from the standpoint of laboratory work, is mathematically to deduce the map directly from the lengths of the A-, B-, and (A + B)-fragments. Constructing the map from this information, however, is a more formidable mathematical problem. We refer to this problem as the double digest problem, or DDP.[9-12] Specifically, we are given a piece of DNA of length L, together with three unordered list of lengths:

- $(a_1, \ldots, a_n)$ produced by cutting at site for enzyme A
- $(b_1, \ldots, b_m)$ produced by cutting at site for enzyme B
- $(c_1, \ldots, c_t)$ produced by cutting at sites for both

A solution consists of locations for sites compatible with these data. (More formally, a solution consists of permutations of the three lists such that every partial sum of the form $a_1 + \ldots + a_i$ or $b_1 + \ldots + b_j$ equals a partial sum of the form $c_1 + \ldots + c_k$.) Finding a solution is the DDP. Usually, all solutions are desired; we call this the complete DDP.

B. Complexity of the Double Digest Problem

We have stated the DDP in a rather idealized form, ignoring certain problems which arise in practice: (1) length measurements entail error (roughly proportional to the true fragment length); (2) if several fragments of similar size are produced, they will migrate to the same position in the gel and may be incorrectly recorded as one fragment; and (3) small fragments may be missed entirely.

Even in its idealized form, the DDP may be surprisingly hard. When we introduce such complications as measurement error (as we shall momentarily), further difficulties arise.

1. Computational Complexity of DDP

One measure of the difficulty of a problem is its worst case computational complexity.[13] A problem is said to lie in P if it can be solved in a polynomial number of steps (i.e., polynomial in the number of bits in the input). It is said to lie in NP if a proposed solution can be verified in a polynomial number of steps.[13] It is widely believed that NP contains problems that cannot be solved in a polynomial number of steps, i.e., that $P \neq NP$. The hardest problems in NP are said to be NP-complete, meaning that the existence a polynomial-time solution for the problem would imply the existence a polynomial-time solution for all problems in NP.

It is not hard to see that DDP is an NP-complete problem,[11] since DDP obviously includes as a special case a problem already known[13] to be NP-complete: the partition problem. In the partition problem, one is given integers $a_1, \ldots, a_m$ and asked whether there exists a subset $S \subset T = \{1, \ldots, m\}$ such that

$$\sum_{i \in S} a_i = \sum_{\in T-S} a_i$$

This is simply the DDP in the case when enzyme B produces two fragments of equal length. Thus, one cannot reasonably hope for a solution to DDP which is efficient in all cases.

2. Number of Solutions to the DDP

Another difficulty with the DDP is that the number of solutions grows at least exponentially with the length of the interval studied. A simple heuristic argument makes this easy to see.

Suppose that enzymes A and B cut at any given site independently with probability p_A and p_B, respectively. With probability $p_A p_B$, a position will be a site for both enzymes; call such a site a coincidence. (This is unrealistic in that sites for A and B never exactly coincide. However, it is justified by the facts that DNA segment lengths are never measured precisely and two enzyme sites can be very close together. Thus, approximate coincidences do occur at about this frequency.) The ends of the DNA segment should also be considered coincidences. Segments of the restriction map between consecutive coincidences may be freely permuted. Since a segment of length L will have roughly $s \approx p_A p_B L$ such segments, there should be at least about $s! > \exp(p_A p_B L)$ restriction maps compatible with the data.

Using the Kingman subadditive ergodic theorem, Goldstein and Waterman[11] make this argument precise, showing that the number of solutions to the DDP grows as $\exp(\gamma p_A p_B L)$ for some $\gamma \geq 1$, with probability 1 and in the mean. Consequently, the average case complexity of the complete DDP is exponential (since there are exponentially many solutions to find).

3. How Hard Is DDP in Practice?

Asymptotically, DDP seems depressing. In practice, however, things may not be so bleak for reasonable values of L, the length of the DNA segment. The behavior of DDP for small values of L has not yet been carefully studied.

Empirically good algorithms may thus exist for L in the range relevant to biologists. Indeed, this is certainly true for some values of L, since molecular biologists make restriction maps of plasmids in this manner by hand.

To pursue this thought, a more positive interpretation of the previous section is that double digest restriction mapping should only be attempted for segments small enough that coincidences will be rare. In practice, this should depend on the accuracy with which fragment lengths can be measured. Apparent coincidences should occur roughly every $1/\alpha p_A p_B$ nucleotides, where α is the "characteristic accuracy" with which lengths can be measured. Given two enzymes with six base recognition sites ($p_A \approx p_B \approx 1/4096$) and measurement accuracy to within about 50 bases, coincidences should only occur roughly every 333,000 bases. Enzymes with four base recognition sites will produce smaller fragments, which can be measured more accurately, say to within ten bases; coincidences will then occur roughly every 6500 bases.

If approximate coincidences are indeed the fundamental problem, this argument suggests that DDP becomes hard when L increases beyond some rough threshold L_0, depending on p_A, p_B, and α. For $L \ll L_0$, the average case complexity is perhaps relatively easy.

Restriction mapping of longer fragments might then best be accomplished by using three (or more) enzymes in all pairwise combinations (since three way coincidences are rarer than two way coincidences, etc.). We define the analogous multiple digest problem (MDP): given all single and double digests for k enzymes, make a restriction map compatible with the data. I pose the following problem: find $L_0 = L_0(k)$ such that MDP for k enzymes is "easy" for $L < L_0$, where L_0 will depend on the frequency with which the enzymes cut and the accuracy of measurement. An answer to this would offer useful prescriptive advice for how many enzymes to use in restriction mapping of longer stretches of DNA. This may become especially relevant as it becomes practical to study and clone fragments of megabase length.

C. Algorithms for the Double Digest Problem

With the above caveats in mind, we survey a few algorithms that have been suggested for DDP.

1. Exhaustive Search Over All Permutations

The first program to be widely used was that of Pearson.[12] In the case of two enzymes, where enzymes A and B yield a and b fragments, respectively, Pearson proposed looking at all a!b! possible permutations. For each arrangement, one computes the lengths $d_1' \leq \ldots \leq d_k'$ of the hypothetical double digest fragments that would arise. They are compared to the actual double digest lengths $d_1 \leq \ldots \leq d_k$ using a chi-squared-like criterion

$$E = \sum (d_k - d_k')^2/d_k$$

as a measure of goodness of fit.

Unfortunately, the approach is completely impractical for large L or for more than two enzymes. A more serious objection is that because of measurement error, the correct order of fragments for the single digest might not give the correct order of fragments in the double digests. An example is given in Figure 1.

2. Branch and Bound

Durand and Bregere[9] proposed a branch and bound procedure for forming the permutations required by Pearson. They proceed from left to right, adding to the leftmost fragment and rejecting (bounding) a partially constructed permutation when there is no double digest fragment to match within acceptable error.

To its credit, the approach incorporates errors and can handle multiple enzymes. Unfortunately, the margins of error snowball as the permutations are built; at some point, they become so large that bounding is no longer possible.

3. Bottom Up Assembly

Fitch et al.[10] proposed an approach involving finding all solutions to all the equations of the form

$$(A_i) \sum_{j \in S} c_j = a_i \text{ for some set S}$$

$$(B_i) \sum_{j \in T} c_j = a_i \text{ for some set T}$$

Because they infer the single digest fragment lengths by adding the component double digest fragments (rather than inferring double digest fragment lengths by subtracting the single digest lengths), the approach is much more robust to measurement error (see Figure 1). This realization was a very important contribution of this work.

Unfortunately, the authors are not specific about how to obtain all solutions to the required equations in a computationally efficient manner; this is important since the problem is in general NP-complete.

4. Growing Point Method

Blattner et al.[40] adopt a similar approach to avoiding the most serious effects of measurement error, but go a step further by suggesting an heuristic, back-tracking approach to finding solutions. Starting at the left end, a partial map is assembled consisting of an initial portion of the ordering for the A-, B-, and (A + B)-fragments. A new fragment is added to whichever of the three right termini lags furthest behind, after which consistency with the other partial maps is tested.

5. Simulated Annealing on Single Digest Fragments

Goldstein and Waterman[11] explored a rather recent combinatorial optimization technique called simulated annealing.[14] Simulated annealing is motivated by classical thermodynamics. For any possible ordering of the single digest fragments, one defines an "energy function", which measures how close the ordering comes to explaining the double digest data. (For example, the chi-squared-like statistic mentioned earlier would suffice.) Using a fixed value of a control parameter T called "temperature", one randomly permutes single digest fragments in such a way that the probability distribution over the possible ordering tends to the Boltzmann distribution at T (using a procedure introduced by Metropolis et al.[15]). One then lowers the temperature slowly toward zero. If this "cooling" is slow enough, the "lowest energy state" (i.e., the best fit solution) is obtained, just as it is in actual physical systems.

Simulated annealing has shown promise in such famous NP-complete problems as the traveling salesman problem. Unfortunately, although Goldstein and Waterman's application performs well when fragment sizes are measured exactly, it performs poorly[41] when measurement errors are introduced. The basic flaw seems to be that small errors in single digest measurements may completely distort the predicted lengths of the double digest fragments, as shown in Figure 1.

IV. CONSIDERATIONS IN CONSTRUCTING A LIBRARY

In order to correctly design DNA libraries, it is important to know about the distribution of fragments obtained from partial digestion with a restriction fragment.

Libraries consist of fragments of DNA which are cloned into a bacterial virus, plasmid, or other DNA molecule (generically called a "vector") capable of autonomous replication in a host cell. In general, the vector has a restriction site into which one can insert and propagate DNA fragments of length L with $S_{min} \leq L \leq S_{max}$ (the limits depending on the vector). DNA from the desired source is prepared by partially digesting it with the appropriate restriction enzyme and then ligating into the vector to form the "library".

Several questions arise:

1. **Infinite library problem** — what fraction of the genome can *in principle* be cloned in this way? That is, what fraction is contained in *some* partial digest fragment of length L with $S_{min} \leq L \leq S_{max}$?
2. **Finite library problem** — what fraction of the genome will in fact be cloned as a function of the degree of partial digestion and the size of the library?

The answers to these questions yield extremely practical advice to molecular biologists. They were worked out in two important papers by Seed,[5,16] whose approach we follow here. We suppose that restriction sites for the enzyme occur at independently and at random, with probability p.

A. Infinite Library Problem

The infinite library problem can be cast mathematically as follows. For an arbitrary nucleotide, the set A of distances to restriction sites to the left of the nucleotide is a random subset of the positive integers, with positive integers occurring independently with probability p. Similarly, for the set B of distances to sites located to the right of the nucleotide. The probability $P_\infty(p)$ that the nucleotide can be cloned in an infinite partial digest library is just the probability that $(A+B) \cap [S_{min},S_{max}] \neq \{ \}$.

The problem seems deceptively simple. Indeed, for $S_{min} = 0$ (say, cloning into a plasmid, which has no lower bound on insert), it is easy to show that

$$P_\infty(p) \approx 1 - e^{-pS}(1 + pS)$$

where $S = S_{max}$. In general, however, no closed form expression is known for $P_\infty(p)$ when $S_{min} \neq 0$. Seed provided the upper and lower bounds for $P_\infty(p)$:

$$P_x^-(p) < P_x(p) < P_x^+(p)$$

with

$$P_x^-(p) \approx \exp[-p(L + 1/2\Delta)(1 - e^{-p\Delta})]$$

and

$$P_x^+(p) \approx \exp[-p(L + 1/2\Delta)(1 - e^{-p\Delta(1 + \exp(-p\Delta))/2})]$$

with $\Delta = S_{max} - S_{min}$. The bounds are close together provided that $p\Delta$ is large, i.e., if the enzyme is likely to cut in a region of length Δ.

B. Finite Library Problem

The second question, the finite library problem, is still more difficult. Seed[16] supplied approximate under- and overestimates, although they are considerably more complicated than those above. The estimates allowed him to investigate the important question of how the extent of digestion affects the fraction of the genome that can be cloned.

The optimal degree of partial digestion is that which produces fragments whose number average length equals the mean insert size $L + \frac{1}{2}\Delta$ of the vector, provided that there is no heterogeneity in the rates which with an enzyme cuts at its various sites. However, Seed showed that the representativeness of the library is only slightly affected by even severalfold underdigestion. By contrast, overdigestion has disastrous consequences. Thus, underdigestion is preferred. (The argument for underdigestion becomes even stronger when one takes account of heterogeneity in cutting rates.)

While the primary issues of library making have been answered by Seed's studies, it would be interesting to know whether the extensive mathematical computations used to obtain the estimates might be simplified in order to gain a more direct, analytic understanding of such a basic problem.

V. MAPPING GENES USING RESTRICTION FRAGMENT LENGTH POLYMORPHISMS (RFLPs)

Recently, restriction enzymes have provided a powerful way to easily recognize variation in DNA sequence and thereby to trace the inheritance of a genetic region in a human pedigree. Exploiting this approach, geneticists have approximately located genes for such disorders as Huntington's disease,[17] cystic fibrosis,[18-20] polycystic kidney disease,[21] and Alzheimer's disease.[22]

A. RFLPs as Genetic Markers

While it has been clear since the rediscovery of Mendel that humans obey the same laws of heredity as other organisms, the study of human genetics has lagged behind genetics in experimental organisms in large part because of the lack of genetic markers whose inheritance can be followed through many generations. In fruit flies, for example, single genes causing curly wings, white eyes, or stubby bristles provide such genetic markers.

In 1980, Botstein et al.[23] suggested that slight variations in DNA sequence between a pair of homologous chromosomes could provide such markers for humans. They postulated that variation might be extensive enough that changes would often fall in restriction sites. In such a case, the lengths of the restriction fragments in a specific region would differ between two individuals or between the paternally and maternally derived homologous chromosomes in a single individual (see Figure 2).

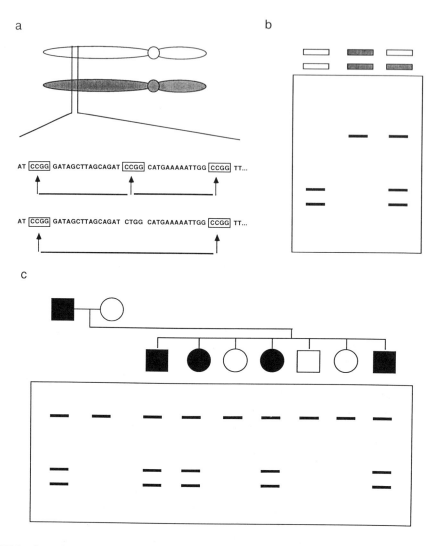

FIGURE 2.   Detection of an RFLP and its use in mapping a disease gene. A small chromosomal region on each of two homologous chromosomes is shown enlarged in a, revealing a single base change in the DNA sequence. The change happens to fall in a site for the restriction enzyme HpaII (which cuts at CCGG). Thus, HpaII will cut this region into two short fragments on the light gray chromosome and into one larger fragment on the dark gray chromosome. The lengths can be visualized via a southern blot. The distinction patterns for two copies of the light gray chromosome, two copies of the dark gray chromosome, and one copy of each is shown in b. Finally, c shows the restriction patterns for various members of a family (father, mother, and seven children). The individuals with darkened symbols have a dominant genetic disease. Note that they have all inherited the light gray allele from the affected father, while none of the unaffected children have done so. This suggests that the region detected by the RFLP lies near the gene causing the disease.

    To find such regions of variation, one would randomly screen DNA clones against restriction-digested DNA from a dozen or so individuals, searching for clones that identify more than one pattern (different variants at a locus are called *alleles* by geneticists). The variations themselves were called restriction fragment length polymorphisms or RFLPs.[23]

    RFLPs were soon shown to be abundant; over 1000 have been found to date and no end is in sight.[24-26] As hoped, random screening of RFLPs has uncovered markers linked to diseases. The basic approach is to find a RFLP with the property that, within each family, the child with a disease usually inherits one allele at the locus while the healthy children do not inherit this allele. (The allele associated with the disease may well vary between families, since the RFLP region and the disease gene have undergone recombination in the general population; only intrafamily correlations are studied.)

Linkage between two genetic loci is formally computed by the method of maximum likelihood. After collecting data on the inheritance of, for example, an RFLP and a dominant genetic disease in several families, one computes the probability $z(\theta)$ that the data would have arisen as a function of the (unknown) probability θ of a recombination between the RFLP and the trait locus; the maximum likelihood estimate of θ^* is used as a measure of the linkage between the loci. The recombination fraction θ varies between 0 and 0.5, representing close physical proximity and complete nonlinkage, respectively. For example, when all relevant inheritance information can be inferred from studying members of the family, one can just count crossovers — instances in which alleles at two loci entered a person through one gamete, but are not passed on together. If there are k crossovers out of n opportunities, then $z(\theta) = \theta^k(1 - \theta)^{n-k}$ and $\theta^* = k/n$.

The odds ratio in favor of linkage as opposed to nonlinkage is $L = z(\theta^*)/z(0.5)$. Usually, human geneticists report $\log_{10}(L)$ is called the LOD score and is additive for data from independent experiments.[27] A LOD score of 3 (i.e., data is 1000 times more likely to have arisen under linkage) is usually taken as the threshold for significance to avoid false positives.[27] The reasoning is roughly as follows: most genetic markers are unlinked to the disease in question, with the excess (based on the genetic length of the human genome) being roughly 50:1. Thus, a 1000:1 odds ratio in favor of linkage from an experiment together with these 50:1 *a priori* odds against linkage yield 20:1 *a posteriori* odds in favor of linkage, or roughly the 5% confidence level. (For an excellent introduction to linkage analysis see Ott.[28])

Linkage analysis would be rather simple, except that often only fragmentary information can be inferred from the data. For example, a healthy individual might be a carrier (heterozygote) for a recessive disease or might even have the disease genotype, but be one of the cases in which the disease state does not manifest itself. An individual's parents might be missing, which would make it difficult to determine which allele at a locus is on the maternally and paternally derived chromosomes. In short, the function $z(\theta)$ may be extraordinarily complex, involving many terms corresponding to the many ways of resolving the uncertainties in the data. Elston and Stewart developed an important algorithm for computing $z(\theta)$ by proceeding recursively up a family tree.

Genetic linkage analysis was developed by such workers as Fisher, Haldane, Morton, and Smith in the middle of this century and predates by far the advent of RFLPs and restriction enzymes. A complete review of this large area is beyond the present scope. Rather, the reader is referred to Ott.[28]

By their abundance, RFLPs both eased the task of finding linkage and have made feasible new analytical methods. This power derives from the ability to construct a complete genetic linkage map of the human (or any other) genome, consisting of RFLPs spaced throughout the length of the genome.

B. Number of RFLPs Needed to Construct a Complete Map

Various research groups, as part of an international collaboration coordinated by the Centre d'Etude du Polymorphisme Humaine (CEPH), are now constructing a complete RFLP linkage map of the human genome. (Similar projects are underway for maize, arabidopsis, and other organisms for which such a map would have research and commercial value. We shall consider the human case, although similar considerations apply to the other cases.)

A rather fundamental mathematical question is to determine how many RFLPs must be found so that every genetic locus will be within a distance of d centiMorgans (cMs) of a mapped RFLP. A cM is a genetic distance in which 0.01 crossovers are expected in any given meiosis; the human genome is estimated to be 3300 cM long. If we require that every locus fall within 10 cM of a RFLP, then each RFLP lies within $c := 20/3300 = 1/165$ of the genome; thus, 165 evenly spaced RFLPs are needed. Of course, in reality, the RFLPs will occur in random positions and thus many more markers will be needed to attain complete coverage.

If we assume that useful RFLPs are distributed uniformly with respect to the genetic length of the genome (see below), then the problem becomes an instance of a problem known in geometric probability:[30,31] covering a set with randomly placed intervals of length 2d. The set studied is usually a circle, but the extension to line segments and unions of line segments (i.e., chromosomes) has also been worked out. These methods were applied to the problem at hand by Lange and Boehnke.[32]

A standard Poisson argument shows that if N RFLPs are available, then an expected fraction equal to $e^{-N/c}$ of the genome will be further than d cM from a RFLP. So, 114 RFLPs would cover half the genome, while 493 RFLPs would cover 95% (assuming the circular model, which is a slight underestimate because of edge effects).

More generally, an entire distribution theory for the number of N of RFLPs is required to completely cover the genome. For example, Lange and Boehnke[32] apply a formula of Flatto and Konheim[31] to show that an expected number of 1273 RFLPs would be required to reach complete coverage with d = 10 cM. Of course, complete coverage is not essential, since a genetic map becomes of great value once, for instance, 90% of the genome is included, which occurs relatively early.

The most serious limitation of the model here is that it assumes a uniform distribution of RFLPs along the genetic length of the genome. While RFLPs can probably be expected to be distributed at random with respect to the DNA base pair length of the genome, there is evidence that crossovers do not occur uniformly with respect to DNA length. For example, there appears to be increased recombination (perhaps two- to fourfold) near the ends of at least certain chromosomes. If so, it may be necessary to study somewhat more RFLPs to overcome the effective selection bias resulting from the nonlinearity between physical and genetic distance.

In any case, however, it seems certain that enough markers will soon be available to construct a complete RFLP map of the human genome. A nearly complete RFLP, covering 95% of the genome, has recently been reported.[26]

C. Algorithms for Constructing a Linkage Map

The mathematical analysis needed for constructing an RFLP map with m loci is rather complex, since the correct order for the m loci must be established (out of m! possible orders) and then m-1 recombination fractions θ_i between consecutive loci must be estimated to produce the maximum likelihood map.

In fact, the process is typically reversed. For each of various candidate orders, the maximum likelihood map is determined; the order giving rise to the ML map with the greatest likelihood is chosen. Thus, we first consider the problem of finding the ML map, given an order for the m genetic loci.

While the traditional Elston-Stewart algorithm[29] is excellent for analysis of two genetic loci, the running time for the analogous computation of $z(\theta_1, \ldots, \theta_m)$ for an m-interval map scales exponentially in m.

When complete information is available for one of the loci, the likelihood function factors into two parts (corresponding to loci to the left and to the right) which may be computed separately in order to reduce computation time.[33]

Recently, Lander and Green[34,42] introduced a general approach to performing the calculation — called Markov reconstruction — that runs in linear time in the number of loci, although the time scales exponentially with the number of individuals in the pedigree. Thus, the algorithm is efficient for construction of multipoint maps in pedigrees of bounded size (probably up to about 20 individuals). Computer programs implementing the algorithm have recently been developed.[34] We sketch the main idea behind the algorithm.

To describe the entire pattern of segregation for a genetic locus in a family with N nonoriginals (individuals with parents in the pedigree), it would suffice to give 2N bits, called the inheritance vector — indicating, for the maternally and paternally derived chromosomes in each nonoriginal, whether the allele at the locus is of grandmaternal or grandpaternal origin. In general, the inheritance vector v_i at a locus M_i is not uniquely determined by the data. (For example, if both parents and their child have genotype a/b, then we cannot determine which parent contributed the "a" allele and which the "b" allele.) However, the Elston-Stewart algorithm for a single locus allows one to compute explicitly the probability distribution of v_i given the data for locus M_i.

Now, if two loci M_i and M_{i+1} are close together, then the corresponding inheritance vectors v_i and v_j will differ in few coordinates. More generally, the inheritance vector at consecutive loci along a chromosome can be viewed as the product of an m-step inhomogeneous Markov chain on the space of all binary 2N-tuples, with a one parameter transition matrix $T(\theta_i)$ on any given step corresponding to the process whereby bits change independently, each with probability θ_i.

Each meiosis involves a draw from the Markov chain. In each case, we have incomplete (and interdependent) information on the state of the Markov chain at the m different loci. Based on this information, we wish to estimate the θ_i.

One can apply the EM algorithm,[34,35] which involves guessing the θ_i using the guessed θ_i as if they were true to determine the expected number of recombinations that occurred, using this expected number as if it were the true number of recombinations to reestimate the θ_i, and so on. Using the Markov chain formulation, it is easy to determine the expected number of crossovers by means of Bayes' theorem, if the θ_i are taken are known. The running time for each iteration is linear in the number of loci. (It is also linear in the size of the support for the various probability distributions at the individual loci; the family must not be so large that these cannot be enumerated. In many practical cases, such as the CEPH families in which human maps are being made, the distributions are small enough to pose no problem. The general case of very large pedigrees and large numbers of loci remains open. It may be possible to use projections of the probability distribution onto certain sets of coordinates and to bound the error from such an approximation, but this area has not yet been pursued.)

Finally, given a fast way to construct the ML map and to determine the associated likelihood, it remains to select the best order for the loci. When the number m of loci is small, exhaustive search is possible. With more loci, one resorts to a true search. Simulated annealing over possible orders has also been tried with some success.

D. Unusual Uses for RFLPs

Once a complete genetic map is available, qualitatively different strategies for mapping diseases become possible. We mention two examples of how to exploit the full information available from a complete RFLP map.[36-38]

1. Simultaneous Search to Find Loci Causing a Heterogeneous Genetic Trait

In most organisms, including humans, the same trait can be caused by mutations at more than one genetic locus. Such a trait is said to be genetically heterogeneous. For example, mutations at any of nine loci will cause yeast to become unable to synthesize the amino acid histidine. In humans, xeroderma pigmentosum and ataxia telangiectasia appear to be heterogeneous traits.

Finding linkage of an RFLP to a heterogeneous trait is difficult, since evidence for linkage in some families (those segregating for a genetic locus near the RFLP) is offset by evidence against linkage in other families (those segregating for an unlinked locus).

One solution is to compute likelihoods for a joint hypothesis — namely, to study all the RFLPs simultaneously and to find a set of two or three candidate loci rather than just a single one that accounts for the inheritance of the trait. The method, called simultaneous search, was introduced by Lander and Botstein;[37] a detailed discussion of the mathematics can be found there. We should note that studying sets of loci increases the number of possible hypotheses (as opposed to single loci), and thus the *a priori* odds in favor of any particular hypothesis is lower. Hence, a higher threshold must be set for significance of the LOD score.[37]

The advantage of the method is most easily seen by the following limiting case: suppose that a trait was caused by mutations at any one of three loci and that three of our RFLPs fell exactly into these genetic positions. This set of three RFLPs would then have the unique property that, while the trait might segregate away from any one or two of the RFLPs in any given family, in no family would it segregate away from all three of the RFLPs. Statistically, detecting tight linkage of the set in all families is easier than detecting tight linkage of just one of the RFLPs in one third of the families (against the background of nonlinkage in the other families).

2. Homozygosity Mapping to Find a Rare Recessive Trait without the Need for Family Studies

For many recessive diseases, it will be difficult to find enough families with multiple affected members to permit linkage analysis to be carried out. The disease may either be quite rare or else those affected may die very young. Most cases will involve only a single affected family member, but this situation is of little or no power in traditional linkage analysis. It would be useful to be able to map genes for such traits without the need for family studies.

One such method, called homozygosity mapping, was introduced by Lander and Botstein.[38] It starts from the observation of Garrod[39] in 1902 that a large proportion of those affected with rare recessive diseases are children of marriages between close relatives. It is now understood, of course, that consanguineous marriages are an excellent way to cause a recessive disease gene to become homozygous by descent.

In homozygosity mapping, one searches the genome for a region in which several consecutive markers are found homozygous in many inbred children affected with the disease; this evidence suggests that the region is frequently homozygous by descent in such children and thus probably contains the disease gene. Mathematically, the significance of finding several consecutive RFLPs homozygous in an inbred child depends on (1) the genetic distance between the RFLPs; (2) the closeness of inbreeding; and (3) the degree of polymorphism of the RFLP, i.e., the chance that it will be homozygous at random in the general population. To evaluate the power of the test, one must compute the likelihood for the segregation data at RFLPs in the region. The required multipoint analysis can be carried out by using the Markov reconstruction algorithm mentioned above. Extensive results are reported by Lander and Botstein.[38]

The power of the method can be illustrated by a limiting case: suppose that we have highly polymorphic RFLPs (ones with many different alleles) very closely spaced throughout the genome and that we examine DNA from an affected child of a first cousin marriage. In the region of the disease gene, the RFLPs will almost certainly be homozygous (which in turn will almost surely indicate homozygosity by descent, since the RFLPs are highly polymorphic). By contrast, RFLPs in some unrelated region will be found homozygous only with probability 1/16 (this being the so-called coefficient of inbreeding for progeny of a first cousin marriage). Thus, finding a stretch of consecutive homozygous RFLPs provides 16:1 odds in favor of the hypothesis that the disease gene is nearby.

If the situation were to be found in three such children, the odds would be 4096:1 in favor

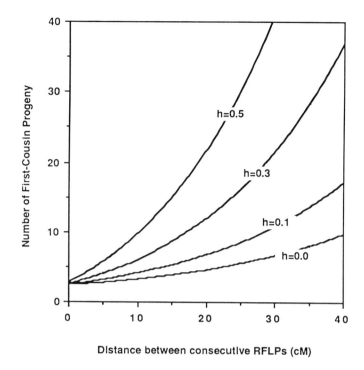

FIGURE 3.   Graph showing the number of unrelated progeny of a first cousin marriage affected with a rare recessive disease needed to map the disease gene, given a complete RFLP linkage map of the human genome. The spacing between consecutive RFLPs varies along the horizontal axis, while the four curves correspond to RFLPs of different degrees of polymorphism (with h denoting the chance that the RFLP is homozygous in a random noninbred individual).

of the disease gene being in the region — well over the 1000:1 odds needed to declare that linkage has been found. Of course, actual RFLPs are not so highly polymorphic nor will they be so closely spaced. Calculations with more realistic spacing of moderately polymorphic RFLPs have been performed. They show between 6 and 15 children may often suffice for finding linkage (see Figure 3). The small numbers required may make homozygosity mapping the method of choice for mapping most rare recessive diseases, as a high density genetic map becomes available.

ACKNOWLEDGMENT

This work was supported by grants from the System Development Foundation and the National Science Foundation.

REFERENCES

1. **Nathans, D. and Smith, H. O.,** Restriction endonucleases in the analysis and restructuring of DNA molecules, *Annu. Rev. Biochem.,* 44, 273, 1975.
2. **Waterman, M. S.,** Frequencies of restriction sites, *Nucleic Acids Res.,* 11, 8951, 1983.
3. **Feller, W.,** *An Introduction to Probability Theory and Its Applications,* 3rd ed., John Wiley & Sons, New York, 1968.

4. **Swartz, M. N., Trautner, T. A., and Kornberg, A.,** *J. Biol. Chem.,* 237, 1961, 1962.
5. **Seed, B.,** Theoretical study of the fraction of a long-chain DNA that can be incorporated in a recombinant DNA partial-digest library, *Biopolymers,* 21, 1793, 1982.
6. **Botchan, M., McKenna, G., and Sharp, P.,** *Cold Spring Harbor Symp. Quant. Biol.,* 38, 383, 1973.
7. **Breen, S., Waterman, M. S., and Zhang, N.,** Renewal theory for several patterns, *J. Appl. Probab.,* 22, 228, 1985.
8. **Griggs, J. R. and Waterman, M. S.,** Interval graphs and maps of DNA, *Bull. Math. Biol.,* 48, 189, 1986.
9. **Durand, R. and Bregere, F.,** An efficient program to construct restriction maps from experimental data with realistic error levels, *Nucleic Acids Res.,* 12, 703, 1984.
10. **Fitch, W. M., Smith, T. F., and Ralph, F. F.,** Mapping the order of DNA restriction fragments, *Gene,* 22, 19, 1983.
11. **Goldstein, L. and Waterman, M. S.,** Mapping DNA by stochastic relaxation, *Adv. Appl. Math.,* in press.
12. **Pearson, W. R.,** Automatic construction of restriction site maps, *Nucleic Acids Res.,* 10, 217, 1982.
13. **Garey, M. R. and Johnson, D. S.,** *Computers and Intractibility: A Guide to the Theory of NP-Completeness,* W. H. Freeman, San Francisco, 1979.
14. **Kirkpatrick, S., Gelatt, C. D., Jr., and Vecchi, M. P.,** Optimization by simulated annealing, *Science,* 220, 671, 1983.
15. **Metropolis, N., Rosenbluth, A., Rosenbluth, M., Teller, A., and Teller, E.,** Equation of state calculations by fast computing machines, *J. Chem. Phys.,* 21, 1087, 1953.
16. **Seed, B., Parker, R. C., and Davidson, N.,** Representation of DNA sequences in recombinant DNA libraries prepared by restriction enzyme partial digestion, *Gene,* 19, 201, 1982.
17. **Gusella, J. F., Wexler, N. S., Conneally, P. M., Naylor, S. L., Anderson, M. A., Tanzi, R. E., Watkins, P. C., Ottina, K., Wallace, M. R., Sakaguchi, A. Y., Young, A. B., Shoulson, I., Bonnilla, E., and Martin, J. B.,** A polymorphic DNA marker genetically linked to Huntington's disease, *Nature (London),* 306, 234, 1983.
18. **Tsui, L. C., Buchwald, M., Barker, D., Braman, J. C., Knowlton, R. G., Schumm, J. W., Eiberg, H., Mohr, J., Kennedy, D., Plesvic, N., Zsiga, M., Markiewica, D., Akots, G., Brown, V., Helms, C., Gravius, T., Parker, C., Rediker, K., and Donis-Keller, H.,** Cystic fibrosis locus defined by a genetically linked polymorphic DNA marker, *Science,* 230, 1054, 1985.
19. **White, R., Woodward, S., Leppert, M., O'Connell, P., Hoff, M., Herbst, J., Lalouel, J. M., Dean, M., and Vande Woude, G.,** A closely linked marker for cystic fibrosis, *Nature (London),* 318, 382, 1985.
20. **Wainwright, B. J., Scambler, P. J., Schmidtke, J., Watson, E. A., Law, H. Y., Farral, M., Cooke, H. J., Eiberg, H., and Williamson, R.,** Localization of cystic fibrosis locus to human chromosome 7cen-q22, *Nature (London),* 318, 382, 1985.
21. **Reeder, S. T., Breuning, M. H., Davies, K. E., Nicholls, R. D., Jarman, A. P., Higgs, D. R., Pearson, P. L., and Weatherall, D. J.,** A highly polymorphic DNA marker linked to adult polycystic kidney disease on chromosome 16, *Nature,* 317, 542, 1985.
22. **St. George-Hyslop, P. H., Tanzi, R. E., Polinsky, R. J., Haines, J. L., Nee, L., Watkins, P. C., Myers, R. H., Feldman, R. G., Pollen, D., Drachman, D., Growdon, J., Bruni,A., Foncin, J. F., Salmon, D., Frommelt, P., Amaducci, L., Sorbi, S., Piacentini, S., Stewart, G. D., Hobbs, W. J., Conneally, P. M., and Gusella, J. F.,** The genetic defect causing familial Alzheimer's disease maps on chromsome 21, *Science,* 235, 885, 1987.
23. **Botstein, D., White, R. L., Skolnick, M. H., and Davis, R. W.,** Construction of a genetic linkage map in man using restriction fragment length polymorphisms, *Am. J. Hum. Genet.,* 32, 314, 1980.
24. **Willard, H., Skolnick, M., Pearson, P. L. and Mandel, J. L.,** *Cytogenet. Cell. Genet.* 40, 360, 1985.
25. **Nakamura, Y., Leppert, M., O'Connell, P., Wolff, R., Holm, T., Culver, M., Martin, C., Fujimoto, E., Hoff, M., Kumlin, E., and White, R.,** *Science,* 235, 1616, 1987.
26. **Donis-Keller, H., Green, P., Helms, C., Cartinhour, S., Weiffenbach, B., Stephens, K., Keith, T. P., Bowden, D. W., Smith, D. R., Lander, E. S., Botstein, D., Akots, G., Rediker, K. S., Gravius, T., Brown, V. A., Rising, M. B., Parker, C., Powers, J. A., Watt, D. E., Kauffman, E. R., Bricker, A., Phipps, P., Muller-Kahle, H., Fulton, T. R., Ng, S., Schumm, J. W., Braman, J. C., Knowlton, R. G., Barker, D. F., Crooks, S. M., Lincoln, S., Daly, M., and Abrahamson, J.,** *Cell,* 51, 3197, 1987.
27. **Morton, N. E.,** Sequential tests for the detection of linkage, *Am. J. Hum. Genet.,* 7, 277, 1955.
28. **Ott, J.,** *Analysis of Human Genetic Linkage* Johns Hopkins University Press, Baltimore, 1985.
29. **Elston, R. C. and Stewart, J.,** A general model for the analysis of pedigree data, *Hum. Hered.,* 21, 523, 1971.
30. **Solomon, H.,** *Geometric Probability,* Society for Industrial and Applied Mathematics, Philadelphia, 1978.
31. **Flatto, L. and Konheim, A. G.,** The random division of an interval and the random covering of a circle, *SIAM Rev.,* 4, 211, 1962.
32. **Lange, K. and Boehnke, M.,** How many polymorphic genes will it take to span the human genome?, *Am. J. Hum. Genet.,* 34, 842, 1982.

33. **Lathrop, G. M., Lalouel, J. M., and White, R. L.,** Construction of human linkage maps: likelihood calculations for multilocus linkage analysis, *Genet. Epidemiol.,* 3, 39, 1986.
34. **Lander, E. S. and Green, P.,** Construction of multi-locus genetic linkage maps in humans, *Proc. Natl. Acad. Sci. U.S.A.,* 84, 2363, 1987.
35. **Dempster, A. P., Laird, N. M., and Rubin, D. B.,** Maximum likelihood from incomplete data via the EM algorithm, *J. R. Stat. Soc. Ser.,* 39, 1, 1977.
36. **Lander, E. S. and Botstein, D.,** Mapping complex genetic traits in humans: new methods using a complete RFLP linkage map, *Cold Spring Harbor Symp. Quant. Biol.,* in press.
37. **Lander, E. S. and Botstein, D.,** Strategies for studying heterogeneous genetic traits in humans by using a linkage map of restriction fragment length polymorphisms, *Proc. Natl. Acad. Sci. U.S.A.,* 83, 7353, 1986.
38. **Lander, E. S. and Botstein, D.,** Homozygosity mapping: a method for mapping recessive genes in humans by studying the DNA of inbred children, submitted.
39. **Garrod, A. E.,** The incidence of alkaptonuria: a study in chemical individuality, *Lancet,* 11, 1616, 1902.
40. **Blattner, A. et al.,** unpublished data.
41. **Waterman, M.,** personal communication.
42. **Lander, E. S., Green, P., Abrahamson, J., Barlow, A., Daly, M., Lincoln, S., and Newburg, L.,** MAPMAKER: an interactive computer package for constructing genetic linkage maps of experimental and natural populations, *Genomics,* 1, 174, 1987.

Chapter 3

SEQUENCE ALIGNMENTS

Michael S. Waterman

TABLE OF CONTENTS

I. INTRODUCTION

When two or more sequences are displayed with one sequence written over another, the resulting configuration is known as an alignment of the set of sequences. These displays are very common in molecular biology as they communicate information about proposed common evolution or function of the nucleotide positions found in any given column of an alignment. Sequence alignments are frequently obtained in an ad hoc manner, and simply written down in a way that makes the result "look good". Sometimes this means that important but implicit criteria have been satisfied. No mathematical approach devoid of deep biological intuition could hope to compete with this method. What is to be hoped for is that, over a long period of cooperation, mathematical and biological scientists can make explicit some of the biological insights. However, alignments that are pleasing to the eye of the scientist may not have much merit beyond that. The commonly used phrases "aligned so as to maximize homology" and "gaps inserted in order to maximize homology" might conceal a fairly confused attempt to maximize matches and minimize gaps. It is often not clear what has been attempted and "homology" is left undefined. In these cases, an explicit optimization function is an advantage, both for checking whether the alignment is optimal and for discussing the desirability of the optimization function itself.

One of the first mathematical questions concerns how difficult the problem of sequence alignment really is. A naive approach to the problem is to systematically list all alignments, evaluating each one. Alas, even for the two sequence case, when gaps are allowed, there are a huge number of alignments, and this exhaustive approach succeeds on only the smallest of problems. Section II will give an account of what is known about the combinatorics of alignments. The message is that alignment is a difficult problem!

Next, Section III turns to the problem of aligning two sequences by dynamic programming methods. This problem has received more mathematical attention than any other in molecular sequence analysis and the length of Section III reflects this. Computer science has studied the same problem under the description of the string edit problem; the problem statement is to find the minimum number of changes (substitutions, insertions, deletions, inversions) to convert one string (sequence, file, or word) into another. This problem has often been studied in many different forms and a book[1] has appeared on dynamic programming approaches to the problems of sequence comparison. In the present chapter, Section III.D on most similar segments is probably the most useful dynamic programming algorithm for current problems in biology, and some new developments are reported. A program written in C for the similar segments algorithm appears in the Appendix. Both similarity and distance methods are given for aligning two sequences. Methods for producing the optimal and near optimal alignments are described.

Many very interesting problems involve more than two sequences. Section IV gives dynamic programming approaches to the several sequence problem. Line geometries, a recent method employing ideas from the geometry of geodesics, are described and illustrated. While the line geometry approach is practical, it is likely to fail when the sequences are processed using the most unrelated sequences first. Line geometries handle the sequences in a given order, not simultaneously. Another dynamic programming method is presented that does not suffer from this shortcoming although it is prohibitively expensive in terms of time storage.

It will have escaped few readers that alignment is closely related to consensus. While the methods for consensus patterns do not instantly solve the problem of aligning several sequences, Section V describes an important new and practical approach. Based on the consensus word algorithm,[2] these techniques can align many long sequences in reasonable time and storage. Many problems in biology involve more than two sequences.

One of the major tasks facing a sequence analyst is that of comparing new sequences with all, or a major portion of, a large data base. The most successful algorithms for that problem are based on hashing the data base, hashing the new sequence, and then comparing hash tables. Section VI treats these issues.

Finally suppose that these or some other methods have produced an alignment of interest to the scientist. Section VII discusses how the alignment might be examined for statistical significance. Some mathematics has recently been worked out that solves several aspects of this problem. Extreme value theory has been employed to derive the so-called log(n) distribution.[3,4] that gives the statistical distribution of the best matching segments between two or more long sequences.

Recently in Waterman,[5] methods of sequence comparison were reviewed and organized. Many references of that paper do not appear in this chapter. Here, the goal is to more fully describe some major methods of sequence alignment and not to provide a review.

II. THE NUMBER OF ALIGNMENTS

In this section, a combinatorial treatment of sequence alignments is given. Biology provides the motivation for aligning sequences and for considering how difficult alignment is. It is then a mathematical task to estimate the number of sequence alignments. The results are applicable to biology in a negative sense; they assure one that a huge number of possible alignments exist and that direct enumeration is hopeless. The two-sequence case is handled first.

Notation is important here. Let $\mathbf{a} = a_1a_2 \ldots a_n$ and $\mathbf{b} = b_1b_2 \ldots b_m$ be two sequences of length, n and m. One way to think of alignment is that an alignment is produced when null elements, ϕ, are inserted into the sequences; the new sequences must be of the same length, L. Then the two sequences are written, one over the other. $\mathbf{a} = a_1a_2 \ldots a_n$ becomes, with the insertion of ϕ, $\mathbf{a}^* = a_1^*a_2^* \ldots a_L^*$ while $\mathbf{b} = b_1b_2 \ldots b_m$ becomes $\mathbf{b}^* = b_1^*b_2^* \ldots b_L^*$. The subsequence of $\mathbf{a}^*$ or $\mathbf{b}^*$ whose elements are not equal to ϕ is the original sequence. The alignment is

$$a_1^*a_2^* \ldots a_L^*$$
$$b_1^*b_2^* \ldots b_L^*$$

To see this process, let $\mathbf{a} = $ ATAAGC and $\mathbf{b} = $ AAAAACG. To obtain an alignment, one of many possibilities is to set $\mathbf{a}^* = \phi$ATAAGCϕ and $\mathbf{b}^* = $ AAAAAϕCG. For example $b_1^* = $ A, $b_6^* = \phi$, and $b_7^* = $ C while $b_1 = $ A, $b_6 = $ C and $b_7 = $ G. The alignment is written

$$\mathbf{a}^* = \phi\text{ATAAGC}\phi$$
$$\mathbf{b}^* = \text{AAAAA}\phi\text{CG}$$

Here $b_1^* = $ A is said to be inserted into the first sequence or deleted from the second, depending on the point of view. $a_2^* = $ A matches $b_2^* = $ A while $a_3^* = $ T and $b_3^* = $ A constitutes a mismatch.

The problem of this section is to find how many ways can $_{b^*}^{a^*}$ be written. No alignment terms $_\phi^\phi$ are allowed as there is no point in matching two deletions. This makes it clear that $\max[n,m] \leq L \leq n + m$. The case $L = n + m$ comes, e.g., by first deleting all a_i and then deleting all b_j:

$$a_1a_2 \ldots a_n\phi\ \phi \ldots \phi$$
$$\phi\ \phi \ldots \phi\ b_1b_2 \ldots b_m$$

Combinatorial insight comes by recognizing that alignments of these two sequences can end in exactly one of three ways

$$
\begin{array}{lll}
\ldots \; a_n & \ldots \; a_n & \ldots \; \phi \\
\ldots \; \phi & \ldots \; b_m & \ldots \; b_m
\end{array}
$$

where $\begin{smallmatrix}a_n\\\phi\end{smallmatrix}$ corresponds to an insertion/deletion of a_n, $\begin{smallmatrix}a\\b\end{smallmatrix}$ corresponds to a match or mismatch of a and b, and $\begin{smallmatrix}\phi\\b_m\end{smallmatrix}$ corresponds to an insertion/deletion of b_m. Note that the fate of the unseen bases (those not displayed) is not specified. Define

$$f(i,j) = \text{number of all possible alignments of one sequence of}$$
$$\text{i letters with another of j letters}$$

The above three cases imply

$$f(n,m) = f(n - 1,m) + f(n - 1,m - 1) + f(n,m - 1)$$

This follows because, for example, the first term corresponding to deleting a_n can obtain with the number of alignments of $a_1 \ldots a_{n-1}$ and $b_1 \ldots b_m$, which is $f(n-1,m)$.

The author obtained the above recursion equation and with P. R. Stein determined that it specified the Stanton-Cowan numbers.[6] Then Stein communicated the problem of asymptotics to H. T. Laquer who obtained the following theorem in 1981.[7]

Theorem 1 — Let f(n,m) be defined as above. Then

$$f(n,n) \approx (1 + \sqrt{2})^{2n+1}\sqrt{n}$$

as $n \to \infty$, where $c(n) \approx d(n)$ means $\lim_{n \to \infty} c(n)/d(n) = 1$.

Two sequences of length 1000, then have

$$f(1000,1000) \approx (1 + \sqrt{2})^{2001}\sqrt{1000} = 10^{767.4\ldots}$$

alignments! There are approximately 10^{80} elementary particles in the universe; Avogadro's number is on the order of 10^{23}

If it is agreed not to count

$$
\begin{array}{llll}
C\phi & \text{and} & \phi C \\
\phi G & & G\phi
\end{array}
$$

as distinct, the situation improves (slightly). Let g(n,m) denote this smaller number of alignments. $\begin{smallmatrix}\phi\\b_m\end{smallmatrix}$ has three possibilities

$$
\begin{array}{lll}
\ldots \; a_n \; \phi & \ldots \; \phi \; \phi & \ldots \; a_n\phi \\
\ldots \; b_{m-1}b_m & \ldots \; b^{m-1}b_m & \ldots \; \phi \; b_m
\end{array}
$$

while $\begin{smallmatrix}a_n\\\phi\end{smallmatrix}$ has

$$
\begin{array}{lll}
\ldots \; a_{n-1}a_n & \ldots \; a_{n-1}a_n & \ldots \; \phi \; a_n \\
\ldots \; b_m \; \phi & \ldots \; \phi \; \phi & \ldots \; b_m\phi
\end{array}
$$

The new version of the recursion equation is

$$g(n,m) = g(n - 1,m) + g(n,m - 1) + g(n - 1,m - 1) - g(n - 1,m - 1)$$

substracting the double count. The result is given in the next theorem, where the asymptotics are derived from Stirling's formula.[8]

Table 1
BEHAVIOR OF $h(b,n) \approx \gamma_b n^{-1/2} D_b^n$, THE NUMBER OF ALIGNMENTS OF TWO SEQUENCES OF LENGTH n WITH MATCHED BLOCKS OF LENGTH AT LEAST b

b	D_b	γ_b
1	5.8284	0.57268
2	4.5189	0.53206
3	4.1489	0.54290
4	4.0400	0.55520
5	4.0103	0.56109
10	4.0001	0.56183
. . .		
∞	4.0000 . . .	$0.56419 \ldots = \pi^{-1/2}$

Theorem 2 — If g(n,m) is defined as above, $g(0,0) = g(0,1) = g(1,0) = 1$, and $g(n,m) = \binom{n+m}{n}$. If $n = m$,

$$g(n,n) = \binom{2n}{n} \approx 2^{2n}(4\sqrt{n\pi})^{-1}, \quad \text{as } n \to \infty$$

Two sequences $n = m = 1000$ have $g(1000,1000) \sim 10^{600}$ alignments so that direct search is still impossible.

It is possible to further reduce the number of alignments by requiring matches and mismatches to occur in blocks of length at least b without interruptions by deletions. The motivation for this is that biologists sometimes reject alignments with small groups of matches. The counting scheme of Theorem 1 is readopted with this new requirement. The following theorem appears in Griggs et al.[9] where it is derived via generating functions.

Theorem 3 — Let $h(b,n)$ be the number of alignments of two sequences of length n where matches must occur in blocks of length at least $b \geq 1$. Define $\Phi(x) = (1-x)^2 - 4x(x^b - x + 1)^2$, and let ρ be the smallest real root of $\Phi(0) = 0$. Then

$$h(b,n) \approx (\gamma_b n^{-1/2}) D_b^n, \quad \text{as } n \to \infty$$

where $D_b = \rho^{-1}$ and

$$\gamma_b = (\rho^b - \rho + 1)(-\pi\rho\Phi'(\rho))^{-1/2}$$

Notice that $b = 1$ has $h(1,n) = f(n,n)$. Table 1 shows the behavior with b. When $b = 2$, for example,

$$h(2, n) \approx (0.53206)n^{-1/2}(4.5189)^n$$

More than two sequences is bound to make the problem more complicated, greatly increasing the number of alignments. The question is to determine how many more alignments. Recently, Griggs et al.[10] have provided an answer which is given in the next theorem. The methods of proof are the most difficult of any required so far, using a saddle point techinque.

Theorem 4 — Let $f_k(n)$ be the number of alignments of k sequences of length n. For a fixed $k \geq 2$,

$$\lim_{in \to \infty} \frac{\ell n\, f_k(n)}{n} = \ell n\, c_k$$

where

$$c_k = (2^{1/k} - 1)^{-k} \approx \frac{1}{\sqrt{2}}\left[\frac{k}{\ell n(2)}\right]$$

For our use notice that

$$f_k \cong c_k^n = (2^{1/k} - 1)^{-nk}$$

$$\approx 2^{-n/2}\left(\frac{k}{\ell n(2)}\right)^n$$

For $n = 1000$ and $k = 3$, $f_3(1000) \cong 10^{1755}$.

III. DYNAMIC PROGRAMMING ALIGNMENT OF TWO SEQUENCES

Needleman and Wunsch[11] wrote a paper titled "A general method applicable to the search for similarities in the amino acid sequence of two proteins". It was surely unknown to the authors that their method fit into a broad class of algorithms introduced by Richard Bellman under the name dynamic programming. Their paper has had a great deal of influence in biological sequence alignment. Its great advantage is that an explicit criterion for optimality of alignment is stated, as well as efficient method of solution given. Insertions, deletions, mismatches (negative similarity), and matches (positive similarity) were allowed in the alignments.

During early 1970s, Stan Ulam and some other mathematicians became interested in defining a distance $D(\mathbf{a},\mathbf{b})$ on sequences. The minimum distance alignment was defined to be an alignment with the smallest weighted sum of mismatches, insertions, and deletions. The advantage of a distance was the construction of a metric space on the space of sequences:

1. $D(\mathbf{a},\mathbf{b}) = 0$ if and only if $\mathbf{a} = \mathbf{b}$.
2. $D(\mathbf{a},\mathbf{b}) = D(\mathbf{b},\mathbf{a})$ (symmetry).
3. $D(\mathbf{a},\mathbf{b}) \leq D(\mathbf{a},\mathbf{c}) + D(\mathbf{c},\mathbf{b})$ for any $\mathbf{c}$ (triangle inequality).

The emphasis on sequence metrics came from the fact that a matrix of sequence distances was often used to construct an evolutionary tree. P.H. Sellers[12] gave a dynamic programming algorithm, very similar to that of Needleman and Wunsch, to calculate the distance.

The historical order is reversed here. Distance methods are described in Section III.A, with similarity methods in Section III.B. As mentioned in the introduction, we find similarity to be the most satisfactory. All problems known to be solvable with distance methods can be solved with similarity methods. However, in Section III.D, a similarity solution is given that has no distance counterpart. Still, the metric space associated with a distance makes it worthwhile to present distance methods. Section III.C shows several simple modifications to solve related problems such as best fit of a short sequence into a long one. Section III.D studies the important problem of locating segments of two sequences which are unexpectedly similar, although the full sequences might not have a good alignment. New results are given here for this problem. Section III.E closes with a recent modification of the dynamic programming algorithms that allows all alignments near the optimal to be produced.

A. Distance Alignment

The sequences $\mathbf{a} = a_1 a_2 \ldots a_n$ and $\mathbf{b} = b_1 b_2 \ldots b_m$ are written over the alphabet

{A,C,G,T}. Any finite alphabet will of course work here. In particular the 20-letter, amino acid, alphabet of proteins, or the purine/pyrimidine alphabet for DNA can be used. Let $d(a,b)$ be a distance on the alphabet and let $g(a)$ be the positive cost of a gap of the letter "a". The distance $d(a,b)$ represents the cost of a mutation of a into b. If $d(a,b)$ is extended so that $d(a,\phi) = d(\phi,a) = g(a)$, then define

$$D(\mathbf{a},\mathbf{b}) = \min \sum_{i=1}^{L} d(a_i^*,b_i^*)$$

where the minimum is extended over all alignments of **a** with **b**. Seller's result[12] can be summarized in the next Theorem.

Theorem 1 — If $\mathbf{a} = a_1a_2 \ldots a_n$ and $\mathbf{b} = b_1b_2 \ldots b_m$, define $D_{i,j} = D(a_1a_2 \ldots a_i, b_1b_2 \ldots b_j)$. Also set

$$D_{00} = 0, D_{0,j} = \sum_{k=1}^{j} d(\phi,b_k), \quad \text{and} \quad D_{i,o} = \sum_{k=1}^{i} d(a_k,\phi)$$

Then

$$D_{i,j} = \min\{D_{i-1,j} + d(a_i,\phi), D_{i-1,j-1} + d(a_i,b_j), D_{i,j-1} + d(\phi,b_j)\} \tag{1}$$

If $d(.,.)$ is a metric on the alphabet, then $D(.,.)$ is a metric on the set of finite sequences.

Proof — We verify Equation 1 with reasoning similar to that for verifying the recursion equation for $f(n,m)$ in Section II. The alignment of $a_1 \ldots a_i$ and $b_1 \ldots b_j$ can end in one of three ways

$$
\begin{array}{ccc}
\ldots a_i & \ldots a_i & \ldots \phi \\
\ldots \phi & \ldots b_j & \ldots b_j
\end{array}
$$

If the optimal alignment ends in $\begin{smallmatrix} a_i \\ \phi \end{smallmatrix}$, the cost must be $D_{i-1,j} + d(a_i,\phi)$ since the initial part of the alignment must itself be optimal and align $a_1 \ldots a_{i-1}$ with $b_1 \ldots b_m$.

If the optimal alignment ends in $\begin{smallmatrix} a_i \\ b_j \end{smallmatrix}$ the cost must be

$D_{i-1,j-1} + d(a_i, b_j)$ since $a_1 \ldots a_{i-1}$ and $b_1 \ldots b_{j-1}$ must be optimally aligned

The case $\begin{smallmatrix} \phi \\ b_j \end{smallmatrix}$ is identical in reasoning with the case $\begin{smallmatrix} a_i \\ \phi \end{smallmatrix}$.

The optimal alignment has least cost of these three possibilities and Equation 1 is proven. Another statement of Equation 1 is

$$D_{i,j} = \min\{D_{i-1,j} + g, D_{i-1,j-1} + d(a_i,b_j), D_{i,j-1} + g\}$$

when g is a constant gap cost, $g = d(\phi,a) = d(a,\phi)$. These algorithms have computation cost proportional to nm, $O(nm)$.

To illustrate the algorithm, we align two *Escherichia coli* tRNA sequences, threonine tRNA (sequence **a**; GenBank name ECOTRTACU) and valine tRNA (sequence **b**; GenBank name ECOTRV1). The algorithm has $d(a,b) = 2$, if $a \neq b$, and $g = 2.5$. Entries in the matrix in Table 2 are multiplied by 10 to allow use of integer arithmetic. Table 2 shows the matrix for the 5' (left) ends of the sequences. There are 72 optimal alignments, one of which is shown next. Portions of the alignment common to all 72 alignments are boxed.

Table 2

DISTANCE MATRIX FOR ALIGNMENT OF THREONINE tRNA (a) WITH VALINE tRNA (b)

	G	G	T	G	A	T	A	T	G	G	A	G	T	G	A	G	A	C	C	T	C	A	A	G
G	0	25	50	75	100	125	150	175	200	225	250	275	300	325	350	375	400	425	450	475	500	525	550	575
C	25	20	45	70	95	120	145	170	195	220	245	270	295	320	345	370	395	420	445	470	475	500	525	550
T	50	45	40	45	70	95	120	145	170	195	220	250	275	300	325	350	375	400	425	450	450	475	500	525
G	75	60	45	40	65	90	115	140	165	170	195	225	250	275	300	325	350	375	400	425	425	450	475	500
A	100	75	70	65	45	70	95	120	145	170	195	220	245	270	295	320	345	370	395	400	425	420	450	475
T	125	100	65	70	70	45	70	95	120	145	170	195	220	245	270	295	320	345	370	395	370	395	420	445
A	150	125	95	70	65	70	45	70	95	120	145	170	195	220	245	270	295	320	345	345	345	370	395	420
T	175	150	120	115	90	65	70	45	70	95	120	145	170	195	220	245	290	295	320	320	320	345	370	395
A	200	175	145	140	115	70	85	70	70	95	95	145	170	195	215	240	265	290	295	320	295	320	345	370
G	225	200	170	145	140	95	70	95	70	70	95	120	145	170	195	220	245	270	295	270	295	295	320	345
C	250	225	195	170	165	120	95	70	95	95	120	145	170	170	195	220	245	270	245	270	265	290	295	320
A	275	250	220	195	170	145	120	95	70	95	70	120	145	170	170	195	220	245	270	245	240	265	290	295
G	300	275	250	225	200	170	145	120	95	70	95	70	95	120	145	170	195	220	245	270	245	240	265	290
T	325	300	275	250	225	190	170	145	120	95	90	95	70	95	115	140	165	190	215	240	265	240	215	240
G	350	325	300	275	245	220	195	170	145	120	95	70	95	70	90	115	140	165	190	215	240	265	240	215
T	375	350	325	300	270	245	220	195	170	145	120	95	90	95	90	115	140	165	190	195	220	245	240	240
G	400	375	350	325	295	270	245	220	195	170	145	120	115	90	115	90	115	140	165	190	215	220	215	240
T	425	400	375	350	320	295	270	245	220	195	170	165	140	115	90	115	90	115	140	165	190	215	240	215
G	450	425	400	375	345	320	295	270	245	215	190	165	140	140	115	140	115	140	115	140	165	190	215	210
A	475	450	425	390	370	345	320	295	270	240	215	190	165	165	140	165	140	165	140	165	140	165	190	215
G	500	475	445	440	390	370	345	315	290	265	240	215	190	190	165	190	165	190	165	190	165	190	165	190
A	525	500	470	465	415	390	370	340	315	290	265	240	215	215	190	215	190	215	190	215	190	215	190	215
C	550	535	490	485	460	415	390	365	340	315	290	265	240	240	215	240	215	240	215	240	215	240	215	240
C	575	560	510	505	480	440	415	390	365	340	315	290	265	265	240	265	240	265	240	265	240	265	240	265
C	600	560	535	530	505	460	440	415	390	365	340	315	290	290	265	290	265	290	265	290	265	290	265	290
A	625	590	585	535	510	485	465	440	415	390	365	340	315	315	290	315	290	315	290	315	290	315	290	315
C	650	635	585	580	555	510	485	460	440	415	390	365	340	340	315	340	315	340	315	340	315	340	365	340
C	675	660	610	605	580	535	510	485	460	435	410	390	365	365	340	365	340	365	390	365	390	365	390	365
C	700	660	635	610	585	560	535	510	485	460	435	410	390	390	365	390	415	390	415	390	415	390	415	390
T	725	710	660	635	620	585	560	535	510	485	460	435	415	440	415	440	415	440	415	440	440	465	440	415
G	750	735	685	660	635	610	585	560	535	510	485	460	435	455	460	485	460	485	460	485	465	490	465	440
G	775	760	710	685	660	635	610	585	560	535	510	485	460	480	485	510	485	510	505	510	490	505	490	465
T	800	785	735	710	685	660	635	610	585	560	535	510	535	535	535	535	535	535	560	560	530	555	515	515
G	825	790	765	740	715	690	665	640	615	590	565	540	560	585	560	585	560	585	560	585	580	580	565	540
A	850	835	790	765	740	720	695	665	640	615	640	665	640	610	635	610	635	610	635	610	635	590	565	565
G	875	860	815	790	770	745	720	690	665	640	665	690	665	635	660	635	660	635	660	685	660	635	610	605
G	900	875	845	820	795	770	745	720	695	670	695	715	685	685	685	710	685	710	685	710	685	660	635	605

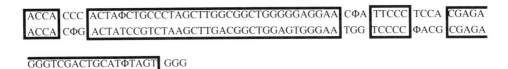

GGGTCGACTGCATΦTAGT GGG
TGGTTGACTCGATATAGT CΦG

To obtain all optimal alignments there are two techniques. The first involves saving pointers at each (i,j). The pointers show which of $(i-1,j)$, $(i-1,j-1)$ and $(i,j-1)$ are involved with the optimal $D_{i,j}$. Then, when $D_{n,m}$ is found, the pointers are followed to produce alignments. The second technique is to ask, at each (i,j) on an optimal path, which of $(i-1,j)$, $(i-1,j-1)$, or $(i,j-1)$ are optimal by recomputing the three terms. The alignments in these cases are produced by depth first search with stacking, where the stacks are managed by last in-first out. This is usually referred to as a traceback. Table 2 can be used to illustrate these alignment procedures.

Frequently in sequence evolution, gaps of several adjacent bases are not the sum of single base gaps but the result of one event. It is thus sometimes required to weight these multiple gaps differently from summing single gap weights. Let g_k be the gap weight for a gap of k bases. It is reasonable that $g_k \leqq kg_1$ holds. In Waterman et al.,[13] an algorithm was given for this case.

Theorem 2 — Set $D_{i,j} = D(a_1, \ldots a_i, b_1 \ldots b_j)$, $D_{0,0} = 0$, $D_{0,j} = g_j$, $D_{i,0} = g_i$. Then

$$D_{i,j} = \min\{D_{i-1,j-1} + d(a_i,b_j), \min_{1\leq k\leq j}\{D_{i,j-k} + g_k\},$$
$$\min_{1\leq \ell\leq i}\{D_{i-\ell,j} + g_\ell\}\}$$

The computation time of this algorithm is $\Sigma_{i,j}(i+j) = O(n^2m + nm^2)$, or $O(n^3)$ if n = m. For sequences of length 1000 or more, it is important to reduce this running time. This was accomplished by Gotoh[14] for this case of g_k linear.

Theorem 3 — Let $g_k = \alpha + \beta(k-1)$ for constants α and β. Set $E_{0,0} = F_{0,0} = D_{0,0} = 0$, $E_{i,0} = D_{i,0} = g_i$, and $F_{0,j} = D_{0,j} = g_j$. If $E_{i,j}$ and $F_{i,j}$ satisfy

$$E_{i,j} = \min\{D_{i,j-1} + \alpha, E_{i,j-1} + \beta\}$$

and

$$F_{i,j} = \min\{D_{i-1,j} + \alpha, F_{i-1,j} + \beta\}$$

then

$$D_{i,j} = \min\{D_{i-1,j-1} + d(a_i,b_j), \quad E_{i,j} \quad, \quad F_{i,j}\}$$

This gives an O(nm) running time for linear gap weights. If g_k is concave, such as $g_k = \alpha + \beta\log(k)$, then Waterman[15] gives an algorithm with a more complex algorithm. Miller and Myers[47] give a $O(n^2\log n)$ algorithm for g_K concave. If g_k is convex, an O(nm) algorithm is easier to obtain than when g_k is concave. However, convex gap functions seems an unlikely situation in biology.

B. Similarity Alignment

Now take s(a,b) to be a similarity measure on the alphabet. That is, we must have s(a,a) > 0 for all a. For some (a,b) pairs, it is necessary that s(a,b) < 0. The idea is that similarity (e.g., matching a with a) is rewarded by a positive score while aligning dissimilar letters is penalized by a negative score. Let $-\hat{g}(a)$ be the gap penalty associated with a. ($\hat{g}$ is used to distinguish this function from the gap weight of distance alignment.) Set $s(a,\phi) = s(\phi,a) = -\hat{g}(a)$. Then define the similarity of **a** and **b** by

$$S(\mathbf{a},\mathbf{b}) = \max \sum_{i=1}^{L} s(a_i^*, b_i^*)$$

where the maximum is over all alignments. The theorem of Needleman and Wunsch is
Theorem 1 — If $\mathbf{a} = a_1 a_2 \ldots a_n$ and $\mathbf{b} = b_1 b_2 \ldots b_m$, define

$$S_{i,j} = S(a_1 a_2 \ldots a_i, b_1 b_2 \ldots b_j). \quad \text{Also set } S_{00} = 0,$$

$$S_{0,j} = \sum_{k=1}^{j} s(\phi, b_k), \quad \text{and} \quad S_{i,0} = \sum_{k=1}^{i} s(a_k, \phi). \quad \text{Then}$$

$$S_{i,j} = \max\{S_{i-1,j} + s(a_i, \phi), S_{i-1,j-1} + s(a_i, b_j), S_{i,j-1} + s(\phi, b_j)\}$$

If $\hat{s}(a,\phi) = \hat{s}(\phi,a) = -\hat{g}$, for all a,

$$S_{i,j} = \max\{S_{i-1,j} - \hat{g}, S_{i-1,j-1} + s(a_i, b_j), S_{i,j-1} - \hat{g}\}$$

This theorem is proved exactly as was Theorem 1, Section III.A.

To illustrate the similarity algorithm, we align the same sequences as above, *E. coli* threonine tRNA and *E. coli* valine tRNA. We use a single gap algorithm and choose the parameters $s(a,a) = +1$, $s(a,b) = -1$ if $a \neq b$, and $\hat{g} = 2$. In Theorem 4 it is shown that for these parameters, the set of optimal similarity alignments is identical to that for the distance optimal alignments with the parameters of Table 2. Table 3 shows the matrix (S_{ij}) for the 5' (left) ends of the sequences.

The multiple gap case is covered by the next theorem. Gap penalty $\hat{g}_k$ is again assumed to be a function of gap length k.
Theorem 2 — Set $S_{i,j} = S(a_1 a_2 \ldots a_i, b_1 b_2 \ldots b_j)$, $S_{0,0} = 0$, $S_{0,j} = -\hat{g}_j$, $S_{i,0} = -\hat{g}_i$. Then

$$S_{i,j} = \max\{S_{i-1,j-1} + s(a_i, b_j), \max_{1 \leq k \leq j}\{S_{i,j-k} + \hat{g}_k\},$$

$$\max_{1 \leq \ell \leq i}\{S_{i-\ell,j} + \hat{g}_\ell\}\}$$

The following result obtains the O(nm) running time for the case of linear gap weights.
Theorem 3 — Let $\hat{g}_k = \alpha + \beta(k-1)$ for constants α and β. Set $E_{0,0} = F_{0,0} = S_{0,0} = 0$, $E_{i,0} = S_{i,0} = -\hat{g}_i$ and $F_{0,j} = S_{0,j} = -_{g_j}$. If

$$E_{i,j} = \max\{S_{i,j-1} - \alpha, E_{i,j-1} - \beta\}$$

$$F_{i,j} = \max\{S_{i-1,j-1} - \alpha, F_{i-1,j} - \beta\}$$

then

$$S_{i,j} = \max\{S_{i-1,j-1} + s(a_i, b_j), E_{i,j}, F_{i,j}\}$$

The parallels between the formulas for distance and similarity alignment lead to a natural question. When are similarity and distance algorithms equivalent? This question was an-

Table 3

SIMILARITY MATRIX FOR ALIGNMENT OF THREONINE tRNA (a) WITH VALINE tRNA (b)

The body of this page is a large numerical similarity (alignment) matrix. The left‑hand axis (Threonine tRNA, a) is labelled, top to bottom, by the nucleotide sequence:

G C T G A T A T A C C C A A T G G G A A G C C C T T G T A A G G A G G T A A G G G T G A G

The top axis (Valine tRNA, b) is labelled by the nucleotide sequence:

G G G T G A T G G C A C G A T C T C A G C T G A C G G G G A A C A C T C

The matrix cells contain the computed alignment scores. The first (leftmost) column, read top to bottom, runs:

1, −1, −3, −5, −7, −9, −11, −13, −15, −17, −19, −21, −23, −25, −27, −29, −31, −33, −35, −37, −39, −41, −43, −45, −47, −49, −51, −53, −55, −57, −59, −61, −63, −65, −67, −69, −71, −73, −75, −77, −79, −81, −83, −85, −87

and the first (top) row runs:

1, −1, −3, −5, −7, −9, −11, −13, −15, −17, −19, −21, −23, −25, −27, −29, −31, −33, −35, −37, −39, −41, −43, −45, −47, −49, −51, −53, −55, −57

swered by Smith and Waterman[16] and Fitch et al.[17] When full sequences are aligned by distance (similarity), there is a similarity (distance) algorithm that gives the same set of optimal alignments. That is, finding similarity and distance alignments are dual problems.

Theorem 4 — Let a similarity measure be given with s(a,b) and gap penalties $\hat{g}_k$ and a distance measure be given with d(a,b) and gap weight g_k. Assume there is a constant c, $0 \leq c \leq \max_{a',b'} d(a',b')$ such that $s(a,b) = c - d(a,b)$ and $\hat{g}_k = g_k - (kc)/2$. Then an alignment is similarity optimal if and only if it is distance optimal.

Proof — For simplicity, the proof uses the single gap case ($g_k = \infty$ for $k \geq 2$). Now by elementary counting

$$n + m = 2\#\text{matches} + \#\text{gaps}$$

obviously holds. Using this simple equation,

$$D(\mathbf{a},\mathbf{b}) = \min\left\{ \sum_{\text{matches}} d(a,b) + g_1 \#\text{gaps} \right\}$$

$$= \min\left\{ \sum_{\text{matches}} c - \sum_{\text{matches}} s(a,b) + g_1 \#\text{gaps} \right\}$$

$$= \min\left\{ c(n + m)/2 - \sum_{\text{matches}} s(a,b) + (g_1 - c/2)\#\text{gaps} \right\}$$

$$= c(n + m)/2 - \max \sum_{\text{matches}} s(a,b) - (g_1 - c/2)\#\text{gaps} \right\}$$

Notice that

$$D(\mathbf{a},\mathbf{b}) + S(\mathbf{a},\mathbf{b}) = c(n + m)/2$$

so "large distance" is "small similarity". After seeing this equivalence, it is surprising that there are problems with a simple similarity algorithm for which no equivalent simple distance algorithm exists. This situation arises in Section D.

C. Fitting One Sequence into Another

Next the algorithms are modified to solve a new problem: the best fit of a "short" sequence into a "larger" sequence. An example of when this might be of interest is in locating a regulatory pattern in a nucleotide sequence, such as TATAAT in a bacterial promoter. The algorithm finds where the short pattern approximately appears in the longer sequence.

First consider the problem of fitting $\mathbf{a} = a_1 a_2 \ldots a_n$ into $\mathbf{b} = b_1 b_2 \ldots b_m$. For the purpose of visualizing the problem think of n as much smaller than m. (The relative sizes of n and m are irrelevant to the mathematics.) The problem is to find i and j ($i \leq j$) such that

$$S(\mathbf{a}, b_i b_{i+1} \ldots b_{j-1} b_j) = \max_{k \leq \ell} S(\mathbf{a}, b_k b_{k+1} \ldots b_{\ell-1} b_\ell)$$

This problem is simply solved. We just use the similarity algorithm of Theorem 1, Section III.B. with $S_{0,j} = 0$ for all j. Then the required j is found by

$$S(\mathbf{a}, b_i \ldots b_j) = \max_{1 \leq j \leq m} S(n,j)$$

and i is found by tracing back beginning at (n,j) (instead of n,m)). The same procedure works with distance, as first shown by Sellers.[18,19]

To illustrate this algorithm, we take as sequence *b* the *E. coli* promoter sequence of lacI.[20] In *E. coli* promoter sequences, the -10 signal or pattern TATAAT is well known to have functional significance. The designation -10 refers to the distance to the left (5′) of the mRNA start. We take **a** = TATAAT. As above s(a,a) = 1, s(a,b) = -1 if a $\neq$ b, and $\hat{g} = 2$. The matrix (S(i,j)) is shown in Table 4. Searching the last row of the matrix gives two solutions of $\max_{1 \leq j \leq 58} S(6,j) = 2$, at (6,13) and (6,43). The pattern at (6,43) has the alignment

TATAAT

CATGAT

and is CATGAT in the promoter sequence, the canonical -10 pattern. The pattern at (6,13) has the alignment

TATAAT

TCGAAT

with TCGAAT in the promoter sequence, an equally good fit.

This illustrates the utility of the algorithm, in that it locates the putative -10 signal CATGAT in lacI. It also emphasizes the difficulty of promoter signal analysis by finding an equally good pattern TCGAAT 30 bases 5′ of the -10 pattern.

D. Identification of Similar Segments

Surprising relationships have been discovered between sequences that overall have little similarity. See Weiss,[21] Doolittle et al.[22] and Naharro[23] for accounts of some unexpected long matching segments between viral and host DNA. The subject of this subsection is a dynamic programming algorithm to find these similar segments. This is probably the most useful dynamic programming algorithm for current problems. For a mathematical statement of the problem, it is necessary to assume a similarity function s(a,b). The object is to find

$$\max_{\substack{1 \leq i \leq j \leq n \\ 1 \leq k \leq \ell \leq m}} S(a_i a_{i+1} \dots a_{j-1} a_j, b_k b_{k+1} \dots b_{\ell-1} b_\ell)$$

This amounts to $\binom{n}{2}\binom{m}{2}$ sequence alignment problems, and a new algorithm must be devised.

While Sellers[18,19] began the work on problems of this type, his problem formulations were based on distance functions and his algorithms involved forward and backward recursions, each recursion requiring a matrix. Although later[24] similarity functions are recommended by Sellers, those algorithms still involve intersection of path graphs and are quite complex. The similarity formulation given above was presented by Smith and Waterman and is solved in a straightforward way. Define $H_{i,j}$ to be the maximum similarity of two segments ending at a_i and b_j:

$$H_{i,j} = \max\{0; \quad S(a_x a_{x+1} \dots a_i, b_y b_{y+1} \dots b_j): \quad 1 \leq x \leq i, 1 \leq y \leq j\}$$

A recursion similar to those given for the similarity problems discussed above is obtained for H.[25]

Theorem 1 — Set $H_{i,0} = H_{0,j} = 0$ for $1 \leq i \leq n$ and $1 \leq j \leq m$. Then

Table 4

MATRIX FOR BEST FIT OF TATAAT INTO THE *E. COLI* PROMOTER OF lacI

	G	A	C	A	C	C	A	T	C	G	A	A	T	G	G	C	G	A	A	A	C	C	T*	T	C	G	C	G	G	T	A	T	G	G	C	A	T	G	A	T	A	G	C	G	C	C	C	C	G
T -1	-1*	-1	-1	-1	-1	-1	-1	1	-1	-1	-1	-1	1	-1	-1	-1	-1	-1	-1	-1	-1	-1	1*	1	-1	-1	-1	-1	-1	1	-1	1	-1	-1	-1	-1	1	-1	-1	1	-1	-1	-1	-1	-1	-1	-1	-1	-1
A -3	-1	0	-1	0	-1	-1	0	-1	0	-1	0	0	-1	-1	-2	-2	-1	0	0	0	-1	-1	-1	0	0	-1	-1	-2	-2	-1	2	0	-1	-2	-2	0	-1	-1	0	-1	0	-1	-1	-1	-1	-1	-1	-1	-2
T -5	-2	-1	-1	-1	-1	-2	-1	1	-1	-1	-1	-1	1	-1	-1	-2	-2	-2	-1	-1	-1	-2	0	0	-1	-1	-2	-3	-3	-1	0	3	1	-1	-3	-2	1	-1	-1	1	-1	-1	-2	-2	-2	-2	-2	-2	-2
A -7	-3	-1	-1	-1	-2	-2	-1	-1	0	-2	0	0	-1	0	-2	-2	-3	-1	-1	0	-2	-2	-1	-1	-1	-2	-2	-3	-4	-4	0	1	2	0	-2	-2	-1	0	0	-1	2	0	-1	-2	-2	-3	-3	-3	-3
A -9	-5	-2	-2	-1	-2	-3	-1	-2	-1	-1	-1	1	-1	-1	-1	-3	-3	-2	0	0	-1	-3	-3	-2	-2	-3	-3	-3	-5	-5	-3	0	1	1	-1	-1	-3	-1	1	-1	0	1	-1	-1	-2	-2	-4	-4	-4
T -11	-7	-4	-3	-3	-2	-3	-3	0	-2	-3	-2	-1	2*	0	-2	-2	-4	-3	-2	-1	-1	-2	-2	-2	-3	-3	-4	-4	-4	-4	-4	-2	0	0	0	-2	0	-2	-1	2*	0	-1	-2	-2	-4	-5	-5	-6	-6

$$H_{i,j} = \max\{0, H_{i-1,j-1} + s(a_i,b_j), \max_{1 \le k \le i}\{H_{i-k,j} - \hat{g}_k\}$$

$$\max_{1 \le \ell \le j}\{H_{i,j-\ell} - \hat{g}_\ell\}\}$$

Of course, single or linear gaps can be treated as discussed above (see Gotoh[14]). A traceback from (i,j) satisfying

$$H_{i,j} = \max_{\substack{1 \le k \le n \\ 1 \le \ell \le m}}[H_{k,\ell}]$$

will give a maximum similarity segment. What about other highly similar segments?

The following procedure finds one alignment from the highest score and then continues to find the next-best alignment with no matches or mismatches of its alignment in common with those already output. The original algorithm[25] stopped after the maximum segments were output and the algorithm given here is new.[26]

When calculating the matrix H, stack all (i,j,Y) with $Y = H_{i,j}$ and $H_{i,j} \ge C = $ cutoff value. The stack is ordered by $>$ where $(i,j,H_{i,j}) > (k,\ell,H_{k,\ell})$ if

i) $H_{i,j} > H_{k,\ell}$

or ii) $H_{i,j} = H_{k,\ell}$ and $i + j < k + \ell$

or iii) $H_{i,j} = H_{k,\ell}$, $i + j = k + \ell$, and $i < k$

During tracebacks for some stack entry, we only output one alignment. For this one additional concept is needed, that of minimum length alignment. Define the length of an alignment beginning at (p,q) and ending at (i,j) to be $|i+j-(p+q)|$. We only output minimum length alignments, although this is entirely a matter of choice.

The algorithm begins with the top (i,j,Y), i.e., the largest under ">", and that alignment is output. Next we must find the next largest scoring alignment that has no matches or mismatches in common with those already output. The simple concept of recomputing the matrix, not allowing matches or mismatches already used, is employed. This does involve more calculation. As the elements below and to the right of an alignment's end (i.e., (i,j)) must be recomputed, each succeeding alignment takes n*m/4 matrix entry recomputations on the average. While this might be worth the cost because of simplicity, much more efficient algorithms can be given in the cases of single and linear gaps.

Take the single insertion and deletion case, and let (k,ℓ) be the upper leftmost position of a match. (The alignment must end in a match or it is not optimal.) The new matrix N satisfies

$$N_{i,j} = H_{i,j}, \quad i < k \quad \text{and} \quad j < \ell$$

Define $N_{k,\ell}$ by

$$N_{k,\ell} = \max\{0, N_{k-1,\ell} - g_1, N_{k,\ell-1} - g_1\}$$

Note that the match ending the alignment is not allowed. Consider the row (k,j), $\ell<j$. Recompute each entry $j = \ell + 1, \ell + 2, \ldots$ until $H_{k,j} = N_{k,j}$. Then it is clear that $H_{k,\ell} = N_{k,\ell}$ for the rest of the row. Similar considerations hold for the remainder of the alignment. Note that on each row and column it is necessary to go at least to the position that was necessary for the preceding row or column. By this device a much more efficient algorithm is obtained. If an alignment has length L the recomputation required is approximately L^2 and if several alignments are output the recomputation is proportional to $\Sigma_i L_i^2$.

```
      A  G  T  C  C  G  A  G  G  G  C  T  A  C  T  C  T  A  C  T  G  A  A  C
C     0  0  0 10 10  0  0  0  0  0 10  0  0 10  0 10  0  0 10  0  0  0  0 10
C     0  0  0 10 20  1  0  0  0  0 10  1  0 10  1 10  1  0 10  1  0  0  0 10
A    10  0  0  0  1 11 11  0  0  0  0  1 11  0  1  0  1 11  0  1  0 10 10  0
A    10  1  0  0  0  0 21  2  0  0  0  0 11  2  0  0  0 11  2  0  0 10 20  1
T     0  1 11  0  0  0  1 12  0  0  0 10  0  2 12  0  1  0  2 12  0  0  1 11
C     0  0  0 21 10  0  0  0  3  0 10  0  1 10  0 22  2  1 10  0  3  0  0 11
T     0  0 10  1 12  1  0  0  0  0  0 20  0  0 20  2 32 12  0 20  0  0  0  0
A    10  0  0  1  0  3 11  0  0  0  0 30 10  0 11 12 42 22  2 11 10 10  0
C     0  1  0 10 11  0  0  2  0  0 10  0 10 40 20 10  2 22 52 32 12  2  1 20
T     0  0 11  0  1  2  0  0  0  0  0 20  0 20 50 30 20  2 32 62 42 22  2  0
A    10  0  0  2  0  0 12  0  0  0  0 30 10 30 41 21 30 12 42 53 52 32 12
C     0  1  0 10 12  0  0  3  0  0 10  0 10 40 20 40 32 12 40 22 33 44 43 42
T     0  0 11  0  1  3  0  0  0  0  0 20  0 20 50 30 50 30 20 50 30 24 35 34
G     0 10  0  2  0 11  0 10 10 10  0  0 11  0 30 41 30 41 21 30 60 40 20 26
C     0  0  1 10 12  0  2  0  1  1 20  0  0 21 10 40 32 21 51 31 40 51 31 30
T     0  0 10  0  1  3  0  0  0  0  0 30 10  1 31 20 50 30 31 61 41 31 42 22
T     0  0 10  1  0  0  0  0  0  0  0 10 21  1 11 22 30 41 21 41 52 32 22 33
G     0 10  0  1  0 10  0 10 10 10  0  0  1 12  0  2 13 21 32 21 51 43 23 13
C     0  0  1 10 11  0  1  0  1  1 20  0  0 11  3 10  0  4 31 23 31 42 34 33
A    10  0  0  0  1  2 10  0  0  0  0 11 10  0  2  0  1 10 11 22 14 41 52 32
G     0 20  0  0  0 11  0 20 10 10  0  0  2  1  0  0  0  1  2 32 21 32 43
T     0  0 30 10  0  0  2  0 11  1  1 10  0  0 11  0 10  0  0 11 12 23 12 23
A    10  0 10 21  1  0 10  0  0  2  0  0 20  0  0  2  0 20  0  0  2 22 33 13
C     0  1  0 20 31 11  0  1  0  0 12  0  0 30 10 10  0  0 30 10  0  2 13 43
```

A

```
      A  G  T  C  C  G  A  G  G  G  C  T  A  C  T  C  T  A  C  T  G  A  A  C
C     0  0  0 10 10  0  0  0  0  0   0*  0*  0 10   0  0 10   0  0 10  0  0  0 10
C     0  0  0 10 20  1  0  0  0  0  10*  0*  0*10   1 10   1  0 10  1  0  0  0 10
A    10  0  0  0  1 11 11  0  0  0   0   1*  0*  0*  1  0   1 11  0  1  0 10 10  0
A    10  1  0  0  0  0 21  2  0  0   0   0  11*  0*  0* 11   2  0  0 10 20  1
T     0  1 11  0  0  0  1 12  0  0   0  10   0   2*  0*  0*10   0  2 12  0  0  1 11
C     0  0  0 21 10  0  0  0  3  0  10   0   1  10   0*  0*  0*  1*10  0  3  0  0 11
T     0  0 10  1 12  1  0  0  0  0   0  20   0   0  20   0*  0*  0*  0*20  0  0  0  0
A    10  0  0  1  0  3 11  0  0  0   0  30  10   0  11*  0*  0*  0*  0*11*10 10  0
C     0  1  0 10 11  0  0  2  0  0  10   0  10  40  20 10   2*  0*  0*  0*  0* 2* 1 20
T     0  0 11  0  1  2  0  0  0  0   0  20   0  20  50 30  20   0*  0*  0*  0*  0* 0* 0*
A    10  0  0  2  0  0 12  0  0  0   0  30  10  30  41 21  30*10*  0*  0*10*10* 0*
C     0  1  0 10 12  0  0  3  0  0  10   0  10  40  20 40  32  12  40*20*  0*  0* 1*20*
T     0  0 11  0  1  3  0  0  0  0   0  20   0  20  50 30  50  30  20  50*30*10* 0* 0*
G     0 10  0  2  0 11  0 10 10 10   0   0  11   0  30 41  30  41  21  30 60 40*20* 0*
C     0  0  1 10 12  0  2  0  1  1  20   0   0  21  10 40  32  21  51 31 40 51 31 30*
T     0  0 10  0  1  3  0  0  0  0   0  30  10   1  31 20  50  30  31 61 41 31 42 22
T     0  0 10  1  0  0  0  0  0  0   0  10  21   1  11 22  30  41  21 41 52 32 22 33
G     0 10  0  1  0 10  0 10 10 10   0   0   1  12   0  2  13  21  32 21 51 43 23 13
C     0  0  1 10 11  0  1  0  1  1  20   0   0  11   3 10   0   4  31 23 31 42 34 33
A    10  0  0  0  1  2 10  0  0  0   0  11  10   0   2  0   1  10  11 22 14 41 52 32
G     0 20  0  0  0 11  0 20 10 10   0   0   2   1   0  0   0   1   2 32 21 32 43
T     0  0 30 10  0  0  2  0 11  1   1  10   0   0  11  0  10   0   0 11 12 23 12 23
A    10  0 10 21  1  0 10  0  0  2   0   0  20   0   0  2   0  20   0  0  2 22 33 13
C     0  1  0 20 31 11  0  1  0  0  12   0   0  30  10 10   0   0  30 10  0  2 13 43
```

B

FIGURE 1.   Maximum similarity segment analysis of two sequences. Here s(a,a) = 1, s(a,b) = −1 if a ≠ b, and ĝ = 2. In Figure 1A, the initial matrix is shown. Tracing back from the maximum entry 6.2 produces the alignment given in the text. In Figure 1B, the matrix is shown with recomputed entries with * to the right. Now the maximum entry is 6.1.

A computer program written in C for this algorithm is given in the Appendix. The program is also available on tape or disk from the author. To illustrate the algorithm, we set s(a,a) = 1, s(a,b) = −0.9, if a ≠ b, and ĝ = 2. Two sequences are compared and Figure 1A gives the matrix H($\times$ 10), where the best matching segments are

CCAATCTACT
CTACTCTACT

with score 6.2. The matrix N($\times$ 10) is shown in Figure 1B where the recomputed entries are shown with * to the right. For this step, the best matching segments are

CTACTACTGCT
CTACTϕCTACT

with score 6.1.

E. Near Optimal Alignments

The optimal alignments depend on the input sequences and the algorithm parameters. The weights assigned to mismatches and gaps are determined by experience. An effort is made to use biological data to infer meaningful values. Of course, in addition to assigning weights, there are sometimes unknown constraints on the sequences that cause the correct alignment to differ from the optimal alignment given by an algorithm. Hence, it is of some interest to produce all alignments with score (distance or similarity) within a specified distance of the optimum score. Recently, Waterman[27] and Byers and Waterman,[28] presented a new algorithm which accomplishes this. The algorithm has been previously presented for the distance algorithm. In this chapter, it is given for the similarity algorithm.

To be explicit, let $S = (S_{i,j})$ be the single gap similarity matrix with

$$S_{i,j} = \max\{S_{i-1,j-1} + s(a_i,b_j),\ S_{i-1,j} - \hat{g},\ S_{i,j-1} - \hat{g}\}$$

The task is to find all alignments with score within $e > 0$ of the optimum value $S_{n,m}$. All optimum alignments are included.

At position (i,j) assume a traceback from (n,m) to $(0,0)$ is being performed that can result in an alignment with score greater than or equal to $S_{n,m} - e$. The score from (n,m) to but not including (i,j) is T_{ij}. T_{ij} is the sum of the possibly nonoptimal alignment weights to reach (i,j). From (i,j), as usual, three steps are possible: $(i-1,j)$, $(i-1,j-1)$, and $(i,j-1)$. Each step is in a desired alignment if and only if

$$T_{ij} - \hat{g} + S_{i-1,j} \geqq S_{n,m} - e$$

$$T_{ij} + s(a_i,b_j) + S_{i-1,j-1} \geqq S_{n,m} - e$$

$$T_{ij} - \hat{g} + S_{i,j-1} \geqq S_{n,m} - e$$

respectively. Multiple near-optimal alignments can be produced by stacking unexplored directions. Of course, multiple insertions and deletions can be included.

A study of sequence alignment sensitivity to weights and multiple insertions or deletions has been carried out by Fitch and Smith.[29] The sequences displayed below are chicken hemoglobin mRNA sequences, nucleotides 115-171 from the β chain (upper sequence) and 118-156 from the α chain (lower sequence):

```
UUUGCGUCCUUUGGGAACCUCUCCAGCCCCACUGCCAUCCUUGUCACACGGCAACCCCAUGGUC
UUUCCCCACUUCG    AUCUUUGUCACAC                GGCUCCGCUCAAAUC
```

This alignment is presumed correct from the analysis of the many known amino acid sequences for which such RNA sequences code.

With a distance function, using a mismatch weight of 1 and a multiple insertion or deletion function $x_k = 2.5 + k$, where k is the length of the insertion or deletion, the correct alignment is found among the 14 optimal alignments. (This is region Q of the Fitch and Smith paper.) To indicate the size of neighborhoods in this example, there are 14 alignments within 0% of the optimum, 14 within 1%, 35 within 2%, 157 within 3%, 579 within 4%, and 1317 within 5%.

A mismatch weight of 1 and a multiple insertion or deletion function $2.5 + 0.5k$ is in region P of Fitch and Smith; accordingly, the correct alignment is not in the list of the two optimal alignments. This example illustrates the sensitivity of alignment to weighting functions.

IV. DYNAMIC PROGRAMMING ALIGNMENT OF MULTIPLE SEQUENCES

Many sequence alignment problems involve more than two sequences. The straightforward generalization of our two-sequence alignment algorithm to R sequences has complexity to $O(2^R n^R)$ when comparing length n sequences. For R = 3 this is frequently not practical and for R > 3, n must be *very* small. In Section IV.B these algorithms are discussed with some recent improvements. In the next section, IV.A, a geometrical approach, also based on dynamic programming, to these problems is presented.

A. Line Geometries

For this section a new, simple representation of sequences is required. It arises from consideration of a column in an alignment of several sequences. For example, the column

$$\begin{aligned}
\text{seq1} &\quad \ldots \text{ A } \ldots \\
\text{seq2} &\quad \ldots \text{ A } \ldots \\
\text{seq3} &\quad \ldots \text{ T } \ldots \\
\text{seq4} &\quad \ldots \text{ A } \ldots \\
\text{seq5} &\quad \ldots \phi \ldots
\end{aligned}$$

is frequently summarized as the "consensus" letter A. Much information is lost in this summary, and our representation of the column is with the "letter" $a = (p_A, p_C, p_G, p_T, p_\phi)$. For example, p_A represents the proportion of A in the given column. In this example $p = (3/5, 0, 0, 1/5, 1/5) = (0.6, 0, 0, 0.2, 0.2)$. Of course, usual sequences can be represented in this format by using $C = (0,1,0,0,0)$ etc. To compare two "letters" $a = (p_A, p_C, p_G, p_T, p_\phi)$ and $b = (q_A, q_C, q_G, q_T, q_\phi)$, the well-known metric

$$d(a,b) = \left(\sum_i w_i |p_i - q_i|^\alpha \right)^{1/\alpha}$$

is used, where w_i are weighting factors and $\alpha \geq 1$ is a constant. We have found in examples that w_ϕ needs to be larger than the other w_i; certainly ϕ plays a quite different role from A, C, G, or T.

The distance $D(\mathbf{a}, \mathbf{b})$ or similarly $S(\mathbf{a}, \mathbf{b})$ between two sequences $\mathbf{a} = a_1 a_2 \ldots a_n$ and $\mathbf{b} = b_1 b_2 \ldots b_n$ is computed by dynamic programming as above even though the sequence elements are themselves vectors. Associated with $D(\mathbf{a}, \mathbf{b})$ is an optimal alignment.

$$a_1^* a_2^* \ldots a_L^*$$

$$b_1^* b_2^* \ldots b_L^*$$

Now, for this alignment, define $\mathbf{c}(\lambda) = \lambda \mathbf{a} \oplus (1-\lambda)\mathbf{b}$ by $c_i(\lambda) = \lambda a_i^* + (1-\lambda)b_i^*$. The last "+" is simple vector addition. It is not surprising that $\mathbf{c}(1/2)$ is midway between $\mathbf{a}$ and $\mathbf{b}$. In fact, much more is true.

Theorem 1 — Let $\mathbf{c}(\lambda) = \lambda \mathbf{a} \oplus (1-\lambda)\mathbf{b}$ where $0 \leq \lambda \leq 1$. Then

$$D(\mathbf{a},\mathbf{b}) = D(\mathbf{a}, \mathbf{c}(\lambda)) + D(\mathbf{c}(\lambda), \mathbf{b})$$

$$D(\mathbf{a}, \mathbf{c}(\lambda)) = (1-\lambda)D(\mathbf{a},\mathbf{b}),$$

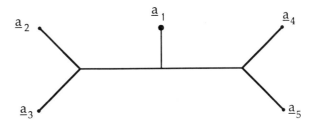

FIGURE 2. Tree relating $\mathbf{a}_1$ (*E. coli*), $\mathbf{a}_2$ (*B. stearo*), $\mathbf{a}_3$ (*H. volcanii*), $\mathbf{a}_4$ (*D. discoideum*), and $\mathbf{a}_5$ (*S. cerevisiae*).

and

$$D(c(\lambda_1),c(\lambda_2)) = |\lambda_1 - \lambda_2|D(\mathbf{a},\mathbf{b})$$

This theorem is proved in Waterman and Perlwitz.[30]

This technique was devised to align several sequences, but it does not always behave well on sets of sequences. Methods of finding "center of gravity" sequences were studied and did not always converge rapidly. However, if the sequences are related by a given phylogenetic tree, useful alignments can be produced by use of "$\oplus$".

As an example of this alignment algorithm, consider the tree of Figure 2 with the associated 5 sequences. Alignment is performed by using the tree to suggest the order of sequence alignment:

$$\mathbf{b} = \frac{1}{5}\,a_1 \oplus \frac{4}{5}\left[\frac{1}{2}\left(\frac{1}{2}\,\mathbf{a}_2 \oplus \frac{1}{2}\,\mathbf{a}_3\right) \oplus \frac{1}{2}\left(\frac{1}{2}\,\mathbf{a}_4 \oplus \frac{1}{2}\,\mathbf{a}_5\right)\right]$$

The deletion term needs a heavier penalty than A,C,G,T:

$$d(a,b) = \sum_{i\in\{A,C,G,T\}} |p_i - q_i| + 4|p_\phi - q_\phi|$$

The resulting $\mathbf{b}$ is used to obtain an overall alignment by aligning each of $\mathbf{a}_1, \ldots \mathbf{a}_5$ with $\mathbf{b}$. The result given below is identical with Woese et al.,[31] who obtain it in Table 31 of their analysis of 16S-like rRNAs.

E. coli ($\mathbf{a}_1$)	CAACCCUUAUCCφUUUGUAACUCAAAGGAGGAAUGUUGGGA
B. stearo ($\mathbf{a}_2$)	CAACCCUCGCCUφCUAGUCACUCUAGAGGGGAAGGUGGGGA
H. volcanii ($\mathbf{a}_3$)	AGACCCGCACUUφCUAAUUACAUUAGAAGGGAAGGAACGGG
D. discoideum ($\mathbf{a}_4$)	AGACCUCGACCUGCUAACCUUCUUAGAGGGGAAGUCCGAGG
S. cerevisiae ($\mathbf{a}_5$)	AGACCUUAACCUACUAAACUUCUUAGAGGGGAAGUUUGAGG

B. Generalization of the Two-Sequence Algorithm

For a straightforward extension of the two-sequence algorithm to more sequences, some notation is first set. There are R sequences, $\mathbf{a} = a_1a_2 \ldots a_n$, $\mathbf{b} = b_1b_2 \ldots b_m$, $\ldots$, $\mathbf{r} = r_1r_2 \ldots r_o$. The algorithm comes from considering an alignment of $a_1 \ldots a_i$; $b_1 \ldots b_j$; $r_1 \ldots r_x$. The last column of the alignment will appear as

$$\epsilon_1 a_i$$

$$\epsilon_2 b_j$$

$$\ldots$$

$$\epsilon_k r_x$$

where $\epsilon_i = 0$ or 1 and $0 \cdot a = \phi$. If $\epsilon = (\epsilon_1, \ldots \epsilon_R) \neq \mathbf{0}$, it is required that there are $2^R - 1$ such columns. Recall that for $R = 2$ there are $2^2 - 1 = 3$ terms to optimize. Here, if a "distance" function is defined on R variables, the formula extends to

$$D_{i,j,\ldots,x} = \min_{\epsilon \neq 0} [D_{i-\epsilon_1,j-\epsilon_2,\ldots x-\epsilon_R} + d(\epsilon_1 a_i, \epsilon_2 b_j, \ldots, \epsilon_k r_x)\}$$

This formula appeared in Waterman et al.,[13] and has computational complexity proportional to $O(2^R n^R)$ where the sequences are assumed to have length n. Storage takes $O(n^R)$. Carrillo and Lipman[48] have improved the complexity of these algorithms with a branch and bound technique.

A deeper analysis by Sankoff[32] appeared earlier. Sankoff assumes that the sequences are related by a given phylogenetic tree. His algorithm constructs sequences for each interior node of the tree and produces an alignment of the R sequences at the exterior nodes along with the (N) sequences $(X_1, X_2, \ldots X_N)$ constructed for the interior nodes. Sankoff and Cedergren[33] give an excellent account of this procedure. The dynamic programming step is given by

$$D_{i,j,\ldots,x} = \min_{\epsilon \neq 0} D_{i-\epsilon_1,j-\epsilon_2,\ldots x-\epsilon_R} + \min \begin{matrix} \epsilon_1 a_i \\ \epsilon_2 a_j \\ \ldots \\ \epsilon_R r_x \\ X_1 \\ \ldots \\ X_N \end{matrix} \qquad (55)$$

The second minimum is to indicate that $X_1 \ldots X_N$ have been chosen for the interior nodes in such a way as to minimum number of mutations along the tree. A generalization of Fitch's parsimony method[34] is used here and takes N steps. The computation requires $O(2^R n^R N)$ steps. $R = 3$ is nearly the largest practical R and Sankoff has devised an iterative method, which works with groups of three sequences, to build up a solution for larger problems. Altschul and Lipman[49] have extended Carrillo and Lipman[48] to align multiple sequences with a given tree.

V. CONSENSUS ALIGNMENT OF MULTIPLE SEQUENCES

As Section IV illustrates, dynamic programming methods have generally not been found practical for more than two sequences. It is natural to ask whether methods for finding consensus patterns can be applied to find alignments, which are in a real sense consensus patterns themselves. Usually, it will be reasonable to limit the amount of shifting one sequence can have, relative to the others. That is, the alignment

$$\text{sequence 1} \ldots a_i$$

$$\text{sequence 2} \ldots b_j$$

$$\ldots$$

$$\text{sequence r} \ldots r_x$$

is only allowed when $|i-j|, \ldots |i-x|, |j-x|, \ldots$ are all less than, or equal to, some bound. It is feasible to set the bound equal to sequence length and, therefore, to allow unrestricted shifting. The object of this section is to use the algorithm for consensus words to make a useful, practical, alignment algorithm (see the chapter on consensus patterns[2]). This algorithm is presented in a recent paper.[35]

To conform with the conventions of the previous chapter, the object is to find consensus words w, k letters in length, where the window width is W. This means the maximum shift between matched words is $W-k$. The bound on $|i-j|, \ldots, |i-x|, |j-x|, \ldots$ is thus $W-k$. The window at position i appears as:

Position

$$i+1 \ldots i+W$$

sequence 1 $\ldots$ $a_{i+1}a_{i+2} \ldots a_{i+}W$

sequence 2 $\ldots$ $b_{i+1}b_{i+2} \ldots b_{i+}W$

$\ldots$

sequence R $\ldots \ldots$ $r_{i+1}r_{i+2} \ldots r_{i+}W$

window width $=$ W

A neighborhood of, say, less than, or equal to, 2 mismatches is specified for matching words, and a score $s_w(v)$ is given to a word v in the neighborhood of w, where $0 \leq s_w(v) \leq 1$. Define the maximum scoring word in the window of sequence i to be v_i so that v_i best matches w. Then the score of w in the sequence set is

$$S(w) = \sum_{i=1}^{R} \max_{V}\{s_w(v)\} = \sum_{i=1}^{R} s_w(v_i)$$

A consensus word w* is one satisfying

$$S(w^*) = \max_w S(w)$$

where w ranges over all k-letter words.

An illustration of the location of such a consensus word is given next, where only the window is displayed.

Position
i

sequence 1 $\ldots..v_1\ldots...$
sequence 2 $\ldots\ldots\ldots.$
sequence 3 $v_3\ldots\ldots..$
$\ldots$ $\ldots\ldots\ldots.$
sequence R $\ldots\ldots..v_R\ldots$
W

The words v_i are in the neighborhood of w. Here, sequence 2 fails to have a word v_2 in the neighborhood of w.

Define a partial order on consensus words by their location in the sequences as follows: $w^{(1)} < w^{(2)}$ if the occurrence of $w^{(1)}$ in sequence i is to the left of (and not overlapping) the occurrence of $w^{(2)}$ in sequence i, for all $i = 1, 2 \ldots R$. If $v_i^{(1)}$, $v_i^{(2)}$ mark the individual sequence patterns, respectively, in sequence i, then the order appears as

$$\ldots\ldots.v_1^{(1)}\ldots v_1^{(2)}\ldots\ldots\ldots$$
$$\ldots\ldots.v_2^{(1)}\ldots\ldots.v_2^{(2)}\ldots.$$
$$\ldots\ldots\ldots\ldots\ldots\ldots\ldots.v_3^{(1)}\ldots.$$
$$\ldots\ldots\ldots\ldots\ldots\ldots\ldots\ldots\ldots\ldots$$
$$\ldots\ldots\ldots.v_R^{(1)}\ldots v_R^{(2)}\ldots\ldots$$

An optimal alignment A, is one that satisfies

$$S(A) = \max_{A'} S(A') = \max_{A'} \sum_{w_1 < w_2 < \ldots} S(w_i)$$

In general, it is not known how to find S(A). However, one version of the problem can be solved exactly.

Let $w_1|w_2$ mean that consensus words w_1 and w_2 can be found in nonoverlapping windows:

$$\ldots\ldots.v_1^{(1)}\ldots\ldots\ldots\ldots\ldots.v_1^{(2)}\ldots\ldots$$
$$\ldots\ldots\ldots.v_2^{(1)}\ldots\ldots\ldots\ldots\ldots\ldots$$
$$\ldots\ldots.v_R^{(1)}\ldots\ldots\ldots\ldots.v_R^{(2)}\ldots\ldots$$

The modified optimization problem is to find the alignment A, satisfying

$$R(A) = \max_{A'} R(A') = \max_{A'} \sum_{w_1|w_2|\ldots} R(w_i)$$

A simple recursion for R is easily given which is linear in sequence length. Define R_i to be the value of R for the set of sequences ending with column i. Then

$$R_i = \max\{R_{j-1} + S(w_{j,i}):i = W + 1 \leq j \leq i\}$$

where $w_{j,i}$ is the consensus word with the window from column j to column i.

If much shifting is taking place in the optimal alignment A associated with S(A), then the alignment A* in R(A*) is unsatisfactory and overlapping windows must be considered. To overcome this difficulty in a practical way, find

$$\hat{T}_i = \max\{\hat{T}_{j-1} + \hat{S}(w_{j,i}):i - W + 1 \leq j \leq i\}$$

where $\hat{S}(w_{i,j})$ is the largest score for a consensus word in the window of width W, such that all occurrences of $w_{j,i}$ are to the right of the matches in $\hat{T}_{j-i}$. While this algorithm is not guaranteed to find S(A), it is much more useful than R(A) for most problems. In addition, it is practical for the alignment of many sequences, while dynamic programming is not.

Another hierarchical algorithm is to find the maximum scoring word w in the entire sequence, $\max_{1 \leq i;w'} S_i(w') = S(w)$, and to realign the sequences on w. This breaks the set into two shorter blocks. The same procedure can be reapplied, recursively, to produce an alignment.

VI. DATA BASE SEARCHES

In summer 1988, there were approximately 20×10^6 bp of data in GenBank, a nucleic acid data base, containing approximately the same data which is in the EMBL data base in Heidelberg. The data represent nearly 5600 nucleotide sequences, at an average of approximately 900 to 1000 bp per sequence (see Chapter 1). When a new DNA sequence is determined, there are usually some sequence comparisons suggested by the nature of the sequence. If the new sequence is a coding region for a rat immunoglobin (Ig), running the new sequence against all known mammalian Ig sequences is a natural thing to do. However, in addition to these sorts of comparisons, there is increasing interest in seeing if any un- expected relationships show up when the sequence is run against all mammalian DNA or all eukaryotic DNA. The search need not stop even there. Ribosomal RNA structures have been preserved across all life forms.[31] There seems to be some homology between ribosomal proteins from rat and *E. coli*[37]). Therefore, it is not unreasonable to just run the new sequences against the entire data base and see if any unexpected matches show up.

If the search for a match between a new sequence of 10^3 bp and a data base of 6×10^6 bp were performed with the dynamic programming algorithm of Section III.D, then the running time is proportional to $6 \times 10^9 = (10^3) (6 \times 10^6)$. On a VAX 11/780, this might take a day or more of CPU time. With increasing computer capacity, this should not be too disturbing, but it indicates that such a venture is not to be lightly undertaken.

One response to this important problem has been to utilize the computer science technique of hashing to obtain information about possible regions of high matching. The first use of hashing in molecular biology was made by Dumas and Ninio.[38] The method was later utilized by Wilbur and Lipman[39] and Karlin et al.[40] in developing their own approaches to sequence comparisons.

The basic method begins with a choice of word size, say k letter words. Then a DNA sequence $\mathbf{a} = a_1 a_2 \ldots a_n$ is transformed to a sequence of integers by associating each k triple, $a_i a_{i+1} \ldots a_{i+k-1}$, with one of the integers $0, 1, \ldots 4^k - 1$. For example, let

$$\hat{a} = \begin{cases} 0, & \text{if } a = A \\ 1, & \text{if } a = C \\ 2, & \text{if } a = G \\ 3, & \text{if } a = T \end{cases}$$

Then define

$$x_i = \hat{a}_i \cdot 4^{k-1} + \hat{a}_{i+1} \cdot 4^{k-2} + \ldots + \hat{a}_{i+k-2} \cdot 4^1 + \hat{a}_{i+k-1} \cdot 4^0$$

Notice that $x_{i+1} = x_i \cdot 4 + \hat{a}_{i+k} \bmod 4^k$, so that these transformations can be rapidly made.

To continue with a numerical example, let $\mathbf{a} = $ TAGAGCA. With $k = 2$, $4^k = 16$ and

$$x_1 = 3 \cdot 4 + 0 = 12$$
$$x_2 = 12 \cdot 4 + 2 \bmod 16 = 2$$
$$x_3 = 2 \cdot 4 + 0 \bmod 16 = 8$$
$$x_4 = 8 \cdot 4 + 2 \bmod 16 = 2$$
$$x_5 = 2 \cdot 4 + 1 \bmod 16 = 9$$
$$x_6 = 9 \cdot 4 + 0 \bmod 16 = 4$$

and $\mathbf{a} = (12)(2)(8)(2)(9)(4)$.

Next, lists are made of locations of all occurrences of the integers $0, 1, \ldots, 4^k - 1$. In our numerical example, there are only five nonempty lists

$$0 : \phi$$

$$1 : \phi$$

$$2 : 2,4$$

$$3 : \phi$$

$$4 : 6$$

$$\ldots : \phi$$

$$8 : 3$$
$$9 : 5$$

$$\ldots : \phi$$

$$12 : 1$$

$$\ldots : \phi$$

Another approach is to keep a list of positions of the first occurrences of $0, 1, \ldots, 4^k - 1$. In place of the x_i at those locations, are pointers to the next occurrences of the associated integer. In either case, storage is $O(n)$ and the hashing can be performed in time $O(n)$.

Next, two methods, both due to Wilbur and Lipman, which allow use of this information in sequence comparison.

A. A Regions Method

The algorithm described here appears in Wilbur and Lipman. Define a region r by $(v;i,j)$ where v is a word of length k which begins at position i in **a** and position j in **b**.

Define $r_1 = (v_1;i_1,j_1) < r_2 = (v_2;i_2,j_2)$ if $i_1 + k - 1 < i_2$ and $j_1 + k - 1 < j_2$. Set $r_0 = (\phi;0,0)$ as a least element and $r^* = (\phi;n,m)$ as a greatest element. $\Gamma = (r_1 r_2, \ldots r_i)$ is a path if $p < q$ implies $r_p < r_q$. The score of path Γ is given by

$$\text{score}(\Gamma) = \sum_{k=1}^{\ell} s(r_k) - \sum_{k=1}^{\ell-1} g(i_{k+1} - |w_k| - i_k - 1, j_{k+1} - |w_k| - j_k - 1)$$

where $s(\cdot)$ is a similarity score for region r_k, like $|w_k|$, and $g(\cdot,\cdot)$ is a gap penalty. Then

$$\text{score}(\mathbf{a},\mathbf{b}) = \max\{\text{score}(\Gamma): \Gamma \text{ is a path from } r_0 \text{ to } r_*\}.$$

The algorithm makes two lists of regions: L^-, ordered by $<$ and L^+, ordered by the usual order $<<$ of best scores from r_0 to the region listed in L^+.

$$\gamma = \text{score } (r_u) - g(i_q - |w_{r_u}| - i_u - 1, j_q - |w_{r_u}| - j_u - 1) + s(r_q) > \text{score}(r_q)$$

If there is no region r_u in L^+ below r_q under $<$ with a score greater than score $(r_q) - s(r_q)$, or if the inequality cannot be satisfied, go to (C)

(B) Set score $r_q = \gamma$ and go to (A)
(C) Remove r_q from L^- and insert it in L^+ under $<<$.
     If $L^- \neq \phi$, go to (A).

Changes can be made to this algorithm to give maximum scoring segments. A more practical algorithm is given next.

B. Rapid Similarity Searches

The method described here is due to Wilbur and Lipman[39] and was extended, especially for protein data base searches, by Lipman and Pearson.[41] Recently, Pearson and Lipman[50] have modified their earlier work to DNA sequences. Each of the 4^k words w, of length k, can be located in each sequence, and the positions of the word w in **a** can be considered to match the **b** positions of w. Each such match, say position i in **a** and position j in **b**, has an associated offset $i - j$. The offsets or diagonals with a large number of matches are candidates for good matching regions. This technique is not so rigorous as the dynamic programming methods but it is a great deal faster. In fact, searches of the entire DNA data base can be accomplished on an IBM PC and several groups have programmed this algorithm.

VII. THE STATISTICAL DISTRIBUTION OF ALIGNMENT SCORES

Much has been written about the statistical distribution of distance and similarity scores. In this section, we focus attention on the statistical distribution of the scores of maximum similarity segments (see Section III.D), when the scores are computed for random sequences. The idea is that when the sequences satisfy some model of randomness, such as uniform and independent bases, there is a resulting distribution of maximum similarity segment scores. The scientist can use this distribution to ascertain whether the scores from real, biological sequences are, in the statistical sense, significantly larger than those from random sequences. Of course, there is little agreement about the appropriate model of randomness. Fortunately, as we discuss in Section VII.B, the distribution of maximum similarity segment scores for real, unrelated biological sequences coincides with that of independent, identically distributed sequences of the same composition.

Although simulations are often recommended to determine statistical significance, there are several drawbacks to this approach. First of all, it is expensive in terms of computer time. Also, it often requires more time from the scientist to set up and process the simulations. Frequently, the simulations fail to give the desired results. If statistical significance of a real sequence matching is to be estimated and that significance is α, then $1/\alpha$ simulations must, on the average, be run before seeing a result as extreme as in the real sequences. When α = 0.0001, a not unreasonable case, we must do on the order of 10,000 runs. While simulations are often unavoidable, they are not ideal.

Recently, however, some new results in probability theory give very precise answers to certain problems that arise in practice. These are discussed in the subsections on the "log(n) law". What is less well-understood, is that the log(n) law and another equally special result give guidance on what to expect for the distribution of any maximum similarity algorithm. There are only two behaviors of expected similarity score with sequence length: either proportional to sequence length or to logarithm of sequence length. This result, along with a table of means and variances, is given in Section VII.C on expected behavior.

A. The Log(n) Law
Erdos and Renyi[42] proved in 1970 that the length R_n of the longest run of heads in independent coin tosses with P(Heads) = p grows like $\log_{1/p}(n)$:

$$P\left(\lim_{n \to \infty} \frac{R_n}{\log_{1/p}(n)} = 1\right) = 1$$

If our sequences are perfectly aligned

$$a_1 \, a_2 \, ... \, a_n$$
$$b_1 \, b_2 \, ... \, b_n$$

this mathematical result provides the answer to questions about longest match. Simply write H if $a_i = b_i$, T if $a_i \neq b_i$ and calculate

$$p = p_A^2 + p_{KC}^2 + p_G^2 + p_T^2$$

The length of the longest match is the length of the longest head run. Notice that we assume the distributions of the sequences are identical. The results stated here hold if the sequences have base distributions that are "not too different".

When the sequences are allowed to shift relative to one another, the answer changes. Now matches can include offsets such as

$$a_1 \ a_2 \ \ldots \ a_{n-j+1} \ \ldots \ a_n$$
$$b_1 \ b_2 \ \ldots \ b_j \ b_{j+1} \ldots \ b_n$$

It has been shown[43] that shifting doubles the growth of the longest match length M_n:

$$P\left(\lim_{n\to\infty} \frac{M_n}{\log_{1/p}(n)} = 2\right) = 1$$

Much more precise results have been obtained. With $\mathbf{a} = a_1 a_2 \ldots a_n$ and $\mathbf{b} = b_1 b_2 \ldots b_m$, it is required below that $\log(m)/\log(n) \to 1$. The expectation (mean) of M, the longest match length including k mismatches, is approximately

$$E(M) \cong \log(qmn) + k\log\log(qmn) + k\log(q/p) - \log(k!) + \gamma \log(e) - 1/2$$

where $q = 1-p$, $\log = \log_{1/p}$ and $\gamma = 0.577 \ldots$ is the Euler-Mascheroni constant. The variance is approximately

$$Var[M(n,m)] \cong [\pi \log(e)]^2/6 + 1/12$$

In the case of $k = 0$,

$$E(M) \cong \log(qmn) + \gamma \log(e) - 1/2$$

While it might seem natural to perform the normal approximation at this point, that is not correct! The tail behavior of the distribution is extreme value which has exponential tails. The correct procedure can be found in Theorem 2 of Arratia et al.[4] Results closely related to these were first announced for repeats in a single sequence, with $k = 0$, and minor differences in constants, by Karlin et al.[3] The more general case stated here is from Arratia et al.[4] As discussed in Chapter 6, these formulas can be extended to study the longest match common to R of N sequences. Instead, here we pursue generalizations that allow less exact matching.

B. A Data Base Study

In Smith et al.,[45] the following similarity and gap functions are used:

$$s(a,a) = 1$$
$$s(a,b) = -0.9 \quad \text{if } a \neq b$$
$$w(1) = 2$$
$$w(k) = \infty \quad \text{if } k \geqq 2$$

to study maximum similarity segment scores from real, biological sequences. While the log(n) law appears useful for a fixed number of mismatches, what is the distribution of

$$S(\mathbf{a},\mathbf{b}) = \max_{\substack{I \subset \mathbf{a} \\ J \subset \mathbf{b}}} S(I,J)$$

for a similarity function such as that specified above? Here, I and J denote contiguous segments of sequence.

In the study cited above, all pairwise comparisons were made with a set of 204 vertebrate and eukaryotic DNA sequences and complements for a total of $\binom{204}{2} = 20{,}706$ comparisons. The results display remarkable linear behavior with $\log_{1/p}(nm)$. The best fit of the data, after adjusting for outliers by techniques of robust statistics, is

$$\hat{S} = 2.5 \log_{1/p}(nm) - 8.99$$

This fit of real sequence data is identical to the fit of simulated sequences reported below.

Therefore, allowing insertions and deletions does not change the $\log(nm)$ growth, although the slope is certainly changed. Note that $\log(nm) = \log(n^2) = 2 \log n$ if $n = m$.

C. Linear and Logarithmic Behavior

Let μ be the non-negative mismatch penalty and δ the non-negative deletion penalty for the maximum segment similarity; measure S and write $S = S(\mu,\delta)$ to indicate this dependence. The goal of this section is to give information about the probability distribution of $S(\mu,\delta)$ for all $\mu \geq 0$, $\delta \geq 0$. It was only recently that anything was learned about these questions and much work remains for mathematicians to complete the theory.[46] Still, the broad outlines have been established and the results are both theoretically and practically of interest.

Now for two random sequences of length n,

$$S(\infty,\infty) \cong 2 \log(n)$$

by the above discussion. In contrast, if no penalty is associated with unmatched bases, it is known[33] that

$$S(0,0) \cong c \cdot n$$

where c is a constant. While the precise distribution of $S(\infty,\infty)$ is known, even the value of $c = c(0,0)$ has eluded probabilists for more than 10 years. It has recently been shown that this contrasting behavior between linear and logarithm growth is general. There is a one-dimensional curve through $[0,\infty]^2$, such that the behavior is linear on one side of the curve and logarithmic on the other.[46] Let R(0) be the region containing (0,0) and R(∞) the region containing (∞,∞). Then the theorem is that

$$S(\mu,\delta) \approx c(\mu,\delta) \cdot n \quad \text{if} \quad (\mu,\delta) \in R(0)$$

and

$$S(\mu,\delta) \approx d(\mu,\delta) \cdot \log(n) \quad \text{if} \quad (\mu, \delta) \in R(\infty)$$

Table 5 gives means and variances for a large simulation. In this simulation, 28 independent pairs of sequences were generated of lengths $2^7, 2^8, \ldots, 2^{12}$ where $p_A = p_C = p_G = p_T = 1/4$. At each (μ,δ) of Table 5 and for each of the $28(6) = 168$ pairs of sequences, $S(\mu,\delta)$ was calculated. In the region R(0), (which contains all of column $\mu = 0.50$), a linear fit was made to the data for each pair (μ,δ). In Table 5, the triple

Table 5
SLOPES, INTERCEPTS, AND STANDARD DEVIATIONS FOR S(μ,δ) IN THE LINEAR, R(0), AND LOGARITHMIC, R(∞), REGIONS

δ\μ	0.25	0.50	0.75	1.00	1.25	1.50	2.00	2.50	3.00	3.50	4.00	4.50	5.00
0.25	-2.86	-2.82	-2.82	-2.82	-2.82	-2.82	-2.82	-2.82	-2.82	-2.82	-2.82	-2.82	-2.82
	0.51	0.48	0.48	0.48	0.48	0.48	0.48	0.48	0.48	0.48	0.48	0.48	0.48
	5.14	5.73	5.73	5.73	5.73	5.73	5.73	5.73	5.73	5.73	5.73	5.73	5.73
0.50	-2.05	-2.03	-1.73	-1.18	-1.18	-1.18	-1.18	-1.18	-1.18	-1.18	-1.18	-1.18	-1.18
	0.42	0.38	0.34	0.30	0.30	0.30	0.30	0.30	0.30	0.30	0.30	0.30	0.30
	5.64	6.30	6.78	7.25	7.25	7.25	7.25	7.25	7.25	7.25	7.25	7.25	7.25
0.75	-0.93	-0.47	0.03	1.01	2.47	4.53	4.53	4.53	4.53	4.53	4.53	4.53	4.53
	0.35	0.29	0.24	0.20	0.16	0.13	0.13	0.13	0.13	0.13	0.13	0.13	0.13
	5.60	6.24	6.66	7.29	7.82	8.63	8.63	8.63	8.63	8.63	8.63	8.63	8.63
1.00	-0.19	1.54	2.53	4.49	7.79	11.88							
	0.31	0.22	0.16	0.11	0.07	0.03							
	5.63	6.07	6.65	6.99	7.08	7.07							
1.25	0.77	2.92	6.45	9.98			-4.13	-3.08	-3.08	-3.08	-3.08	-3.08	-3.08
	0.28	0.18	0.10	0.04			1.85	1.64	1.64	1.64	1.64	1.64	1.64
	5.79	5.70	6.53	6.63			1.63	1.49	1.49	1.49	1.49	1.49	1.49
1.50	1.60	4.13	8.95		-6.48	-3.93	-2.34	-2.01	-2.03	-2.03	-2.03	-2.03	-2.03
	0.25	0.15	0.06		2.21	1.76	1.46	1.38	1.36	1.36	1.36	1.36	1.36
	5.83	5.63	6.13		1.75	1.41	1.33	1.22	1.20	1.20	1.20	1.20	1.20
2.00	2.75	6.70		-5.09	-2.14	-1.40	-1.60	-1.50	-1.42	-1.36	-1.29	-1.29	-1.29
	0.21	0.09		1.95	1.44	1.27	1.23	1.20	1.18	1.17	1.16	1.16	1.16
	5.19	5.99		1.71	1.35	1.27	1.20	1.14	1.12	1.10	1.10	1.10	1.10
2.50	3.98	9.52	-9.10	-2.94	-1.52	-1.19	-1.23	-1.21	-1.22	-1.18	-1.15	-1.14	-1.13
	0.19	0.06	2.69	1.58	1.30	1.20	1.15	1.14	1.13	1.12	1.12	1.11	1.11
	5.25	5.66	2.24	1.44	1.26	1.22	1.14	1.09	1.05	1.04	1.03	1.02	1.01
3.00	5.11	12.02	-6.20	-2.45	-1.46	-1.24	-1.11	-1.08	-1.05	-1.02	-1.00	-0.99	-0.97
	0.17	0.04	2.21	1.47	1.26	1.18	1.12	1.11	1.09	1.09	1.08	1.08	1.08
	5.08	5.32	2.00	1.37	1.23	1.20	1.14	1.08	1.05	1.03	1.02	1.00	1.00
3.50	6.23	14.25	-5.40	-2.00	-1.31	-1.21	-1.06	-1.02	-0.98	-0.94	-0.91	-0.90	-0.89
	0.16	0.02	2.07	1.40	1.23	1.17	1.11	1.10	1.08	1.07	1.07	1.07	1.07
	4.82	5.17	1.93	1.36	1.24	1.20	1.13	1.06	1.03	1.01	1.00	1.00	1.00
4.00	7.25		-5.28	-1.80	-1.24	-1.20	-1.05	-1.01	-0.98	-0.94	-0.91	-0.90	-0.90
	0.15		2.03	1.37	1.22	1.17	1.11	1.09	1.08	1.07	1.07	1.06	1.06
	4.96		1.91	1.37	1.23	1.19	1.12	1.05	1.02	1.01	1.00	1.00	1.00
4.50	8.06		-5.23	-1.74	-1.21	-1.19	-1.04	-0.99	-0.95	-0.92	-0.89	-0.89	-0.89
	0.14		2.01	1.36	1.21	1.16	1.11	1.09	1.07	1.07	1.06	1.06	1.06
	5.20		1.89	1.33	1.22	1.17	1.10	1.04	1.02	1.00	1.00	1.00	1.00
5.00	8.65		-5.26	-1.71	-1.19	-1.18	-1.02	-0.97	-0.92	-0.90	-0.88	-0.88	-0.88
	0.13		2.01	1.35	1.21	1.16	1.10	1.09	1.07	1.07	1.06	1.06	1.06
	5.44		1.87	1.31	1.21	1.16	1.09	1.03	1.02	1.01	1.01	1.00	1.00

$$a$$
$$b$$
$$s$$

in region R(0) means that

$$S(\mu,\delta) = a + b{\cdot}n$$

with standard deviation s; while for (μ,δ) in region $R(\infty)$, the triple means that

$$S(\mu,\delta) = a + b\log_2(n)$$

with standard deviation s.

These means and variances can be used for estimates of statistical significance. Above, it was noted that $S(\infty,\infty)$ has exponential tails, not the tails of the normal distribution. We conjecture that all of region $R(\infty)$ has exponential tails, but that is by no means established mathematically. Moreover, convergence to extreme value distributions is usually very slow, so that except for $S(\infty,\infty)$, it is unclear what constants to use. To further complicate the situation, in R(0), knowledge beyond linear behavior is completely lacking. Still, it is possible to use the present state of knowledge to obtain useful information.

For illustration, consider *E. coli* threonine tRNA and *E. coli* valine tRNA. Both sequences are 76 in length. To be consistent with the analysis of these sequences in Section III.A, take $\mu = 1$ and $\delta = 2$. A computer sequence comparison yields $S(1,2) = 24 - 1(7) - 2(1) = 15$. This is the score of the longest boxed portion of the alignment in III.A. The pair (1,2) is in $R(\infty)$ and Table 5 gives $a = -5.09$, $b = 1.95$, and $s = 1.71$. Therefore,

$$a + b\log_2(n) = -5.09 + 1.95\log_2(78) = 7.0935$$

and

$$S(1,2) = 15 = 7.1665 + 4.624(1.71)$$

so that S(1,2) is 4.624 standard deviations above the mean.

If additional information is required about the significance, Chebyshev's inequality can be used, as in Smith et al.[45] This conservative result, valid for all probability distributions, is that the probability of $|S(\mu,\delta) - \text{mean}| \geq \lambda$ is less than, or equal to, $(s/\lambda)^2$. In our example, $\lambda = (4.581)s$ and the statistical significance of our result is therefore no larger than $(1/4.581)^2 = 0.0477$.

APPENDIX

```
/* code for finding segments from two sequences with maximum similarity */
/* Michael S. Waterman and Mark Eggert */
/* see "A NEW ALGORITHM FOR BEST SUBSEQUENCE ALIGNMENTS
       WITH APPLICATION TO TRNA-RRNA COMPARISONS
       Michael S. Waterman and Mark Eggert, Journal of Molecular
       Biology (1987) 197,723-728 */

#include "maxsegs.h"

/* sequence lengths */
int m, n;

/* sequences as arrays of characters */
char *x, /* x[1]...x[m] */
     *y; /* y[1]...y[n] */
```

```
/* score cells as arrays of arrays of short integers */
short
    **F, /* F[0][0]...F[1][n] */
    **S; /* S[0][0]...S[m][n] */

int maxantidiag; /* maximum antidiagonal of traceback end */
int maxS, maxSi, maxSj; /* maximum score and its location */
int maxi; /* maximum i of traceback end */
int force; /* flag to force reporting maximum score */

/* weighting constants for SIMPLE match/mismatch score */
int match, delta; /* s(a,b)=match if a==b
                          delta if a!=b */

/* weighting constants for LINEAR insertion/deletion score */
int alpha, beta; /* w(k)=alpha+beta*(k-1) */

/* cutoff, tracebacks are not done from cells with scores below this value */
int cutoff;

/* structure for cell information */
typedef struct {int i, j} cellinfo;

/* array of cell structures to be ordered */
cellinfo *list;

/* number of cell structures in array */
int listcount;

/*****************************************************************************/
/* maxsegs() is the entry point after all initialization is done           */
/* BEFORE maxsegs() is called:                                             */
/* match, delta, alpha, beta and cutoff must be assigned                   */
/* x and y must be loaded with the sequences to be compared                */
/* m and n must be assigned the sequence lengths                           */
/* the score arrays must be initialized thus:                              */
/* S[i][0]==0 for all i                                                    */
/* F[0][j]==0 for all j                                                    */
/* S[0][j]==0 for all j                                                    */
/*****************************************************************************/

maxsegs()
{
        make_S();
        trace();
}

#define FAST_REG

/* load score cells with pre-traceback values */

make_S()
{
        register int i, j;
        /* register to hold x[i] */
        register char cx;
        /* registers to make array access easier */
        register short E, *Sp, *Fp=F[0], *bFp=F[1], *sFp;

        maxS=0;
        listcount=0;

        for (j=1; j<=n; ++j)
                Fp[j]=0;
        /* recursive S for LINEAR weighting */
        for (i=1; i<=m; ++i)
        {
                E=0;
                sFp=Fp;
                Fp=bFp;
                bFp=sFp;
                Sp= S[i];
                cx=x[i];
                for (j=1; j<=n; ++j)
                {
                        /* E[i][j] == max { 0, max over k {S[i][j-k]-w(k)} } */
                        E=max(0,
```

```
                                          Sp[j-1]-alpha,
                                          E-beta);

                          /* F[i][j] == max { 0, max over k {S[i-k][j]-w(k)} } */
                          Fp[j]=max(0,
                                          S[i-1][j]-alpha,
                                          bFp[j]-beta);

                          Sp[j]=max(S[i-1][j-1]+s(cx, y[j]),
                                          (int)Fp[j],
                                          (int)E);

                          if (Sp[j]>maxS)
                          {
                                  maxS=Sp[j];
                                  maxSi=i;
                                  maxSj=j;
                          }
                          if (Sp[j]>=cutoff)
                          {
                                  list[listcount].i=i;
                                  list[listcount].j=j;
                                  ++listcount;
                          }
                  }
          }
}

/* match/mismatch score */

int s(a, b) char a, b;
{
        if (a==b)
                return(match);
        else
                return(delta);
}

/* deletion/insertion score */
int w(k) int k;

{
        return(alpha+beta*(k-1));
}

/* recalculation variables */
int lasti, lastj;
/* If row j is being analysed
   all cells from cell[lasti][j-1] to cell[m][j-1] are unchanged. */
/* If column i is being analysed
   all cells from cell[i-1][lastj] to cell[i-1][n] are unchanged. */

/* Cellorder returns a value of type RELATION. The RELATION type, and its values
   BEFORE, SAME_AS and AFTER are defined in max_segs_defs. The cellorder code
   compares two cell structures, item1 is "cellorder(&item1, &item2)" item2. Our
   program uses this, but its use is hidden in the sorting code */

RELATION cellorder(item1, item2) cellinfo *item1, *item2;
{
        /* order by cell's content */
        if (S[item1->i][item1->j]>S[item2->i][item2->j])
                return(BEFORE);
        if (S[item1->i][item1->j]<S[item2->i][item2->j])
                return(AFTER);

        /* order by distance of cell's antidiagonal from origin */
        if ((item1->i+item1->j)<(item2->i+item2->j))
                return(BEFORE);
        if ((item1->i+item1->j)>(item2->i+item2->j))
                return(AFTER);

        /* order by cell's position on cell's antidiagonal */
        if (item1->i<item2->i)
                return(BEFORE);
        if (item1->i>item2->i)
                return(AFTER);
```

```
        /* same content, same position on same antidiagonal */
        return(SAME_AS);
}

/* make tracebacks */
trace()
{
        int i, j, k;
        int scorei, scorej, scoreS;

        /* enqueue qualifying cells */
        /* if the highest is too low */
        printf("maxS is %d\n", maxS);
        if (maxS<cutoff)
        {
                if (force)
                {
                        list[listcount].i=maxSi;
                        list[listcount].j=maxSj;
                        ++listcount;
                        cutoff=0;
                }
        }
        else
        {
        /* sort array with an algorithm following cellorder's behavior: */
        /* sort(pointer to array, number of objects in array) */
                sort(list, listcount);
        }
        /* start traceback at each queued entry,
           taking entries from "top" of array */
        /* this allows us to easily sort remaining entries
           indexed 0 to listcount-1 */
        while (--listcount>=0)
        {
                scorei=list[listcount].i;
                scorej=list[listcount].j;
                scoreS=S[scorei][scorej];
                /* check if entry is OK */
                if (scoreS>=cutoff)
                {
                        maxantidiag=0;
                        maxi=m;
                        /* finds "shortest" traceback */
                        findnode(scorei, scorej);
                        lasti=lastj=0;
                        /* if this traceback succeeds... */
                        if (plot(scorei, scorej))
                        {
                                /* recalculate scores off end of traceback */
                                redoscores(scorei, scorej);
                                /* print the alignment in */
                                /* a form the user likes  */
                                diagnostic_stuff(scorei, scorej, scoreS);
                                /* resort list */
                                sort(list, listcount);
                        }
                }
                else
                        /* if the top entry is too low, all are too low */
                        break;
        }
}

BOOLEAN plot(i, j) int i, j;
{
        int k, l;

        /* stop at zeros, return TRUE if this is shortest */
        if (i+j<maxantidiag)
                return(FALSE);
        if (S[i][j]==0)
        {
                if (i+j==maxantidiag&&i==maxi)
                        return(TRUE);
                else
```

```
                                      return(FALSE);
                }

        /* check deletion branch */
        for (k=1; k<i; ++k)
        {
                if (S[i-k][j]==0)
                        break;
                else if (S[i][j]==S[i-k][j]-w(k))
                {
                        if (plot(i-k, j))
                        {
                                for (l=k-1; l>=0; --l)
                                {
                                        /* note that cell i-l,j   */
                                        /* is deleted              */
                                        /* output something like   */
                                        /*    x[i-l]               */
                                        /*    -                    */
                                        diag(i-l, j, XDEL);
                                        redoone(i-l, j);
                                        redocolumn(i-l, j);
                                }
                                return(TRUE);
                        }
                }
        }
}

/* check match/mismatch branch */
if (S[i][j]==S[i-1][j-1]+s(x[i], y[j]))
{
        if (plot(i-1, j-1))
        {
                /* note that cell i,j has had match or mismatch        */
                /* produce alignment output something like:            */
                /*    x[i]                                             */
                /*    y[j]                                             */

                /* S is built "left to right"                 */
                /* recursion is "right to left"               */
                /* alignment output occurs on recursion exit */
                /* so it comes out "left to right"            */
                diag(i, j, MATCH);
                if (redoone(i, j))
                {
                        redocolumn(i, j);
                        redorow(i, j);
                }
                return(TRUE);
        }
}

/* check other deletion branch */
for (k=1; k<j; ++k)
{
        if (S[i][j-k]==0)
                break;
        else if (S[i][j]==S[i][j-k]-w(k))
        {
                if (plot(i, j-k))
                {
                        for (l=k-1; l>=0; --l)
                        {
                                /* note that cell i,j-l is deleted */
                                /* output something like           */
                                /*    -                            */
                                /*    y[j-l]                       */

                                diag(i, j-l, YDEL);
                                redoone(i, j-l);
                                redorow(i, j-l);
                        }
                        return(TRUE);
                }
        }
}
}
return(FALSE);
```

```
        }

/* find "shortest" traceback */
findplot(i, j) register int i, j;
{
        register int k, l;
        /* stop if already too low */
        if (i+j<maxantidiag)
                return;
        /* stop at zeros */
        if (S[i][j]==0)
        {
                if (i+j>maxantidiag)
                {
                        maxantidiag=i+j;
                        maxi=i;
                }
                else if (i+j==maxantidiag)
                {
                        if (i>maxi)
                                maxi=i;
                }
                return;
        }

        /* check match/mismatch branch */
        if (S[i][j]==S[i-1][j-1]+s(x[i], y[j]))
                findplot(i-1, j-1);

        /* check deletion branch */
        for (k=1; k<i; ++k)
        {
                if (S[i-k][j]==0)
                        break;
                else if (S[i][j]==S[i-k][j]-w(k))
                        findplot(i-k, j);
        }

        /* check other deletion branch */
        for (k=1; k<j; ++k)
        {
                if (S[i][j-k]==0)
                        break;
                else if (S[i][j]==S[i][j-k]-w(k))
                        findplot(i, j-k);
        }
}

/* find cell common to all tracebacks with minimum i+j */
findnode(i, j) int i, j;
{
        int nodei=i, nodej=j, righti=i, rightj=j, lefti=i, leftj=j;
        int k, leftindex=lefti+leftj, rightindex=righti+rightj;

        /* move down left-most and right-most tracebacks
           until they meet for the last time */
        for (;;)
        {
                /* left side */
                do
                {
                        if (S[lefti][leftj]==0)
                        {
                                break;
                        }
                        /* check deletion branch */
                        for (k=1; k<=lefti; ++k)
                        {
                                if (S[lefti-k][leftj]==0)
                                {
                                        if (S[lefti][leftj]==
                                                S[lefti-1][leftj-1]+
                                        s(x[lefti], y[leftj]))
                                {
                                        --lefti;
                                        --leftj;
                                        leftindex-=2;
```

```
                              }
                              else
                              {
                                      for (k=1; k<leftj; ++k)
                                      {
                                              if (S[lefti][leftj]==
                                                  S[lefti][leftj-k]-w(k))
                                              {
                                                      leftj-=k;
                                                      leftindex-=k;
                                                      break;
                                              }
                                      }
                              }
                              break;
                      }
                      else if (S[lefti][leftj]==S[lefti-k][leftj]-w(k))
                      {
                              lefti-=k;
                              leftindex-=k;
                              break;
                      }
              }
      }
      while (leftindex>rightindex);
      if (S[lefti][leftj]==0)
      {
              if (leftindex>maxantidiag)
              {
                      maxantidiag=leftindex;
                      maxi=lefti;
              }
              else if (leftindex==maxantidiag)
              {
                      if (lefti>maxi)
                              maxi=lefti;
              }
              break;
      }
      /* right side */
      do
      {
              if (S[righti][rightj]==0)
              {
                      break;
              }
              for (k=1; k<=rightj; ++k)
              {
                      if (S[righti][rightj-k]==0)
                      {
                              if (S[righti][rightj]==
                                  S[righti-1][rightj-1]+
                                  s(x[righti], y[rightj]))
                              {
                                      --rightj;
                                      --righti;
                                      rightindex-=2;
                              }
                              else
                              {
                                      for (k=1; k<righti; ++k)
                                      {
                                              if (S[righti][rightj]==
                                                S[righti-k][rightj]-w(k))
                                              {
                                                      righti-=k;
                                                      rightindex-=k;
                                                      break;
                                              }
                                      }
                              }
                              break;
                      }
                      else if (S[righti][rightj]==
                               S[righti][rightj-k]-w(k))
                      {
```

```
                                        rightj-=k;
                                        rightindex-=k;
                                        break;
                                }
                        }
                }
                while (leftindex<rightindex);
                if (S[righti][rightj]==0)
                {
                        if (rightindex>maxantidiag)
                        {
                                maxantidiag=rightindex;
                                maxi=righti;
                        }
                        else if (rightindex==maxantidiag)
                        {
                                if (righti>maxi)
                                        maxi=righti;
                        }
                        break;
                }
                if (lefti==righti)
                {
                        nodei=lefti;
                        nodej=leftj;
                }
        }
        /* now, find the "shortest" path from this node */
        findplot(nodei, nodej);
}

SE(i, j)
        register int i, j;
{
        register int k, m=0, s0;
        register short *Sp=S[i];

        for (k=1; k<j; ++k)
        {
                s0=Sp[j-k];
                if (s0==0)
                        break;
                s0-=w(k);
                if (s0>m)
                        m=s0;
        }
        return(m);
}

SF(i, j)
        register int i, j;
{
        register int k, m=0, s0;

        for (k=1; k<i; ++k)
        {
                s0=S[i-k][j];
                if (s0==0)
                        break;
                s0-=w(k);
                if (s0>m)
                        m=s0;
        }
        return(m);
}

/* return TRUE if further cells will be affected */
BOOLEAN redoone(i, j) int i, j;
{
        int newS;

        /* recalculate matrix at one place */

        /* omit scores from pathways already taken */
        newS=max(readdiag(i, j, MATCH)?0:(S[i-1][j-1]+s(x[i], y[j])),
                readdiag(i, j, XDEL)?0:SF(i,j),
                readdiag(i, j, YDEL)?0:SE(i,j));
```

```
        /* note result */
        if (S[i][j]!=newS)
        {
                S[i][j]=newS;
                return(TRUE);
        }

        /* if further cells will be unaffected, report this */
        if ((i>=lasti)&&(j>=lastj))
        {
                return(FALSE);
        }

        /* report that further cells will be affected */
        return(TRUE);
}

/* recalculate column of matrix */
redocolumn(i, j) int i, j;
{
        int newS;
        int firstj=0; /* j of cell with lowest j of contiguous unchanged cells */

        while (++j<=n)
        {
                /* recalculate S sans previous paths */
                /* readdiag==true if cell[i][j] was MATCHed or XDELed or YDELed */
                newS=max(readdiag(i, j, MATCH)?0:(S[i-1][j-1]+s(x[i], y[j])),
                        readdiag(i, j, XDEL)?0:SF(i,j),
                        readdiag(i, j, YDEL)?0:SE(i,j));

                if (S[i][j]==newS)
                {
                        /* remember lowest cell
                           where all further cells don't change */
                        if (firstj==0)
                                firstj=j;
                        /* when no further cells will change, we're done */
                        if (j>=lastj)
                        {
                                /* remember position for next scan */
                                lastj=firstj;
                                break;
                        }
                }
                else
                {
                        /* note that cell has changed */
                        /* clear j of lowest of contiguous unchanged cells */
                        firstj=0;
                        /* actually change S */
                        S[i][j]=newS;
                }
        }
}

/* recalculate row */
redorow(i, j) int i, j;
{
        int newS;
        int firsti=0;

        while (++i<=m)
        {
                newS=max(readdiag(i, j, MATCH)?0:(S[i-1][j-1]+s(x[i], y[j])),
                        readdiag(i, j, XDEL)?0:SF(i,j),
                        readdiag(i, j, YDEL)?0:SE(i,j));

                if (S[i][j]==newS)
                {
                        if (firsti==0)
                                firsti=i;
                        if (i>=lasti)
                        {
                                /* the first shall be last */
                                lasti=firsti;
                                break;
```

```
                                        }
                        }
                        else
                        {
                                firsti=0;
                                S[i][j]=newS;
                        }
                }
        }
}

/* redo cells off end of traceback */
redoscores(i, j) int i, j;
{
        for (; (++i<=m)&&(++j<=n);)
        {
                /* if cells need to be checked, check */
                if (redoone(i, j))
                {
                        redocolumn(i, j);
                        redorow(i, j);
                }
                else
                {
                        return;
                }
        }
}
```

ACKNOWLEDGMENTS

This work was supported by grants from the System Development Foundation and the National Institutes of Health.

REFERENCES

1. **Kruskal, J. B. and Sankoff, D.,** *Time Warps, String Edits, and Macromolecules: The Theory and Practice of Sequence Comparison,* Sankoff, D. and Kruskal, J. B., Eds., Addison-Wesley, London, 1983.
2. **Waterman, M. S.,** Consensus patterns in sequences, *Mathematical Methods for DNA Sequences,* Waterman, M. S., Ed., CRC Press, Boca Raton, Fla., 1988.
3. **Karlin, S., Ghandour, G., Ost, F., Tavare, S., and Korn, L. J.,** New approaches for computer analysis of nucleic acid sequences, *Proc. Natl. Acad. Sci. U.S.A.,* 80, 5660, 1983.
4. **Arratia, R., Gordon, L., and Waterman, M. S.,** An extreme value theory for sequence matching, *Ann. Stat.,* 14, 971, 1985.
5. **Waterman, M. S.,** General methods of sequence comparison, *Bull. Math. Biol.,* 46, 473, 1984.
6. **Stanton, R. G. and Cowan, D. D.,** Note on a "square functional" equation, *SIAM Rev.,* 12, 277, 1970.
7. **Laquer, H. T.,** Asymptotic limits for a two-dimensional recursion, *Stud. Appl. Math.,* 64, 271, 1981.
8. **Feller, W.,** *An Introduction to Probability Theory and Its Applications,* Vol. 1, 3rd ed., John Wiley & Sons, New York, 1968, 52.
9. **Griggs, J. R., Hanlon, P. J., and Waterman, M. W.,** Sequence alignments with matched sections, *SIAM J. Algorithm Disc. Meth.,* 7, 604, 1986.
10. **Griggs, J. R., Hanlon, P., Odlyzko, A., and Waterman, M. S.,** On the number of alignments of k sequences, *Asian J. Comb.,* in press.
11. **Needleman, S. B. and Wunsch, C. D.,** A general method applicable to the search for similarities in the amino acid sequences of two proteins, *J. Mol. Biol.,* 48, 444, 1970.
12. **Sellers, P.,** Theory and computation of evolutionary distances, *SIAM J. Appl. Math.,* 26, 787, 1974b.
13. **Waterman, M. S., Smith, T. F., and Beyer, W. A.,** Some biological sequence metrics, *Adv. Math.,* 20, 367, 1976.
14. **Gotoh, O.,** An improved algorithm for matching biological sequences, *J. Mol. Biol.,* 162, 705, 1982.
15. **Waterman, M. S.,** Efficient sequence alignment algorithms, *J. Theor. Biol.,* 108, 333, 1984.
16. **Smith, T. F. and Waterman, M. S.,** Comparison of biosequences, *Adv. Appl. Math,* 2, 482, 1981.

17. **Smith, T. F., Waterman, M. S., and Fitch, W. M.,** Comparative biosequence metrics, *J. Mol. Evol.,* 18, 38, 1981.
18. **Sellers, P.,** Pattern recognition in genetic sequences, *Proc. Natl. Acad. Sci. U.S.A.,* 76, 3041, 1979.
19. **Sellers, P.,** The theory and computation of evolutionary distances: pattern recognition, *J. Algorithms,* 1, 359, 1980.
20. **Hawley, D. K. and McClure, W. R.,** Compilation and analysis of *Escherichia coli* promoter DNA sequences, *Nucl. Acids Res.,* 11, 2237, 1983.
21. **Weiss, R.,** Oncogenes and growth factors, *Nature (London),* 304, 12, 1983.
22. **Doolittle, R. F., Hunkapiller, K., Hood, L. E., Devare, S. G., Robbins, K. C., Aaronson, S. A., and Antoniades, H. M.,** Simian sarcomaviruses onc gene v-sis is derived from the gene (or genes) encoding a platelet-derived growth factor, *Science,* 221, 275, 1982.
23. **Naharro, G. K., Robbins, C., and Reddy, E. P.,** Gene product of v-fgr onc: hybrid protein containing a portion of actin and tyrosin-specific protein kinase, *Science,* 223, 63, 1984.
24. **Sellers, P.,** Pattern recognition in genetic sequences by mismatch density, *Bull. Math. Biol.,* 46, 501, 1984.
25. **Smith, T. F. and Waterman, M. S.,** Identification of common molecular subsequences, *J. Mol. Biol.,* 147, 195, 1981a.
26. **Waterman, M. S. and Eggert, M.,** A new algorithm for best subsequence alignments with application to tRNA-rRNA comparisons, *J. Mol. Biol.,* 197, 723, 1987.
27. **Waterman, M. S.,** Sequence alignment in the neighborhood of the optimum with general applications to dynamic programming, *Proc. Natl. Acad. Sci. U.S.A.,* 80, 3123, 1983.
28. **Byers, T. H. and Waterman, M. S.,** Determining all optimal and near-optimal solutions when solving shortest path problems by dynamic programming, *Oper. Res.,* 32, 1381, 1984.
29. **Fitch, W. M. and Smith, T. F.,** Optimal sequence alignments, *Proc. Natl. Acad. Sci. U.S.A.,* 80, 1382, 1983.
30. **Waterman, M. S. and Perlwitz, M.,** Line geometries for sequence comparisions, *Bull. Math. Biol.,* 46, 567, 1984.
31. **Woese, C. R., Gutell, R., Gupta, R., and Noller, H. F.,** Detailed analysis of the higher-order structure of 16S-like ribosomal ribonucleic acids, *Microbiol. Rev.,* 47, 621, 1983.
32. **Sankoff, D.,** Minimal mutation trees of sequences, *SIAM J. Appl. Math.,* 78, 35, 1975.
33. **Sankoff, D. and Cedergreen, R. J.,** *Time Warps, String Edits, and Macromolecules: The Theory and Practice of Sequence Comparison,* Sankoff, D. and Kruskal, J., Eds., Addison-Wesley, London, 1983, 253.
34. **Fitch, W. M.,** Towards defining the course of evolution: minimum change for a specific tree topology, *Syst. Zool.,* 20, 406, 1971.
35. **Waterman, M. S.,** Multiple sequence alignment by consensus, *Nucl. Acids Res.,* 14, 9095, 1986.
36. **Fickett, W. J. and Burks, C.,** Development of a database for nucleic acid sequences, in *Mathematical Methods for DNA Sequences,* Waterman, M. S., Ed., CRC Press, Boca Raton, Fla., 1988.
37. **Lin, A., McNally, J., and Wool, I. G.,** The primary structure of rat liver ribosomal protein L37, *J. Biol. Chem.,* 258, 10664, 1983.
38. **Dumas, J. P. and Ninio, J.,** Efficient algorithms for folding and comparing nucleic acid sequences, *Nucl. Acids Res.,* 80, 197, 1982.
39. **Wilbur, W. J. and Lipman, D. J.,** Rapid similarity searches of nucleic acid and protein data banks, *Proc. Natl. Acad. Sci. U.S.A.,* 80, 726, 1983.
40. **Karlin, S., Ghandour, G., and Foulser, D. E.,** Comparative analysis of human and bovine papalloma viruses, *Mol. Biol. Evol.,* 1, 357, 1984.
41. **Lipman, D. J. and Pearson, W. R.,** Rapid and sensitive protein similarity searches, *Science,* 227, 1435, 1985.
42. **Erdos, P. and Renyi, A.,** On a new law of large numbers, *J. Anal. Math.,* 22, 103, 1970; reprinted in *Selected Papers of Alfred Renyi, 1962-1970,* Vol. 3, Akademiai Kiado, Budapest, 1976, 43.
43. **Arratia, R. and Waterman, M. S.,** An Erdos-Renyi law with shifts, in *Advances in Mathematics,* Vol. 55, Academic Press, New York, 1985, 13.
44. **Karlin, S., Ost, F., and Blaisdell, B. E.,** Patterns in DNA and amino acid sequences and their statistical significance, in *Mathematical Methods for DNA Sequences,* Waterman, M. S., Ed., CRC Press, Boca Raton, Fla., 1988.
45. **Smith, T. F., Waterman, M. S., and Burks, C.,** The statistical distribution of nucleic acid similarities, *Nucl. Acids Res.,* 13(2), 645, 1985.
46. **Waterman, M. S., Gordon, L., and Arratia, R.,** Phase transitions in sequence matches and nucleic acid structure, *Proc. Natl. Acad. Sci. U.S.A.,* 84, 1239, 1987.
47. **Miller, W. and Myers, E. W.,** Sequence comparison with concave weighting functions, *Bull. Math. Biol.,* in press.

48. **Carrillo, H. and Lipman, D.,** The multiple sequence alignment problem in biology, *SIAM J. Appl. Math.,* in press.
49. **Altschul, S. F. and Lipman, D.,** Trees, stars, and multiple biological sequence alignment, *SIAM J. Appl. Math.,* in press.
50. **Pearson, W. R. and Lipman, D. J.,** Improved tools for biological sequence comparisons, *Proc. Natl. Acad. Sci. U.S.A.,* 85, 2444, 1988.

Chapter 4

CONSENSUS PATTERNS IN SEQUENCES

Michael S. Waterman

TABLE OF CONTENTS

I. INTRODUCTION

One of the most difficult pattern recognition problems in sequence analysis is that of locating consensus patterns; its solution is of much importance to molecular biologists. These consensus patterns can occur among a set of sequences or within a single sequence. Sometimes the patterns all have exactly the same letters which occur in identical locations in all sequences of interest; there is little need for sophisticated programs designed to find such obvious features. For example, ACC occurs at the 3′ end of all tRNA molecules, in the same position relative to the acceptor stem. Features such as this one have been conserved over vast amounts of evolutionary time and are, without doubt, essential to the functioning of the organisms. It is more frequently the case, however, that a feature is conserved, but not conserved precisely in location or in pattern. There are different reasons for these various degrees of conservation; one classic example is discussed next.

The famous TATAAT box in bacterial promoters is located approximately 10 bases upstream (5′ or left) from the transcription start site. This 6-letter pattern occurs, however imperfectly, in the −10 region of all bacterial promoters. The variations in location and pattern might lead to skepticism regarding its existence or relevance to function. However, a number of experiments have essentially settled those issues. In Hawley and McClure,[1] the known −10 and −35 patterns were searched for in sequenced bacterial promoters, aligned on, and the consensus patterns refined. These two consensus sequences are known from experimental evidence to contain functional information that affects promoter activity.[1,2] Even after these detailed studies, it is not evident whether other features of DNA promoter sequences affect promoter activity. Other effects might not be as large as those attributed to the −10 and −35 consensus patterns, but still might be very important.

In Section II, we give a method for locating unknown patterns occurring imperfectly in both composition and location in a set of many sequences. The techniques work well on sequence sets such as bacterial promoters, and a subset of the known bacterial promoters is analyzed for illustration. Required for this analysis is a precise definition of consensus sequence specifying the amount of mismatch and/or gap allowed, as well as the amount of shifting permitted. These parameters and the quantity to be optimized are used to define consensus. The number of possible alignments in these sequence sets is enormous. Nonetheless, the techniques work rapidly on most problems of interest.

Next, in Section III, a related problem is considered. While homology in sequence pattern is an important biological feature, the sequence patterns can have other additional properties. Many (but not all) known protein binding sites have an approximate palindromic symmetry and are composed of inverted, complementary repeats. (A palindrome in nucleic acids is a sequence such as ACTGCAGT or TTAGCGGCTAA.) The knowledge that the pattern sought is a palindrome allows us to look more deeply into the sequences and to detect even weaker consensus patterns. A well-known pattern of this type is that found by Pelham[3] in promoters of heat-shock genes in *Drosophila*. The modification of the above method to the search for palindromes is necessary to detect signals or patterns of the strength found in the heat-shock sequences, and these sequences are used to illustrate the analysis.

Repeats in a single sequence have also been of much interest. Exact repeats are the basis of the algorithms of Karlin et al.[4] and Martinez and Sobel,[5,6] and the computer methods to rapidly find exact repeats are usually based on hashing. Hashing techniques do not apply to inexact repeats. Our interest here is in inexact repeats, and a modification of Section II will let us study inexact repeats in Section IV. Of necessity, the search is restricted to smaller patterns, up to 9 to 12 bases in length. While hashing methods are routinely used in data base searches,[7] our methods do not apply to those problems.

Just as palindromes are of interest in the study of regulatory patterns common to a set of sequences, consensus palindromes along a single sequence reveal possible binding sites for a regulatory protein. The patterns are usually weak and quite hard to find by inspection. An algorithm adapting those of Sections II and III to a single sequence is given in Section IV along with application to the GAL1 promoter sequence.

Many weak consensus patterns in molecular biology involve long patterns. For example, the Alu family of repeats involves 300 base patterns, which occur thousands of times in the human genome. The methods used above involve storage of all possible patterns of interest. This approach is impossible for longer patterns. For example, there are $4^{300} \approx 4.1 \times 10^{180}$ patterns of length 300. Other methods, perhaps less optimal, must be developed. A recent approach to these problems is described in Section V.

Whenever a consensus pattern is located, whether by inspection or by computer, the question of statistical significance often arises. Biological significance cannot be equated with statistical significance. However, patterns that are extremely likely to occur in random sequences of similar composition seem unlikely to be biologically significant. We prefer simple models of randomness for doing these calculations. These simple models do not model the real sequences themselves particularly well,[8] but the distribution of matching between unrelated real sequences is modeled very well by that between independent sequences of the same composition.[9] For our purposes here, studying weak matchings between many sequences, the theory of large deviations is very useful. In Section VI, this theory, as well as the log(n) distribution and simulation, is discussed.

II. CONSENSUS WORDS IN MULTIPLE SEQUENCES

As described in the introduction, in this section we study the problem of determining consensus words that occur in a set of sequences, where the occurrences of the words are inexact and differ in location from sequence to sequence. We first give a combinatorial treatment of the number of alignments possible with some constraints on amount of shifting. Then we describe the algorithm we employ to identify consensus patterns. Lastly, to illustrate the analysis, we study a set of bacterial promoters with these methods.

A. Combinatorics

In a direct approach to the problem, the R sequences under consideration can be analyzed for consensus words by placing them into various alignments. For each alignment, the various columns are examined for "consensus" letters. Groups of consensus letters can then be identified as consensus patterns. The goal here is to decide the difficulty in such a straightforward approach to identifying consensus patterns.

Let the initial alignment of R sequences of the same length N be given as:

$$
\begin{array}{llll}
a_{11}a_{12} & \cdots & a_{1N} \\
a_{21}a_{22} & \cdots & a_{2N} \\
\cdots & \cdots & \cdots \\
a_{R1}a_{R2} & \cdots & a_{RN}
\end{array}
$$

The simplest scheme for alternate alignment is to allow shifts of the sequences relative to one another, without any gaps inserted into the sequences. Usually the amount of shifting is limited to a fixed number of bases:

original position: a_{11} $\cdots$ $a_{1,R-k}$ $\cdots$ $a_{1,R}$
shifted by k bases: $a_{1,1}$ $\cdots$ $a_{1,k+1}$ $\cdots$ $a_{1,R}$

If each sequence can be shifted up to k bases, then there are $k + 1$ choices for the positioning of each sequence. Consequently, there are $(k + 1)^R$ of these alignments, since each sequence can be put into k new positions. In our example problem below, there are R = 59 sequences. With only k = 1, there are $(k + 1)^{59} = 2^{59} \approx 5.77 \times 10^{17}$, and no computer could possibly analyze all these alignments directly. The first analysis we perform in subsection C will have k = 3 so that $(3 + 1)^{59} \approx 3.32 \times 10^{35}$.

Additionally, we might want to insert gaps into the sequences. The number of alignments when gaps are allowed greatly increases the numbers obtained above (see Chapter 3[10]). These simple observations about the number of alignments show that a direct approach to consensus pattern identification is impossible. The ideas here apply equally well to the search for consensus palindromes (Section III) or to any situation where the correct sequence alignment is not precisely known.

B. Algorithm

The brute force approach of the last section has another problem in addition to that of combinatorics. There, an analysis could be based on percentages of bases in columns of an alignment. Here, we give an analysis based on the occurrence of k-letter words, and our consensus pattern is some k-letter word. In this way, it is possible to directly study the objects of interest. The algorithm was first presented by Waterman et al.[11]

Fundamental to our analysis is the concept of neighborhood of a word. Suppose k = 6 and w = TATAAT. In the set of 4^k k-letter words, there is one word equal to w, $\binom{6}{1}3 = 18$ words within 1 mismatch of w, and $\binom{6}{2}3^2 = 15 \cdot 9 = 135$ words within 2 mismatches of w.

No. of length 6 words	Mismatches from w = TATAAT
TATAAT	0
AATAAT	1
CATAAT	1
GATAAT	1
TCTAAT	1
TGTAAT	1
TTTAAT	1
TAAAAT	1
TACAAT	1
TAGAAT	1
TATCAT	1
TATGAT	1
TATTAT	1
TATACT	1
TATAGT	1
TATATT	1
TATAAA	1
TATAAC	1
TATAAT	1

The neighborhood of a word is limited by the algorithm to words within a certain number of mismatches, deletions, and insertions of the consensus word. For example, the first analysis of subsection C allows a consensus word to be "found" in a neighborhood of up to 2 mismatches away from the consensus and does not allow any insertions or deletions.

Another parameter that must be specified is W, the window width. W is the number of sequence letters that can be searched for a consensus word of k-letters. This allows shifts of up to k-letters. Below, for example, we search the promoter sequences for words of six letters in a window of 9 bases. If the window is set too wide, statistically insignificant patterns will be found. On the other hand, if a window is too narrow, the true consensus pattern can be missed. There is a balance of pattern length and neighborhood size with window width. As the likelihood of finding an acceptable pattern in random data increases, the window width should be decreased.

We now begin an explicit definition of the algorithm. The window specifies a search of the sequences a_1, a_2, . . . a_R from column j + 1 to column j + W. It is assumed that the sequences have been placed in an initial alignment, simply aligning on right (3′) ends, on left (5′) ends, or on some known biological feature in the data. The window reveals the sequences

Column	j + 1	j + 2	. . .	j + W
Sequence 1	$a_{1,j+1}$	$a_{1,j+2}$	. . .	$a_{1,j+W}$
Sequence 2	$a_{2,j+1}$	$a_{2,j+2}$	. . .	$a_{2,j+W}$
. . . .			. . .	. . . .
Sequence R	$a_{R,j+1}$	$a_{R,j+2}$	. . .	$a_{R,j+W}$

We index the neighborhood of a word w by d = 0,1,2, . . . , where d = 0 indicates the word w, and d = 1 might, for example, indicate the 1 mismatch neighborhood of w. For each sequence $a_{i,j+1}$ . . . $a_{i,j+W}$, let q(i,w,d) = 1 if the best occurrence of w in the ith sequence is as a dth neighbor, and q(i,w,d) = 0, otherwise. We order the neighbors by the penalties given below; let is suffice here that exact (d = 0) is best, d = 1 is next best, etc.

There are several approaches to computing

$$Q(i) = (q(i,w,0), q(i,w,1), ...)$$

In this representation of Q(i), there are 4^k lines, each corresponding to some w. In our program, each k-letter word in the sequence itself is used to produce all neighbors, and these neighbors are used to construct q(i,w,·) for all 4^k words w. This involves storing all 4^k words and finding their best occurrence in $a_{i,j+1}$ . . . $a_{i,j+W}$. We do not directly search the sequence for all the 4^k words but instead use the k-letter sequences in $a_{i,j+1}$ . . . $a_{i,j+W}$ to find the neighbors.

Next set

$$V = \sum_{i=1}^{R} Q(i)$$

$V = (v_{w,d})$ is useful since $v_{w,d}$ is an integer equal to the number of times or lines that w has its best occurrence as a dth neighbor. We are now ready to define the score associated with word w:

$$s_w = \sum_{d \geq 0} \lambda_d v_{w,d}$$

where λ_d is the weight given to having a best occurrence of w as a dth neighbor. The weight λ_d gives the preferences among the neighbors of w. In our program, we use the ratio of matching letters to w and the length of word k. That is

$$\lambda_{exact} = k/k = 1$$

and

$$\lambda_{1\ mismatch} = (k - 1)/k = 1 - 1/k$$

For words of length 6, six occurrences of 1 mismatch neighbors of w is equal in weight to five exact occurrences of w. There is no virtue in this scheme except that of simplicity, and λ_d can be easily changed.

Finally, we define a winning word w to satisfy

$$S(w) = \max_u\{s_u\}$$

Generally, with fixed W and n(d) = number of words in the neighborhood of w, the computation time (for R sequences of length N) is proportional to

$$R(N - W + 1)(W - k + 1)n(d)$$

It is pleasant, for W and n(d) fixed and N much larger than W, that the running time is approximately proportional to RN, so that twice as many sequences take twice the running time, and the same holds true for sequences of twice the original length. The maximum of n(d) is 4^k, but usually we have n(d) much less. For k = 6, 4^6 = 4096 while allowing up to d = 2 mismatches gives n(2) = 1 + 6 + 135 = 154 and d = 3 mismatches gives n(3) = 1 + 6 + 135 + 540 = 682.

Many useful extensions can be made to these ideas. Certainly it is easy to relax the requirement that the consensus letters be contiguous. The positions of the consensus letters relative to one another must be fixed before the search is made. Otherwise, we would be faced with the task of searching over all $\binom{W}{k}$ ways of taking k consensus letters within the window. An algorithm could be devised, but we are not confident that it would be very useful.

When a signal or consensus word is located, the sequences could be aligned on the consensus word and then the sequences studied with this new alignment. We have implemented this feature and have found it quite useful. If two distinct patterns are located (approximately) a fixed distance apart, then aligning on the stronger pattern could allow the weaker pattern to become evident.

Another natural modification that we allow is search in all alphabets. The alternate alphabet most often invoked is the purine/pyrimidine alphabet, {R,Y}, where R = A or G, and Y = C or T. There is some hope of detecting DNA structural patterns by these sub-alphabets.[12] In addition, various k-letter structural motifs might be identified with their k-letter patterns and, with a proper concept of neighborhood, consensus structural patterns could be studied.

Finally, each sequence occurrence could be weighted by another constant, K_i. The definition of V would change to

$$V = \sum_{i=1}^{R} K_i Q(i)$$

Our motivation here is that a measurement of promoter strength, for example, might give a weighting of how much importance we should associate with patterns from each sequence. Unfortunately, we have not yet found an appropriate example to which we can apply this algorithm.

It has occurred to analysts that the signal might really be missing patterns rather than abundant patterns.[12] For these searches, the word of interest has score $\min_u\{s_u\}$, and there is no difficulty in including these searches.

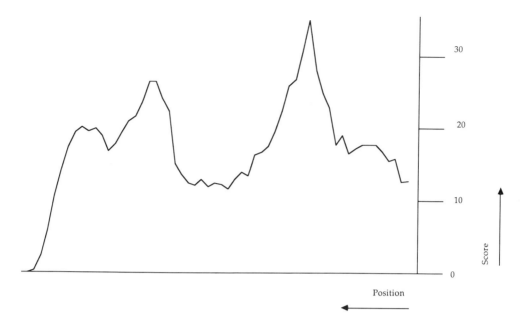

FIGURE 1. Graph of scores of the 59 bacterial promoter sequences that appear, along with their names, in Figure 2. The window width W = 9, the word size k = 6, and the neighborhood is up to mm = 2 mismatches.

C. Bacterial Promoters

The example analyzed in this section consists of 59 *Escherichia coli* promoter sequences originally analyzed by Hawley and McClure.[1] One or two bases were added to the sequences where the sequences are known, with the data taken from the references given by Hawley and McClure.[1] The analysis of this section follows Galas et al.[13] The graph of scores appears in Figure 1, and sequences are presented with their names and the three major consensus patterns in Figure 2; this is discussed in detail later. The sequences are aligned on the trascription start site, which is position 10 in Figure 2. The usual biological indexing would have this position indexed + 1, the numbering increasing to the right; any position to the left of the start of transcription is negative. There is no 0 in the biological scheme of indexing positions. For ease of sequence handling, we number the sequences from + 1, right to left, as indicated in Figure 2.

The first analysis has the window width set at W = 9, with the word size k = 6, and allows a neighborhood of up to 2 mismatches. To index all possible window positions, we take the right-hand edge of the window. The resulting graph appears in Figure 1. The horizontal axis represents window position in the sequences. When a feature of interest is located on a graph, the program allows us to move the window to the position pointed to on the graph. For example, the sharp peak at the right-hand edge of the graph corresponds to the sequence pattern indicated in the right-hand column of Figure 2. The black region indicates the window; notice that it is of width 9. The lower case letters show patterns found to produce the score at the peak. In the right-hand column, the consensus pattern is, approximately (within the neighborhood), the well-known − 10 pattern TATAAT. It occurs exactly 9 times; in 17 sequences, its best occurrence is with 1 mismatch (mm), while in 18 sequences, its best occurrence is with 2 mm. The resulting score is s = 35.17.

The middle column represents the − 35 consensus pattern. In this analysis, the consensus word is w = TTGACA with 4 exact occurrences, 15 with 1 mm and 13 with 2 mm. The $s_{TTGACA} = 26.83$. Aligning on the − 10 pattern does not enhance the − 35 pattern, nor does aligning on the − 35 pattern enhance the − 10 pattern.[13] We conclude that, while the sequence patterns are about 17 bases apart, the pattern spacing is not too closely linked.

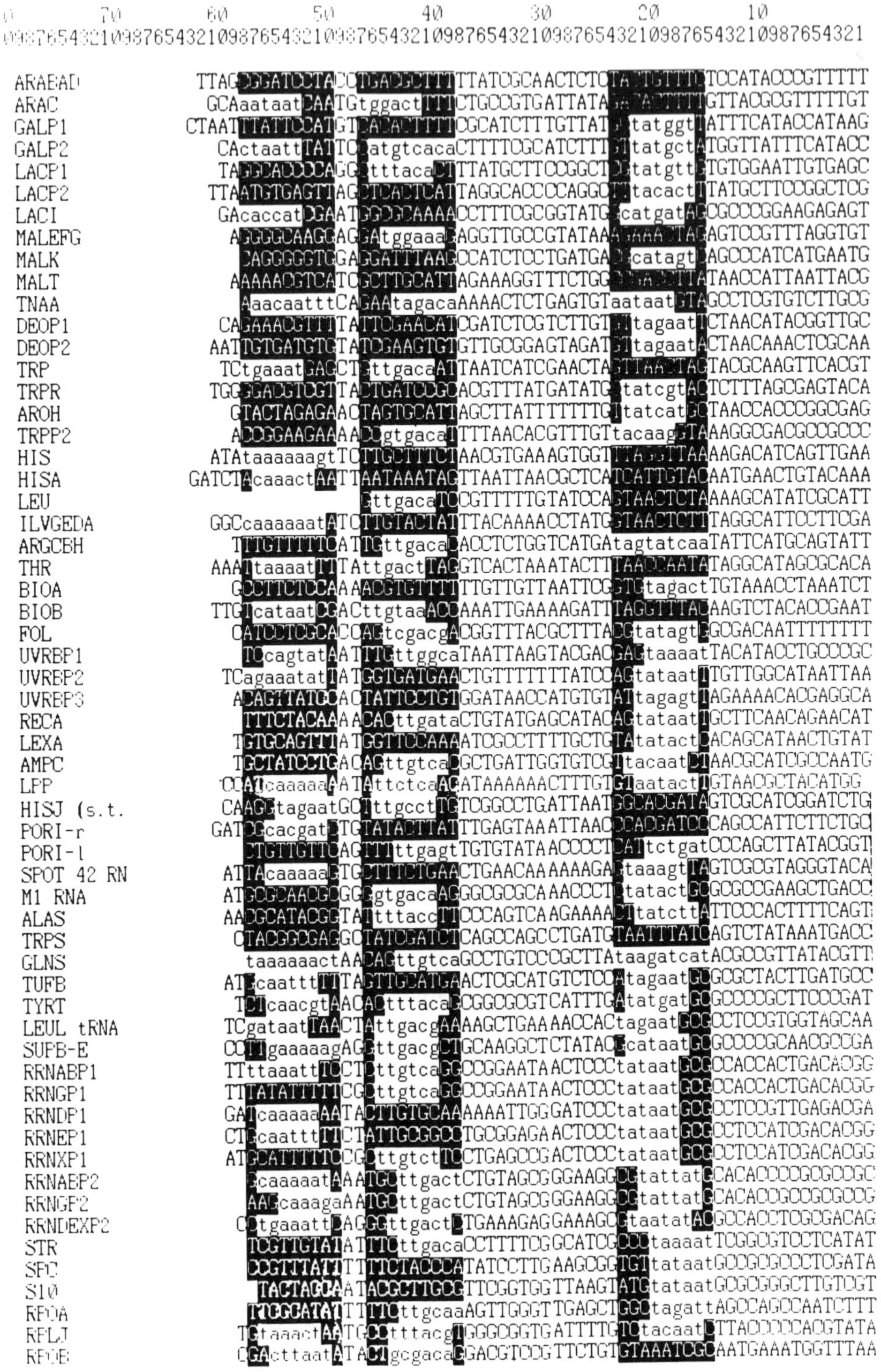

FIGURE 2.   The 59 bacterial promoter sequences analyzed. The three black columns indicate the window locations of the -44, -35, and -10 patterns, with the patterns shown in lower case.

Table 1
C·POLYA·T PATTERNS
IN −44 REGION

A

lpp	CAAAAAAAT
malT	TAAAAAAAC
his	TAAAAAAG
glnS	TAAAAAAC
spoT 42 RNA	CAAAAG
rrnAB P2	CAAAAT
supB − E	GAAAAAG
thr	TAAAT
recA	CAAAC
bioA	CAAAAC
trp P2	GAAAC
hisA	CAAAC
araC	CAAAT
rplJ	TAAAC
tnaA	TAAAC
rrnAB P1	TAAAT
rrnD P1	GAAAT
deo P1	GAAAC
trp	GAAAT
uvrB P2	GAAAT
rrnG P2	GAAAT
rrnDEX P2	GAAAT
hisJ	TAGAAT
uvrB P1	TATAAT
bio B	CATAAT

B

spc	GAAAAAAT
tufB	TAAAAAAT
rpoA	GAAAAAT
rrbG P1	GAAAAAT
rrnE P1	GAAAAAT
rrnX P1	GAAAAAT
thr	TAAAAT
deo P1*	TAAAAC
rrnAB P1*	TAAAAT
lexA	TAAAC
gal 8P2	TAAAT

Note: In column A the sequence patterns are shown, while those sequence patterns with pattern in reverse orientation are shown in column B.

Next, we examine the new pattern found by Galas et al.,[13] approximately at position −44: CAAAAT. In Hawley and McClure, an "A" was noted in this region. The pattern C·polyA·T appears, in forward or reverse orientation, in approximately half this data set (see Table 1 for these explicit sequences). Wu and Crothers[14] and Crothers et al.[15] have presented evidence of an unusual conformation associated with these sequences, a bending of the DNA. The sequence may have functional importance in these promoters. The CRP protein (CAP) alters the conformation in the *lac* control region when it binds to a site just 5' of the −35 region.[16]

This suggests that the role of CAP could be played by sequence conformation in some bacterial promoters.

To see how to set the window and mismatch parameters, we present some graphs in Figure 3. With fixed W and k, let mm increase from 0 to 3. At mm = 0, the signal is small; perhaps the − 10 signal might be suspected, but even that is doubtful. As mm increases to 1 and then to 2, the sequence features become more clear. When mm = 3 the noise of the sequences is beginning to affect the signal. It is even more interesting to vary the window width. At W = k = 6, no shifting is allowed. Then the signals become a little more evident at W = 7 and even clearer at W = 9. Finally, with W = 15 the signals have again become swamped by sequence noise. Much can be learned from sitting at a graphics terminal and varying these parameters.

To illustrate sequence patterns quite invisible to the eye, we take the three alphabet C,T,R = {A,G}. Figure 4 shows the graphs for two runs. Some new patterns appear besides those at − 10, − 35, and − 44. Figure 4A finds at approximately − 23, a pattern TRR which occurs 23 times with W = 6, k = 3, and mm = 0. This is above that expected from random sequences of these compositions. The literature assigns a CAT pattern at + 1, the transcription start site. Here we find CRT occurring 24 times at the transcription start site. In Figure 4B, we have W = 5, k = 4, and mm = 1. The pattern TRRR at − 23 occurs 5 times exactly and 27 times with mm = 1. This is less statistically significant than the k = 3 version of the pattern.

When the program is run on the data set searching for absent patterns, $s^* = \min_w\{s_w\}$, the only features of interest correspond exactly to − 10 and − 35. We interpret this as being due to the occurrence of the − 10 and − 35 consensus words. Nothing new is learned from this analysis.

III. CONSENSUS PALINDROMES IN MULTIPLE SEQUENCES

It is feasible that additional information is available regarding the possible consensus patterns. This knowledge can be used to restrict the set of possible consensus patterns from the 4^k possibilities for k-letter words. Having a smaller set is certainly useful in terms of storage and can help reduce running time if the neighborhood structure is convenient. In addition, detection of a pattern in this reduced set of patterns can be more sensitive.

This section treats one such example, that of palindromes or patterns with reverse complement. Protein binding sites are frequently approximate palindromes, the motivation for these considerations. The example studied in Section III.B is the *Drosophila* heat-shock promoters. In these sequences, the determinant of heat-shock response does not seem to be detectable with the consensus word method of Section II, but some signal does appear when the consensus palindrome method is used.

A. Algorithm

As discussed above, we restrict the set of consensus patterns to palindromes. Specifically, palindromes of length 2k + 1 have the form

$$A_1A_2 \ldots A_kNB_k \ldots B_2B_1$$

where $\bar{B}_i = A_i [\bar{A} = T, \bar{G} = C, \bar{T} = A, \text{ and } \bar{C} = G]$ and N, of course, denotes an arbitrary base. Palindromes of length 2k do not have the N in the middle. Thus, there are 4^k palindromes of length 2k or 2k + 1. The idea here is similar to that for consensus words. Each sequence or word can contribute to the score of a palindrome if it is in the palindrome's neighborhood. Therefore, it is of interest to look at an example, w = TAAGGCTA. Notice that w is not a palindrome and, in fact, no palindrome is 1 mismatch (mm) from w. If the neighborhood allows up to 3 mismatches, then the following neighbors result.

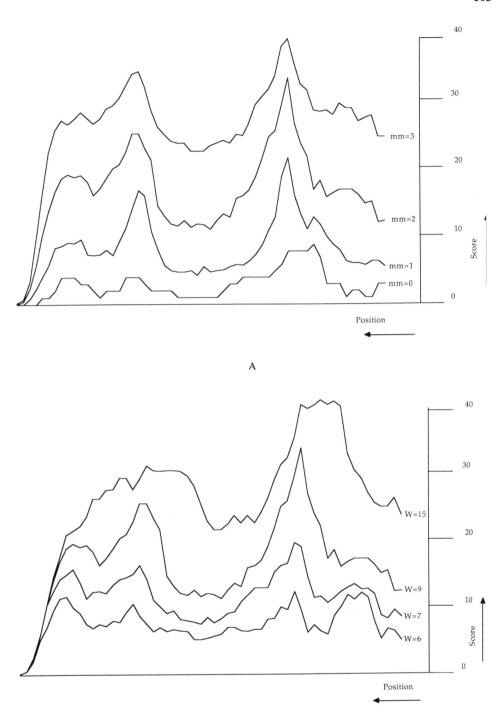

FIGURE 3. A study of the effects of varying algorithm parameters. (A) The mismatch parameter is set at mm − 0,1,2,3 with W = 9 and k = 6. (B) The window width is set at W = 6,7,9,15 with k = 6 and mm = 2.

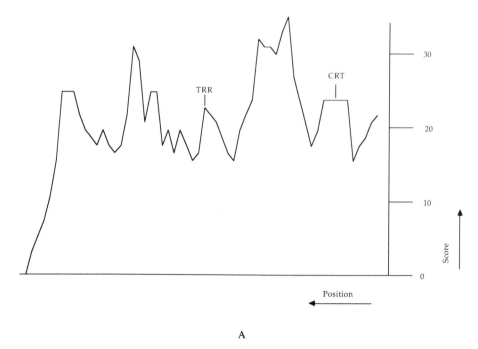

A

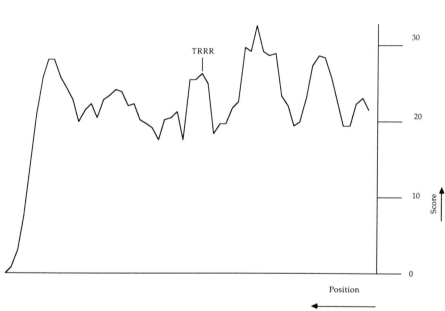

B

FIGURE 4.   Analysis with the alaphabet C,T,R = {A,G}. (A) W = 6, k = 3, and mm = 0. (B) W = 5, k = 4, and mm = 1. A new pattern TRR or TRRR appears at approximately −23.

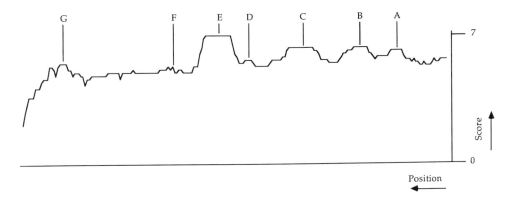

FIGURE 5. Graph for consensus word scores in seven *Drosophila* heat-shock gene promoters. Here w = 20, k = 6, and mm = 2. Scores of some patterns of interest are labeled.

Length 6 palindromes	mm from w = TAAGGCTA
TAAGCTTA	2
TAACGTTA	2
TAGGCCTA	2
TAGCGCTA	2
TAATATTA	3
TAAATTTA	3
TAGTACTA	3
TAGATCTA	3
TATCGATA	3
TACCGGTA	3
TATGCATA	3
TACGCGTA	3
TATGCATA	3

The remainder of setting up the algorithm goes as with the previous algorithm in Section II.B. Let the window and neighborhood be defined. Then let $V = [v_{p,d}]$ be defined by setting $v_{p,d}$ equal to the number of lines a palindrome p has its best occurrence as a dth neighbor. Then the score for p is

$$s_p = \sum_{d \geq 0} \lambda_d v_{p,d}$$

where as before λ_d is the weight given to a dth neighbor occurrence of the palindrome p. The winning palindrome is that with $\max_p \{s_p\}$. The algorithms to accomplish these tasks are similar to those of Section II.B.

B. Heat-Shock Promoters

In higher organisms, there is a collection of genes that are principally expressed at higher temperatures. These genes seem to be stimulated by a number of physiological stresses, one of which is heat. It is natural to study these genes to determine the features that differentiate their control from that of other genes.

In *Drosophila*, these genes are known as heat-shock genes. A number of *Drosophila* heat-shock genes and their 5′ flanking DNA have been sequenced. While there are no patterns which obviously differentiate these sequences, several studies have addressed this issue.[3,17] The consensus pattern suggested by those authors is a weak palindrome. In this section, we study these sequences using the tools described above.

The first approach is by the analysis for consensus word. The sequences are aligned on the start of transcription, approximately position 90 of Figure 6. In Figure 5, we give the graph of scores vs. positions for window width W = 20, word size k = 6, and a neighborhood of up to 2 mm. Clearly, there are some patterns of interest and those appear, along with the sequences, in Figure 6. Patterns (A) and (B) have not been noticed before, while (C), the pattern TTCAAA, 3' of the transcription start site has been described earlier. Pattern (E) is the famous TATAAA box and is almost perfectly aligned with the start of transcription. Pattern (F) would not be noticed, but it appears approximately where the consensus palindrome was noted by Pelham. Finally, we show pattern (G) which is some distance 5' from signals previously noticed.

The Pelham pattern is not located by the consensus word search. For reasons of computer storage, we are unable to use longer words, such as length 14, in that program. The consensus palindrome algorithm allows longer words since there are, for example, 4^7 palindromes of length 14. The window is set at W = 25 and up to 6 mismatches are allowed. Some patterns found by this search for consensus palindromes are shown in Figure 8, with the graph appearing in Figure 7.

The strongest palindrome (C) involves the region near the transcription start site. It is possible to include the TATAAA box in a consensus palindrome (D).

Two other interesting patterns are noticeable, 5' from the TATAAA box. The first of these shown in Figure 9A has not been noticed before. This new palindrome is disjoint from and just 3' of the pattern in Figure 9B, which is approximately the Pelham pattern. In Figure 9C, we show the pattern of Pelham.[3]

IV. CONSENSUS IN ONE SEQUENCE

The algorithms in Sections II and III are designed to find consensus words and palindromes between several sequences where the sequences are in some initial alignment and a fixed amount of shifting is allowed. The motivation for those problems was the determination of consensus protein binding sites. Related motivation exists for studying consensus binding sites in a single sequence. Below, we give algorithms for consensus words and consensus palindromes in a single sequence. The algorithms are applied to study possible binding sites in a yeast regulatory sequence.

A. Algorithms

The sequence being studied is $a = a_1a_2 \ldots a_N$. Initially, we discuss determining k-letter consensus words in the sequence, where the repeating words are not allowed to overlap. Our approach is related to that of the earlier sections.

Set $\lambda_w(v)$ = weight of the word v in the neighborhood of the k-letter word w. For a fixed w, set

$$S_i(w) = \max \left\{ \sum_v \lambda_w(v) \right\}$$

where the maximum is over nonoverlapping words v in $a_1a_2 \ldots a_i$. The idea is to find the largest sum of weights, not allowing the words v to overlap. The winning word w* maximizes $S_N(w)$,

$$S(w^*) = \max_w S_N(w)$$

over the entire sequence $a_1a_2 \ldots a_N$. The approach here is to find $S_N(w)$ for each w. This is easily done by recursion:

$$S_i(w) = \max \{S_{i-1}(w); \quad S_{i-k} + \lambda_w(a_{i-k+1} \ldots a_i)\}$$

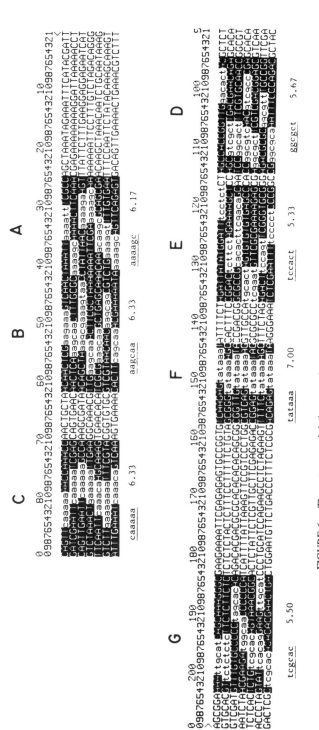

FIGURE 6.   The patterns and their scores that correspond to A through G in Figure 5.

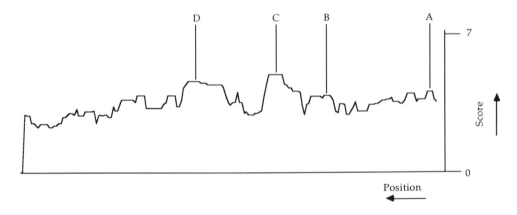

FIGURE 7.   Graph for consensus palindrome scores in seven *Drosophila* heat-shock gene promoters. Here W = 25, palindrome size is 14, and up to mm = 6 are allowed.

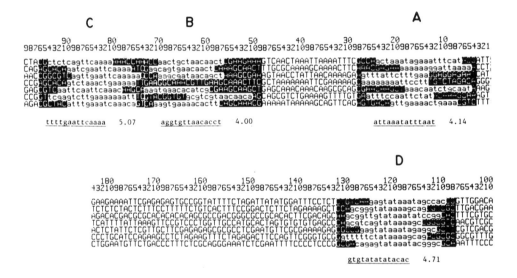

FIGURE 8.   The patterns and scores that correspond to the labels A through D in Figure 7.

If $a_{i-k+1} \ldots a_i$ is in the neighborhood of w, and this is optimal, then $S_i(w)$ equals the second expression within the brackets above. If $a_{i-k+1} \ldots a_i$ is not in the neighborhood of w or if such a pattern is not optimal, then $S_{i-1}(w) = S_i(w)$. This establishes the recursion.

It would appear that $\max_w\{S_N(w)\}$ would take time $4^k \cdot N$ to compute. This number can be reduced, since the $S_i(w)$ need only be updated if $a_{i-k+1} \ldots a_i$ is in the neighborhood of w. Therefore, for every sequence word $a_{i-k+1} \ldots a_i$, we need only update $S_i(w)$ with w in its neighborhood. Therefore, the time complexity of this method is n(d)N, where n(d) is neighborhood size.

It is only the complication of computing neighborhoods that makes the palindrome algorithm distinct from the algorithm just discussed.

B. A Sequence from Yeast

Giniger et al[18] studied the yeast regulatory protein GAL4 which binds to four sites in the sequence UAS_G, to activate transcription of GAL1 and GAL10. The sequence from position 361 to position 486 is presented in Figure 10, along with our analysis. In Figure 10A, we

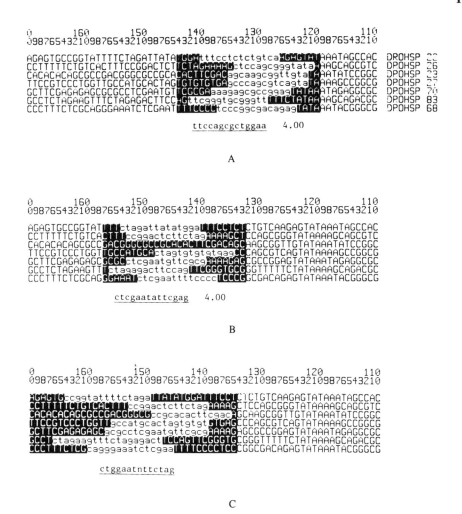

FIGURE 9.   Additional consensus palindromes of interest, just upstream of the TATAAA box.
A is a new pattern just 3′ of the pattern in B, which shows the computer's version of Pelham's
pattern, itself shown in C.

find the best consensus 17-letter palindrome, allowing up to 6 mismatches (out of the 16
letters, excluding the middle letter). The pattern is CGGATGAGNCTCATCCG and achieves
score 2.75 with four occurrences. From 5′ to 3′, the first three patterns coincide with those
of Giniger et al., while the fourth (rightmost) pattern differs in location.

For completeness, we also give a repeats analysis for consensus words in Figure 10B,
with k = 8, allowing 2 mismatches. The consensus pattern CGCCGTCC occurs five times
with score 3.75.

V. LONG CONSENSUS PATTERNS

The consensus algorithms of Sections II, III, and IV depend on storing scores (and other
information) for all patterns of interest. With k-letter words of DNA, this implies that storage
is proportional to 4^k. For k = 10, 4^k = 1,048,576. In the introduction we mention the Alu
family of repeats where k = 300. Obviously, the techniques above, practical for k = 9 to
12 larger, will not be of any use for these problems.

While we do not know, for larger k, of any algorithms guaranteed to be optimal for
computing

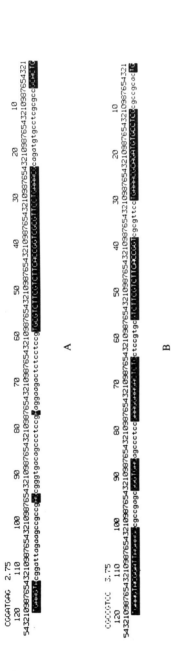

FIGURE 10.   Consensus analysis of the sequence UAS_G. (A) Shows the best consensus k = 17-letter palindrome, allowing up to mm = 6, while B shows the best k = 8-letter consensus repeated word allowing up to mm = 2.

$$\max_w\{s_w\}$$

we do have some useful and practical algorithms to suggest. The following method was developed for a study in progress with Wool, McNalley, and Jones. Our problem is finding the long consensus words among a set of sequences.

Recall that above, in the passage from the set of all k-letter words to the set of all k-letter palindromes, we effectively decreased the size of the set of possible consensus patterns from 4^k to $4^{k/2}$. The simple idea here is to decrease the set of possible consensus words to include only those k-letter words actually occurring in the DNA sequences themselves. That is, our consensus word w must appear exactly somewhere in

$$\begin{matrix} a_{1,1}a_{1,2} & \cdots & a_{1,N} \\ a_{2,1}a_{2,2} & \cdots & a_{2,N} \\ \cdots & \cdots & \cdots \\ a_{R,1}a_{R,2} & \cdots & a_{R,N} \end{matrix}$$

We then look for the best occurrence of w in each sequence. It is guaranteed to occur exactly in at least one sequence. If no insertions or deletions are allowed, searching one sequence for w can be done in time and storage $k(N - k + 1)$. (Actually, using techniques of computer science, this number can be reduced to approximately $N + k$.) However, it is unlikely that in long DNA patterns, insertions and deletions can be ignored. The dynamic programming methods of Chapter 3[10] allow us to find the best fit of w into $a_{i,1} \ldots a_{i,N}$ in time and storage proportional to k.N, allowing insertions and deletions. Thus, the score s_w can be found in R·k·N steps. Still, this must be done for each sequence word, so that the time is proportional to $R^2(N - k + 1)(k)(N)$.

This number is large for many problems, but is not much larger than the time of making all pairwise comparisons, $\binom{R}{2}N^2$. The difficulty of the pairwise comparisons approach is that best matching segments between two sequences might not have any relationship with the consensus word between (say) 60 sequences. This is certainly the case with the bacterial promoters discussed in Section II.

The method can be made adaptive by taking the words matching the consensus w and further refining it, modifying the pattern to one not actually in the data. The procedure is iterated until the pattern does not change.

There is a way to use all pairwise comparisons which does not require us to set word size before the search. The maximum segments algorithm from Chapter 3[10] computes a matrix $H = (H_{ij})$ where H_{ij} is interpreted as the maximum of all subsequences ending in i (from one sequence) matched with a subsequence ending in j from the second sequence. If the first sequence is $\mathbf{a}_1 = a_{1,1} \ldots a_{1,j} \ldots a_{1,N}$, then $\max_j H_{ij}$ gives the best match of $a_{1,\ell} \ldots a_{1,i}$ matching the second sequence for all $\ell \leq i$. We use

$$\sum_{\text{sequences}} \max_j H_{ij}$$

to score subsequences from $\mathbf{a}$ that end at $a_{1,i}$.

Clearly, we have suggested algorithms that are not too efficient. Still, they will often run on available computers in reasonable time and are much more informative than trying to look at the sequences two at a time.

VI. ESTIMATES OF STATISTICAL SIGNIFICANCE

Statistics is useful in sequence analysis to provide clues about what patterns or alignments should be taken seriously. It is by no means our intention to equate biological significance with statistical significance, however, either of these terms might be defined. To use a statistical approach, the sequences must be viewed as following some model of randomness. Then the analyst estimates the likelihood, under the model, of observing some pattern at least as extreme as that actually observed in the sequences. The logic employed is that patterns that are extremely likely to occur in random sequences of similar composition should not be examined as carefully as patterns which are very unlikely to occur. Biology must provide the resolution of these issues; statistics is only a tool to distinguish patterns of possible interest.

We now discuss the issue of what model of randomness to use. Sometimes there is confusion of what actually needs to be modeled. To model the sequences themselves is not the object. If it were, higher order Markov chains, with memory of at least 2, would be required.[8] However, what is really needed is a model of randomness that produces, for example, the same distribution of maximum scores as that obtained from unrelated biological sequences. The distribution of scores from best matching segments between two unrelated biological sequences has been shown to be very well modeled by that from comparing sequences of identical composition with independent and identically distributed bases. See Smith et al.[9] or Chapter 3[10] for discussions of this work. This is the basis for our assumptions of very simple statistical models in this section.

When long sequences are being compared, the recently developed extreme value theory, referred to here as the log(n) distribution, is very useful in assessing the best matching segments between the sequences. Karlin and collaborators[4] have developed a theory which gives the distribution of the longest exact match, common between L or more sequences of length N, with a total of R sequences ($2 \leq L \leq R$). A theory allowing increasing amounts of mismatch (including insertions and deletions) has been developed elsewhere and is discussed in Section VII of Chapter 3.[10] Since the log(n) theory is treated elsewhere in this book, we discuss other approaches here.

A. The Binomial Distribution and Large Deviations

When the sequences are not long enough for the log(n) theory to apply, there is another useful theory to consider. Let α be the probability of a word occurring within the neighborhood of w in a sequence, within the window. We refer to this event as a "success". Here, we give an estimate of the probablity of $n \geq \beta R$ successes where $\beta > \alpha$. The probability of n successes is, by the binomial distribution,

$$\binom{R}{n} \alpha^n (1 - \alpha)^{R-n}$$

and we wish to evaluate

$$\sum_{n \geq \beta R} \binom{R}{n} \alpha_n (1 - \alpha)^{R-n}$$

If R is small, this sum can be directly calculated.

When R is not small, it is necessary that there be enough sequences for the law of large numbers to be valid. The case of the *Escherichia coli* promoters with R = 59 sequences is a good one. The approach we now discuss is from the theory of large deviations and is found in Bahadur[19] and Ellis.[20] Large deviation theory deserves to be more widely applied.

To present the most basic feature of the theory, assume that we have R trials with the probability α of "success" at each trial. Since R is large, the law of large numbers assures us of about αR successes. The central limit theorem gives additional information about the number of successes. The large deviation estimate of this probability is

$$P(\text{at least } \beta R \text{ successes}) \approx e^{-RH(\beta, \alpha)}$$

where

$$H(\beta, \alpha) = \beta \log(\beta/\alpha) + (1 - \beta)\log(1 - \beta)/(1 - \alpha)$$

When $\beta = 1$, $H(\beta,\alpha) = \log(1/\alpha)$ and $e^{-RH(\beta,\alpha)} = \alpha^R$.

How is the large deviation estimate to be used in the case of consensus patterns in *E. coli* promoters? Let us take a window size of $W = 9$, a word size of $k = 6$, and allow up to $mm = 2$ mismatches. The sequences are approximately $N = 60$ bases long. It is assumed that all bases are equally likely, $P(A) = P(T) = P(G) = P(C) = 1/4$, and independent.

The probability that a given pattern appears on a given line with fixed window position

$$\alpha = (W - k + 1) \cdot F \cdot 4^{-k}$$

where F is the neighborhood size. The factor $W - k + 1$ is to allow for the different positions of the word in the window. The probability p that at least βR of the lines have the consensus word w for a *fixed* window position is

$$p = e^{-RH(\beta,\alpha)}, \text{ fixed window position and fixed word}$$

while

$$p = (N - W + 1) e^{-RH(\beta,\alpha)}, \text{ any window position and fixed word}$$

is the probability for some window position. Since the analysis has been done for a fixed word w, we can relax that to any word, any window position by multiplying by 4^k, the number of k-letter words:

$$p = (N - w + 1) 4^k e^{-RH(\beta,\alpha)}, \text{ any window position and any word}$$

For our specific numbers, $k = 6$, $N = 60$, $R = 59$, and $W = 9$, we still need to determine α and β. To calculate α, recall that

$$\alpha = (W - k + 1)F 4^{-k}$$

where F is neighborhood size. Since $F = 154$ for up to 2 mm,

$$\alpha = (9 - 6 + 1)(154)4^{-6}$$

$$= 0.150...$$

In Section II, we found 9 exact occurrences of TATAAT, 17 with 1 mm, and 18 with 2 mm. This makes $\beta = 44/59 \approx 0.746$. Then $H(0.746, 0.150) = 0.890$. For any window position and any word,

$$p = (60 - 6 + 1) 4^6 e^{-59(0.890)} \approx 4.2 \times 10^{-18}$$

Therefore, the TATAAT pattern is extremely unlikely in random sequences.

B. Simulations

The promoter sequences unfortunately are not even close to all being composed of 25% A, etc. The problem is that base composition differs from sequence to sequence. The large deviation theory could be applied for sequences of differing compositions, but that would be difficult. In these cases, we turn to simulation for additional insight, although simulation will never be able to estimate significance levels such as 4.2×10^{-18}.

Not only is the theory of large deviations hard to apply when the sequences have different statistical characteristics, but it only predicts the number of sequences in a neighborhood. We are actually interested in the maximum score of consensus words. For these reasons we employ simulation.

The approach is quite simple; we generate sequences with the same number of A, T, G, and C as the promoter sequences, but put those letters in a random order. Then we run the program to get a sample of the maximum score of consensus words. The entire data set (N = 60 letters) is scanned, with the window in all positions. The value of the maximum in these sequences, with N = 60, w = 9, k = 6, and mm = 2, is approximately 17. The score of TATAAT is, from Section II.C, 35.17.

ACKNOWLEDGMENT

This work was supported by grants from the National Institutes of Health and the System Development Foundation.

REFERENCES

1. **Hawley, D. K. and McClure, W. R.,** Complilation and analysis of *Escherichia coli* promoter DNA sequences, *Nucl. Acids Res.,* 11, 2237, 1983.
2. **Mulligan, M. E., Hawley, D. K., Entriken, R., and McClure, W. R.,** *Escherichia coli* promoter sequences predict *in vitro* RNA polymerase selectivity, *Nucl. Acids Res.,* 12, 789, 1984.
3. **Pelham, H. R. B.,** A regulatory upstream promoter element in the drosophila hsp 70 heat-shock gene, *Cell,* 30, 517, 1982.
4. **Karlin, S., Ghandour, G., Ost, F., Tavare, S., and Korn, L. J.,** New approaches for computer analysis of nucleic acid sequences, *Proc. Natl. Acad. Sci. U.S.A.,* 80, 5660, 1983.
5. **Martinez, H. M.,** An efficient method for finding repeats in molecular sequences, *Nucl. Acids Res.,* 11, 4629, 1983.
6. **Sobel, E. and Martinez, H. M.** A multiple sequence alignment program, *Nucl. Acids Res.,* 14, 363, 1986.
7. **Wilbur, W. J. and Lipman, D. J.,** Rapid similarity searches of nucleic acid and protein data banks, *Proc. Natl. Acad. Sci. U.S.A.,* 80, 726, 1983.
8. **Smith, T. F., Waterman, M. S., and Sadler, J. R.,** Statistical characterization of nucleic acid sequences functional domains, *Nucl. Acids Res.,* 11, 2205, 1983.
9. **Smith, T. F., Waterman, M. S., and Burks, C.,** The statistical distribution of nucleic acid similarities, *Nucl. Acids Res.,* 13, 645, 1985.
10. **Waterman, M. S.,** Sequence alignments, in *Mathematical Methods of DNA Sequences,* Waterman, M. S., Ed., CRC Press, Boca Raton, Fla., 1988.
11. **Waterman, M. S., Galas, D., and Arratia, R.,** Pattern recognition in several sequences: consensus and alignment, *Bull. Math. Biol.,* 46, 515, 1984.
12. **Mengeritsky, G. and Smith, T. F.,** Recognition of characteristic patterns in sets of functionally equivalent DNA sequences, *CABIOS,* 3, 223,1987.
13. **Galas, D. J., Eggert, M., and Waterman, M. S.,** Rigorous pattern-recognition methods for DNA sequences. Analysis of promoter sequences from *Escherichia coli, J. Mol. Biol.,* 186, 117, 1985.
14. **Wu, H. M. and Crothers, D.,** The locus of sequence-directed and protein-induced DNA bending, *Nature (London),* 308, 509, 1984.
15. **Koo, H.-S., Wu, H.-M., and Crothers, D. M.,** DNA bending at adenine·thymine tracts, *Nature, (London),* 320, 501, 1986.
16. **Kolb, A., Spassky, A., Chapon, C., Blazy, B., and Bue, H.,** On the different binding affinities of CRP at the *lac, gal, mal*T promoter regions, *Nucl. Acids Res.,* 11, 7833, 1983.
17. **Pelham, H. R. B. and Bienz, M.,** A synthetic heat-shock promoter element confers heat-inducibility on the herpes simplex virus thymidine kinase gene, *EMBO J.* 11(1), 1473, 1982.

18. **Giniger, E., Varnum, S. M., and Ptashne, M.,** Specific DNA binding of GAL4, a positive regulatory protein of yeast, *Cell,* 40, 767, 1985.
19. **Bahadur, R. R.,** Some limit theorems in statistics, *SIAM,* Philadelphia, 1971.
20. **Ellis, R. S.,** *Entropy, Large Deviations, and Statistical Mechanics,* Springer-Verlag, New York, 1985, 71.

Chapter 5

SOME STATISTICAL ASPECTS OF THE PRIMARY STRUCTURE OF NUCLEOTIDE SEQUENCES

Simon Tavaré and Barton W. Giddings

TABLE OF CONTENTS

I. INTRODUCTION

The formidable volume of DNA sequence data generated in the last decade provides a rich source of data to biochemist, geneticist, and statistician alike. This paper studies some statistical aspects of the primary structure of nucleotide sequences.

We have divided our presentation into three main sections. The first gives a brief introduction to molecular biology of the nucleic acids, followed by some examples from the literature that give a feeling for the types of problems that are addressed. The second section describes some Markov chain methods for assessing the dependence structure that exists in a sequence of nucleotides. Particular emphasis is placed on methods for estimating the order of the Markov dependence. These methods are illustrated with an analysis of the bacteriophage λ genome.

The ordering of the bases in a nucleotide sequence is influenced by both random factors (such as mutation) and deterministic pressures (such as selection). The third part of our paper describes some methods for searching for repetitive or periodic patterns in a sequence. We base our analysis on the discrete Walsh transform and compare it to the more familiar Fourier methods.

Our aim has been to focus on some useful analysis techniques, without going into detail on all the variations on a given theme. The references will provide the interested reader with additional information, both biochemical and statistical, about this fascinating field.

II. STATISTICAL ASPECTS OF DNA SEQUENCES

A. Nucleic Acids — A Brief Review of Molecular Biology

The nucleic acids are of two types. The first, deoxyribonucleic acid (DNA), is composed of deoxyribonucleotides connected by phosphodiester linkages. There are four types of nucleotides in DNA: two purines, adenine (A) and guanine (G), and two pyrimidines, cytosine (C) and thymine (T). DNA may be single-stranded (as in certain single-stranded DNA viruses such as M13 or φX174 or when denatured by heat or alkali), but is usually found as double-stranded molecules. The strands of the double helix are held together by hydrogen bonding between bases on the two strands. A pairs with T form two hydrogen bonds per base pair, while G and C pair to form three bonds.

The second type of nucleic acid is ribonucleic acid (RNA). Like DNA, RNA is composed of nucleotides joined by phosphodiester bonds. The nucleotides of RNA, however, are ribonucleotides (ribose, the sugar component of each RNA nucleotide, has a hydroxyl group at the 2' position, whereas deoxyribose, the sugar component of DNA, does not). Furthermore, uracil (U) replaces T in RNA molecules. RNA molecules are usually single-stranded, although there may be a great deal of intrastrand base pairing.

RNA occurs as one of three types of molecules. In a process known as "transcription", RNA polymerase makes a complementary copy of the genetic information (i.e., the base sequence) of one strand of DNA (called the "sense" strand) which is called messenger RNA (mRNA). The mRNA carries sequence information and serves as the template for the synthesis of proteins by a process known as "translation". Messenger RNA constitutes only about 5% of the total cellular RNA.

The information specifying one amino acid is contained in a "codon", a triplet on the mRNA strand recognized by the second type of RNA molecule, the transfer RNA (tRNA). Since any position on the mRNA strand may be occupied by one of four bases, there are $4^3 = 64$ possible codons but only 20 amino acids. Three of the codons are termination signals. The remaining 61 triplets code for amino acids, which suggests the genetic code is degenerate. The amino acids methionine and tryptophan are, for example, each specified by unique codons, while leucine, arginine, and serine may each be specified by one of six codons.[1] Similarly, the other 15 amino acids are each coded for by any of two, three, or four codons.

The third and most abundant type of RNA, comprising about 80% of all cellular RNA, is the ribosomal RNA (rRNA), an important constituent of ribosomes. The precise function of rRNA is not known, although evidence suggests that it is crucial in binding certain components of protein synthesis (such as tRNA and mRNA) to the ribosome.[2]

In 1977, powerful DNA sequencing techniques were announced by Gilbert and Sanger. The concurrent development of these two important DNA sequencing techniques has fostered the rapid accumulation of sequence data; currently, there are about 20 million bases of information available for analysis. A great deal of statistical analysis has been performed on these sequences; we describe some of them briefly.

B. Some Examples of Statistical Studies of DNA

The rapid development of sequencing techniques required the development of computer programs capable of manipulating, analyzing, and comparing long sequences of data. The proliferation of such software is all too obvious: programs are now available which aid in planning cloning projects,[3] predict secondary structure of tRNA and mRNA,[4] determine whether a sequence is protein-coding or noncoding,[5,6] and search for such signals as promoters.[6,7]

Since the bases on DNA encode the information necessary to make each protein, one could suggest that any heterogeneity exceeding random expectation could be a consequence of the difference in the amino acid composition of the various gene products. Elton[8] tested this idea by selecting 42 protein sequences (32 vertebrate and 10 bacterial) with a total combined length of 5801 amino acids. An arbitrary length (20 residues) of each sequence was used to predict the corresponding DNA sequence. Because of the degeneracy of the genetic code, a given protein sequence may be specified by one of several DNA sequences. Elton predicted the base order of each gene fragment, assuming uniform codon preference and then applied analysis of variance to the set of predictions. He concluded that the data (applying uniform codon weighting) were consistent with the suggestion that DNA sequences within genes approximate "random DNA" from the point of view of heterogeneity.[8]

Data, however, suggest that among possible codon choices there are preferences.[9-13] The amino acid glutamine, for example, may be specified by either CAG or CAA, but the CAG codon occurs with much greater frequency in some genes.[14]

Maniatis et al.[14] suggest that knowledge of degenerate codon preference has an important practical application. When screening cellular mRNA for a specific, rare mRNA corresponding to a desired gene product with a partially determined sequence, one can locate the desired mRNA molecule by constructing oligomers complementary to the gene product. Unfortunately, the degeneracy of the genetic code allows even short amino acid sequences to possess a prohibitively large number of possible DNA coding sequences. Taking advantage of codon preference patterns reduces the number of oligomers likely to specify a given protein sequence and can make the mRNA screening process manageable.

Codon preference has been correlated with levels of gene expression in *Escherichia coli* and yeast.[15-18] A strong correlation exists between codon frequency and the relative abundance of the corresponding tRNA.[17,18] Gribskov et al.[16] suggested that codon preferences can be used to predict the relative level of gene expression and give a method to construct preference plots.

Furthermore, codon preferences and other statistical phenomena may be used to determine the function of a given DNA sequence. A common question when analyzing sequence data is whether the bases are part of a coding section (known as an "exon"). As Staden[19] argued, there are two approaches to this problem: one may either infer a strand is proteincoding from such clues as ribosome binding sites and an absence of stop codons or one may examine the properties of the base sequence and determine if they are consistent with properties known to be associated with coding sequences. One such property is codon preference.

Codons are used with unequal frequency in coding sequences. Fickett[20] noted that oligo-nucleotides (especially single bases) tend to be repeated with a periodicity of three in a protein-coding sequence. Furthermore, such periodicity is absent in noncoding sequences. Coding regions may also be detected using vector Fourier methods.[21] Statistical methods may also be used to determine the reading frame of coding sequence.[22]

Until the development of sophisticated DNA sequencing techniques, only a limited amount of reliable sequence data existed. Among the first nucleic acid data analyzed, therefore, were the base compositions of DNA from various sources. The four nucleotides are not evenly represented in any given sequence, and the base composition varies within and between sequences.[23]

Prokaryotic and eukaryotic DNA sequences also display distinct nearest neighbor patterns. The most basic analyses of nearest neighbor frequencies are the observations of dinucleotide frequencies. Distinct patterns, such as the relative rarity of the CG dinucleotide in eukaryotes[12,24-26] and the preference for PuPu and PyPy pairs* over PuPy and PyPu pairs in eukaryotic DNA[27] have been observed. Nussinov[25-28] has suggested that this preference results from structural considerations, with the homopolymeric dinucleotides (PuPu and PyPy) and other doublets which cause little or no steric strain in the DNA molecule being preferred.

Another example of nucleotide ordering is A clustering in sequences. Nussinov[29] examined long (>1 kb) RNA and DNA sequences for homopolynucleotides. She found that all but one of the sequences (16S rRNA, which does not code for protein, but instead serves a functional role in the ribosome) had fewer single and doubly clustered A than expected. Longer runs of A such as triplets were found more frequently than would be expected from random occurrence. G and C tended to cluster less frequently: single G and C and the doublets GG and CC were present in the analyzed sequences more often than expected, while longer clusters of G and C were observed less frequently than expected. Since a G-C base pair has more hydrogen bonds and, consequently, a higher bond energy than an A-T pair, Nussinov suggested that this clustering may be involved in facilitating the ''unzipping'' of the DNA strands, expediting replication, transcription, and/or translation.

Nussinov[30,31] has also examined DNA sequences near transcription inititation sites. Evidence suggests that eukaryotic transcription factors recognize and bind to certain promoter regions, including the so-called ''CCAAT'' and ''TATA box'' sequences located ''upstream''** from the transcriptional start site. Nussinov, however, has found other oligomers arguably as significant as the CCAAT sequence. Eukaryotic sequences within 500 bP of mRNA initiation sites were analyzed for recurring oligomers. TAT/ATA triplets and ATAT/TATA quartets, for example, occur frequently about 275 bases upstream from the start site with a signal strength twice that of the CAAT sequence at −80.[31]

Statistical evaluations have also been performed on single-stranded nucleic acids. The sequences of the single-strand DNA viruses, for example, contain fewer palindromic regions than expected. Palindromes are sequences which, if in double-stranded nucleic acid, would contain a twofold axis of symmetry, e.g., AGCT; consequently, such sequences can fold up on themselves. In one study, Duggleby[32] found improbably few four and six nucleotide palindromes in the single-stranded DNA phage, ΦX174. Other palindromes occurred with a frequency approximately as expected. Duggleby theorized that this paucity of palindromes might be associated with constraints on the secondary structure of single-stranded DNA viruses.

---

* Pu indicates purine base (A or G), while Py indicates pyrimidine base (C or T).

** ''Upstream'' suggests base positions in the 5′ direction from the transcription initiation site. The locations of bases upstream are described by negative integers, corresponding to the discrete number line with the start site equal to zero. Similarly, ''downstream'' implies base positions in the 3′ direction from the transcription start site. The locations of bases downstream are given by positive integers.

III. MARKOV ANALYSIS OF DNA/RNA SEQUENCES

A. Background

The previous section illustrated many examples of the statistical analysis of nucleotide sequences. Many of these are "local" in nature; they use statistics from nearest neighbor frequencies, codon counts, and so on. The very mechanism by which DNA sequences are produced — sequentially in long chains — suggests that the analysis of such sequences might profitably be carried out within the framework of Markov chain methodology. From a statistical point of view, such analyses seem to fall naturally into two camps.

The first might loosely be called "informational analysis". This draws on statistical machinery developed in the late 1950s by Kullback et al.[33] and others. Erickson and Altman[34] used these techniques to search for patterns in the MS2 genome. Rowe and Trainor,[35] Lipman and Maizel,[36] and Lipman and Wilbur[37] use related methods; see also Konopka[38] for a discussion of the evolutionary implications of information content. The second group corresponds to (statistically) more classical Markov chain analysis. See Elton,[24] Almagor,[39] Blaisdell,[40,41] and Garden,[42] for an example.

We first give a brief synopsis of Markov chain terminology. Let $\mathbf{X} = \{X_n, n = 0, 1, 2, \ldots\}$ denote a stochastic process whose states represent the nucleotides in a given DNA (or RNA) sequence. For definiteness, we label the bases in alphabetic order, so that A = 1, C = 2, G = 3, and T = 4. $\mathbf{X}$ is called a Markov chain of order k if

$$\Pr\{X_{n+1} = i_{n+1} \mid X_n = i_n, \ldots, X_{n-k+1} = i_{n-k+1}, \ldots, X_0 = i_0\}$$
$$= \Pr\{X_{n+1} = i_{n+1} \mid X_n = i_n, \ldots, X_{n-k+1} = i_{n-k+1}\}$$

for all $n \geq k - 1$ and for all choices of states $i_0, i_1, \ldots, i_{n+1}$ from $\{1,2,3,4\}$.* Intuitively, this says that the distribution of the next base in the sequence is determined by the previous k bases, and not by earlier ones. When k = 0, the chain comprises independently distributed bases. When k = 1, we recover the usual first order Markov chain case.

The behavior of the (time homogeneous) process $\mathbf{X}$ is determined by its initial distribution and the transition probabilities $p(i_1, i_2, \ldots, i_k; i_{k+1})$ given by

$$p(i_1, i_2, \ldots, i_k; i_{k+1}) = \Pr\{X_{k+1} = i_{k+1} \mid X_k = i_k, \ldots, X_1 = i_1\} \qquad (1)$$

The aim is to estimate the order k of the model, the transition probabilities $p(i_1, i_2, \ldots, i_k; i_{k+1})$, and then to assess various hypotheses about the DNA sequence(s). Typical among analyses for a single sequence might be testing for independence (k = 0), testing for uniformity of base composition, testing a fit to a hypothesized transition matrix, and testing particular transition probabilities. For a collection of sequences (perhaps derived as subsequences of a given sequence), one is usually interested in finding heterogeneity among the sequences. Within the framework of first order Markov chains, these questions are addressed by Elton.[24] Similar questions in higher dimensions may be studied using standard theory; References 43 and 44 are recommended.

Rather than focus on such detailed questions, our interest will focus on statistical aspects of finding the order of the Markov chain.

B. Finding the Order of a Markov Chain

Suppose that the sequence of interest is of length N. For r = 1,2, . . . let $n(i_1, i_2, \ldots, i_r)$

---

* There may be reasons to consider alphabets other than {A,C,G,T}, for example, {Pu,Py}. For simplicity, we stay with the "nucleotide alphabet". The methods to be described later carry over, with obvious changes, to other choices.

be the number of transitions $i_1 \rightarrow i_2 \rightarrow \ldots \rightarrow i_r$ observed in the sequence. It is a standard result[43,44] that the maximum likelihood estimator of $p(i_1, i_2, \ldots, i_k; i_{k+1})$ is

$$\hat{p}(i_1, i_2, \ldots, i_k; i_{k+1}) = n(i_1, i_2, \ldots, i_k, i_{k+1})/n(i_1, i_2, \ldots, i_k, +) \tag{2}$$

where

$$n(i_1, i_2, \ldots, i_k, +) = \sum_j n(i_1, i_2, \ldots, i_k, j)$$

Notice that in fitting a k-th order Markov chain with m states, there are $p = m^k(m - 1)$ independent parameters to be estimated; in our case m = 4, so that

$$p = 3 \times 4^k \tag{3}$$

This gives p = 3 (k = 0), p = 12 (k = 1), p = 48 (k = 2), p = 192 (k = 3), p = 768 (k = 4), and p = 3072 (k = 5). It is clear from this that very long DNA sequences are required for ''good'' estimation of the transition probabilities under the fully parameterized model of Equation 2. We will return to this problem later.

There have been several methods proposed for estimating the order k of a Markov chain. Because we will later want to compare models which are not nested, we will use information criteria rather than a multiple hypothesis testing framework. Among these is a standard information theory method,[43] Akaike's information criterion (AIC),[42,45,46] and the Bayesian information criterion (BIC).[45,47] To compute the BIC, we evaluate the log-likelihood L of the data

$$L = \sum n(i_1, i_2, \ldots, i_k, i_{k+1}) \, \ell n \, \hat{p}(i_1, i_2, \ldots, i_k; i_{k+1}) \tag{4}$$

the sum being over all $i_1, i_2, \ldots, i_k, i_{k+1}$ for which $n(i_1, i_2, \ldots, i_k, i_{k+1}) > 0$. The BIC for order k is then defined by

$$BIC(k) = -2L + p \ln n \tag{5}$$

where n ($\leq$N) is the number of subsequences from which the counts n($\cdot$) were formed. That k which minimizes BIC(k) is taken as the estimator of the true order of the chain. We use BIC because (unlike AIC) it is a consistent estimator of Markov chain order,[45] and it chooses simpler models.

As noted above, a full Markov chain analysis of high order requires very long data sequences. Because of the inherent heterogeneity of the linear structure of DNA sequences, such long *homogeneous* sequences are rather unusual. The data prevent us from performing precisely the type of analysis that seems most interesting. A class of Markov chain models that combines high order dependence with a small number of parameters could prove useful.

C. Models for High-Order Markov Chains

The class of Markovian models we will use in the present analysis was developed by Raftery.[47] The typical transition probability of the k-th order model is of the form

$$p(i_1, i_2, \ldots, i_k; i_{k+1}) = \sum_{j=1}^{k} \lambda_j \, q(i_j, i_{k+1}) \tag{6}$$

where Q = {q(i,j), $1 \leq i,j \leq 4$} is a row-stochastic matrix whose entries are to be estimated

Table 1
FIVE BIOLOGICALLY INTERESTING
REGIONS

Sequence	Positions	Orientation[a]	Length, N
Late	45000-19600	L→R	23102
Early 2	38220-45000	L→R	6780
Early 1	35040-27581	R→L	7460
Control	38030-33290	R→L	4740
Silent	27580-19601	R→L	7980

[a] If orientation is R→L, sequence is read in reverse complement form.

from the data, and $\lambda_1, \lambda_2, \ldots, \lambda_k$ are k parameters, summing to 1, that must also be estimated. This model may be viewed as a discrete state-space analog of the auto-regressive time series models; one extra parameter is introduced for each extra order after the first.

Notice that when k = 1, this model is identical to the usual first order Markov chain described earlier. The number of parameters to be estimated in the k-th order case is reduced from Equation 3 to

$$p = 11 + k \qquad (7)$$

and so we should be able to look for high order dependence more successfully. The price we pay for this is that the algebraic simplicity of Equation 2 no longer applies, and the maximum likelihood estimates of the parameters must be found by numerically maximizing the log-likelihood

$$L = \sum n(i_1, i_2, \ldots, i_k, i_{k+1}) \ln \left(\sum_{j=1}^{k} \lambda_j \, q(i_j, i_{k+1}) \right) \qquad (8)$$

using a constrained nonlinear optimization algorithm.

The BIC for this model is computed using Equation 5; L is the value of the right-hand side of Equation 8 at the maximum likelihood estimates.

D. Examples

We have chosen the bacteriophage λ as the source of our example. The λ genome was sequenced by Sanger et al.[48] and is 48502 nucleotides in length. The sequence was initially broken into five biolgocially interesting regions, given in Table 1.

The BIC indexes given by Equation 5 were calaculated for each sequence. For comparative purposes, we also include a value of k = −1 which corresponds to the model of independent bases, each with relative frequency 1/4. In this case, there are no parameters to estimate, and the BIC value is

$$BIC(-1) = -2n \ln 4$$

where n is the effective number of observations in the data. In all the results presented here, the sequence comparisons were begun at the 7th base of each sequence, so that n = N − 6 may be calculated from Table 1. The results of this analysis are presented in Table 2.

The BIC criterion indicates first order dependence for the regions Silent, Early 1, Early 2, and Control. We might expect the Silent region to have less "structure" than the others,

Table 2
BIC(k) VALUES FOR BACTERIOPHAGE λ

Sequence	Late	Early 1	Early 2	Control	Silent
k = −1	64036	20667	18782	13125	22109
0	63682	20566	18682	13025	21971
1	63258	20472[a]	18618[a]	12982[a]	21900[a]
2	62349[a]	20648	18743	13218	22026
3	63158	21706	19771	14133	23041
4	67923	26149	24040	18345	27580

[a] Denotes order of chain using the BIC criterion.

Table 3
LOCATION OF LATE REGIONS

Sequence	Positions	Orientation[a]	Length, N
Head	1-8550	L→R	8550
Tail	8550-19600	L→R	11050
Lysis	45000-46430	L→R	1430

[a] If orientation is R→L, sequence is read in reverse complement form.

since λ can propagate without this region.[14] The Late region is clearly identified as having an order of dependence of 2.

Models which are so clearly described by first order chains as those here will not typically be improved by using the high order dependence (HOD) models of Equation 6. We therefore analyzed only the Late region to determine whether the HOD model gives a more parsimonious description of the data. The BIC values are 62927 (k = 2) and 62935 (k = 3), compared to the smallest value of 62349 (k = 2) for the general case (see Table 2). The HOD model of order 2 provides the second best description of the data. That it is not the best means that the second order transition matrix of the best model must have a more complicated structure than is contained in Equation 6. The HOD models should provide better models for sequences such as φX174[42] that exhibit a higher order of dependence than λ.

The low orders of dependence identified in these regions may be due in part to inhomogeneity in the sequences. To examine this further, we broke the late region into three subregions labeled Head, Tail, and Lysis. The locations of these regions are given in Table 3 and the corresponding BIC values in Table 4.

The overall appearance of a second order model is maintained. Remarkably enough, the Lysis region is adequately described by the "completely random" model in which bases are laid down uniformly and at random. The Lysis region is composed of three genes, S, R, and RZ.[48] R and S genes are necessary for lysing the bacterium after the production of progeny phage and so are essential to the propagation of the phage in nature. Naively perhaps, we expected the structure of these genes to be similar to other λ genes (i.e., showing some dependence). Individual gene sequences, however, show the same completely random structure as the entire Lysis region. We conjecture that the variability in the estimated orders of dependence of these coding regions can be attributed to different patterns of codon usage among the genes.

We also examined one of the open reading frames in the Early 2 region, ORF290. Once again, a model of independent bases is adequate. It is tempting to conclude that ORF290

125

Table 4
BIC(k) VALUES FOR
BACTERIOPHAGE λ

Sequence	Head	Tail	Lysis
k = −1	23689	30620	3948[a]
0	23532	30287	3966
1	23352	30152	3997
2	23113[a]	29670[a]	4193
3	24114	30567	5017
4	28439	35070	—

[a] Denotes order of chain using the BIC criterion.

has no coding function, but our experience in the Lysis region (and that of Garden[42] for the replicase gene of MS2) demonstrates that protein coding regions may often appear structureless.

IV. TRANSFORM ANALYSIS OF DNA/RNA SEQUENCES

A. Background

The previous section of this article is devoted to stochastic models for the analysis of the primary structure of one or more stretches of DNA. These methods are useful for finding parsimonious descriptions of stretches of sequence with little *apparent* structure. One interesting feature of eukaryotic DNA is the presence of tandem (or periodic) repeats and interspersed base sequence repeats throughout the genome. Such repeats vary in length from simple dinucleotide periodicities (for example, the dinucleotide AG [repeated 28 times] found upstream from the mouse immunoglobulin G3 constant region gene[49]) to very large tandem repeats; the GNOMIC dictionary[50] is an invaluable compilation of examples of this type. Nucleotide sequences that exhibit repetitive structure cannot usefully be described by the earlier Markov chain models; alternatives are needed.

The presence of periodicities in DNA (or protein) sequences has led several authors to use what might broadly be called Fourier analysis methods to search for such structure. Kubota et al.[51] and McLachlan and Karn[52] use correlation coefficients calculated from sequences when residues are replaced by various quantitative properties of the amino acids, such as hydrophobicity. Liquori and co-workers[21] have introduced several Fourier-analytic methods for studying sequence similarities between proteins of different species. Felsenstein et al.[53] suggested Fourier analysis as a fast technique for computing the fraction of matches between two large nucleic acid sequences. Silverman and Linsker[54] and Trifonov and Sussman[55] use related methods to detect regularities in DNA sequences.

In this section we describe another technique of sequency analysis based on the Walsh transform, that is also applicable to problems involving symbol-sequence periodicities.

B. The Walsh Transform

We first give an inductive definition of the Walsh functions $\{W_n(x), 0 \leq x < 1\}$, $n = 0, 1, \ldots$. We initialize the induction by defining

$$W_0(x) \equiv 1, \quad x \in [0,1)$$

$$W_1(x) = \begin{cases} 1, & x \in [0,1/2) \\ -1, & x \in [1/2,1) \end{cases} \tag{9}$$

and then proceed recursively for n = 1,2, . . . via

$$W_{2n}(x) = \begin{cases} W_n(2x), & 0 \le x < 1/2 \\ (-1)^n W_n(2x - 1), & 1/2 \le x < 1 \end{cases} \tag{10}$$

and

$$W_{2n+1}(x) = \begin{cases} W_n(2x), & 0 \le x < 1/2 \\ (-1)^{n+1} W_n(2x - 1), & 1/2 \le x < 1 \end{cases} \tag{11}$$

The Walsh functions are orthogonal and piecewise constant on $[0,1)$.[56] The even numbered Walsh functions are symmetric about $x = 1/2$ (and play the role of the cosine terms in Fourier series), while the odd-numbered Walsh functions are antisymmetric about $x = 1/2$ (and so play the role of the sine terms in Fourier series). These functions may be used to construct the discrete Walsh transform of the sequence $\mathbf{x} = (x_0, x_1, \ldots, x_{N-1})$. When N is a power of 2 (so that $N = 2^p$ for some positive integer p), the following recipe does the trick.

We define first

$$w(k,j) = W_k(j/N), \quad j = 0, 1, \ldots, N - 1 \tag{12}$$

The Walsh transform of $\mathbf{x}$ is then given by

$$a_k = \frac{1}{N} \sum_{j=0}^{N-1} x_j \, w(k,j), \quad k = 0, 1, \ldots, N - 1 \tag{13}$$

and the inverse transform[56] by

$$x_j = \sum_{k=0}^{N-1} a_k w(j, k), \quad j = 0, 1, \ldots, N - 1 \tag{14}$$

There is an explicit formula for $w(k,j)$.[56] If $j = \sum_{r=0}^{p-1} j_r 2^r$, and $k = \sum_{r=0}^{p-1} k_r 2^r$, then

$$w(k,j) = (-1)^{\sum_{r=0}^{p-1} j_r(k_{p-r} + k_{p-r-1})} \tag{15}$$

from which it readily follows that $w(k,j) = w(j,k)$.

We will use the discrete Walsh transform to hunt for periodicities in DNA sequences. Imagine that our sequence of length $N = 2^p$ is listed as $A_0, A_1, \ldots, A_{N-1}$, where (as in Section III) A_i takes the value 1 if the i-th base is an A; 2, if it is a C; 3, if it is G, and 4 if it is T. We generate four associated sequences $\{x_{ij}, j = 0, 1, \ldots, N - 1\}$ of indicators as follows. For $i = 1, \ldots, 4$, set

$$x_{ij} = \begin{cases} 1, & \text{if } A_j = i, \quad j = 0, 1, \ldots, N - 1 \\ 0, & \text{otherwise} \end{cases} \tag{16}$$

Then form the associated Walsh transforms using Equation 13:

$$a_{ik} = \frac{1}{N} \sum_{j=0}^{N-1} x_{ij} w(k,j), \quad k = 0,1, \ldots, N-1 \tag{17}$$

Notice that a_{io} is the fraction of base i in the sequence.

The power spectrum $\{c_k, k = 0,1, \ldots, N-1\}$ of the sequence x is then defined by

$$c_k = \sum_{i=1}^{4} a_{ik}^2 \tag{18}$$

Notice that from a computational point of view, only three of the transform sequences $\{a_{ik}, k = 0,1, \ldots, N-1\}$ need to be calculated. Since

$$\sum_{i=1}^{4} x_{ij} = 1, \quad j = 0,1, \ldots, N-1$$

it follows that

$$\begin{aligned}
\sum_{i=1}^{4} a_{ik} &= \sum_{i=1}^{4} \left(\frac{1}{N} \sum_{j=0}^{N-1} x_{ij} w(k,j) \right) \\
&= \frac{1}{N} \sum_{j=0}^{N-1} \left(\sum_{i=1}^{4} x_{ij} \right) w(k,j) \\
&= \frac{1}{N} \sum_{j=0}^{N-1} w(0,j) w(k,j) \\
&= \begin{cases} 1, & \text{if } k = 0 \\ 0, & \text{if } k \neq 0 \end{cases}
\end{aligned}$$

the last equality following from orthogonality.

We will now compare the properties of the Walsh power spectrum with the perhaps more familiar Fourier power spectrum, found by replacing Equation 17 with

$$a_{mk} = \frac{1}{N} \sum_{j=0}^{N-1} x_{mj} e^{2\pi i jk/N}, \quad k = 0,1, \ldots, N-1 \tag{19}$$

and the value of c_k in Equation 18 by

$$c_k = \sum_{i=1}^{4} |a_{ik}|^2 \tag{20}$$

There are alternative ways of representing the structure of a DNA sequence other than via the indicator variables used in Equation 16. Silverman and Linsker,[54] for example, use a tetrahedral coordinate representation. The computational algorithm used here to calculate the fast Fourier transform is based on the code of Press et al.[57]

C. Examples

Figures 1 through 3 display the spectra for a 128 bP consensus sequence from the AT-

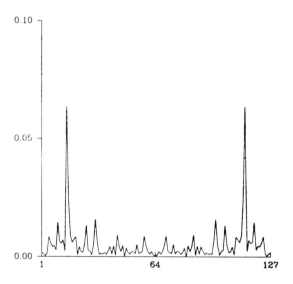

FIGURE 1. Fourier power spectrum for 128 base sequence from *X. laevis* oocyte 5S DNA.

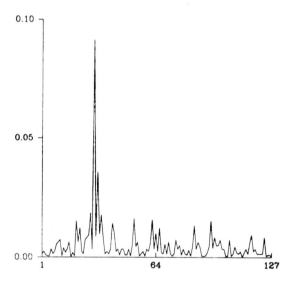

FIGURE 2. Walsh power spectrum for 128 base sequence from *X. laevis* oocyte 5S DNA.

rich spacer region of the 5S DNA of *Xenopus laevis*.[58] Figure 1 illustrates the familiar symmetry of the Fourier power spectrum. The pronounced peak at $k = 16$ shows a periodicity of length 8, corresponding to the simple sequence repeat 8 bases in length.[54,58] In contrast, the Walsh spectrum (Figure 2) is not symmetric; now the peak near $k = 32$ is indicative of a periodic component of length 8. Figure 3 gives the graphs of both transforms, plotted on common axes for comparative purposes. Note that in these plots (and those that follow), the base-frequency information that corresponds to $k = 0$ is not plotted.

The second example is a 128-bP sequence from the human ξ-globin gene[59]; it starts at position 210, in Intron 1. There is a 14 base repeat sequence ACAGTGGGAGGGG repeating (with very little variation) through this region. Notice from Figures 4 and 5 that both power spectra are considerably less well defined, despite the presence of the repeat. There are

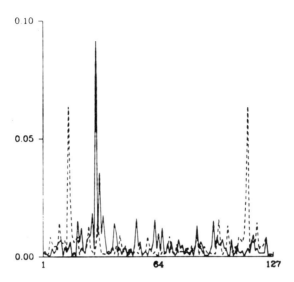

FIGURE 3. Composite of Figures 1 and 2. Dotted lines correspond to Fourier transform and solid lines to the Walsh transform.

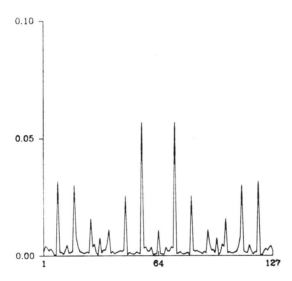

FIGURE 4. Fourier power spectrum for 128 base sequence from human ξ-globin, intron 1.

several reasons for this, among them, the rather repetitive substructure of the repeat and the fact that maximum emphasis of the peaks will occur when the length of the sequence is a multiple of the length of the repeat. Figure 6 gives the superposition of the two graphs.

There are several other comments worth making about use of the discrete Walsh transform in this setting. First, the technique is not limited to the analysis of sequences which have length a power of 2, however, when the length is a power of 2, the computation of the transform coefficients is very simple, both in terms of computational code and speed of execution. The fast Walsh transform requires less storage space than the corresponding fast Fourier transform, and seems to execute about five times faster. On the other hand the Walsh transform is, by its nature, better adapted to hunting for periodicities that are powers of 2

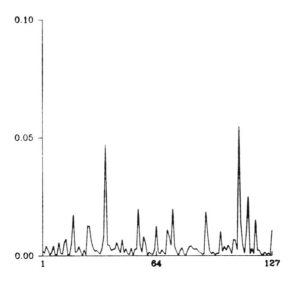

FIGURE 5. Walsh power spectrum for 128 base sequence from human ξ-globin, intron 1.

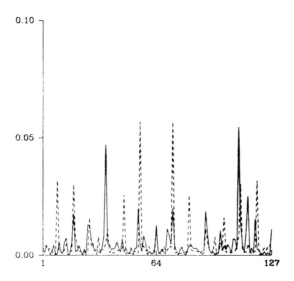

FIGURE 6. Composite of Figures 4 and 5. Dotted lines correspond to Fourier transform and solid lines to the Walsh transform.

in length, and it is not always easy to interpret the form of the power spectrum. Nevertheless, both techniques are a useful augmentation to more traditional oligonucleotide dictionary searches in the hunt for symbol patterns.

ACKNOWLEDGMENTS

This paper forms part of Bart Giddings' Senior Honors thesis at the University of Utah.
Work by Simon Tavaré is supported in part by NSF grant DMS86-08857 and in part by a grant from the System Development Foundation to Michael Waterman.
We would like to thank Jim Keener, Adrian Raftery, and John Roth for useful discussions on some computational and biochemical aspects of this work.

REFERENCES

1. **Freifelder, D.,** *Essentials of Molecular Biology,* Jones & Bartlett Publishers, 1985.
2. **Suzuki, D. T., Griffiths, A. J. F., Miller, J. H., and Lewontin, R. C.,** *An Introduction of Genetic Analysis,* 3rd ed., W. H. Freeman, New York, 1986.
3. **Blumenthal, R. M., Rice, P. J., and Roberts R. J.,** Computer programs for nucleic acid sequence manipulation, *Nucl. Acids Res.,* 10, 91, 1982.
4. **Nussinov, R. and Pieczenik, G.,** Structural combinatorial constraints on base pairing in large nucleotide sequences, *J. Theor. Biol.,* 106, 245, 1984.
5. **Tramontano, A. and Macchiato, M. F.,** Probability of coding a DNA sequence: an algorithm to predict translated reading frames from their thermodynamic characteristics, *Nucl. Acids Res.,* 14, 127, 1986.
6. **Staden, R.,** Graphic methods to determine the function of nucleic acid sequences, *Nucl. Acids Res.,* 12, 521, 1984.
7. **Mulligan, M. E. and McClure, W. R.,** Analysis of the occurrence of promoter-sites in DNA, *Nucl. Acids Res.,* 14, 109, 1986.
8. **Elton, R. A.,** Theoretical models for heterogeneity of base composition in DNA, *J. Theor. Biol.,* 45, 533, 1974.
9. **Miyata, T., Hayashida, H., Yasunaga, T., and Hasegawa, M.,** The preferential codon usages in variable and constant regions of immunoglobulin genes are quite distinct from each other, *Nucl. Acids Res.,* 7, 2431, 1979.
10. **Grantham, R., Gautier, C., Gouy, M., Mercier, R., and Pavé, A.,** Codon catalog usage and the genome hypothesis, *Nucl. Acids Res.,* 8, r49, 1980.
11. **Grantham, R., Gautier, C., and Gouy, M.,** Codon frequencies in 119 individual genes confirm consistent choices of degenerate bases according to genome type, *Nucl. Acids Res.,* 8, 1893, 1980.
12. **Rothberg, P. G. and Wimmer, E.,** Mononucleotide and dinucleotide frequencies and codon usage in poliovirion RNA, *Nucl. Acids Res.,* 9, 6221, 1981.
13. **Modiano, G., Battistuzzi, G., and Motulsky, A. G.,** Nonrandom patterns of codon usage and of nucleotide substitutions in human alpha- and beta-globin genes: an evolutionary strategy reducing the rate of mutations with drastic effects?, *Proc. Natl. Acad. Sci. U.S.A.,* 78, 1110, 1981.
14. **Maniatis, T., Fritsch, E. F., and Sambrook, J.,** *Molecular Cloning: A Laboratory Manual,* Cold Spring Harbor Laboratory, Cold Spring Harbor, N.Y., 1982.
15. **McLachlan, A. D., Staden, R., and Boswell, D. R.,** A method for measuring the non-random bias of a codon usage table, *Nucl. Acids Res.,* 12, 9567, 1984.
16. **Gribskov, M., Devereux, J., and Burgess, R. R.,** The codon preference plot: graphic analysis of protein coding sequences and prediction of gene expression, *Nucl. Acids Res.,* 12, 539, 1984.
17. **Ikemura, T.,** Correlation between the abundance of *Escherichia coli* transfer RNAs and the occurrence of the respective codons in its protein genes, *J. Mol. Biol.,* 146, 1, 1981.
18. **Ikemura, T.,** Correlation between the abundance of yeast transfer RNAs and the occurrence of the respective codons in protein genes, *J. Mol. Biol.,* 158, 573, 1982.
19. **Staden, R.,** Measurement of the effects that coding for a protein has on a DNA sequence and their use for finding genes, *Nucl. Acids Res.* 12, 551, 1984.
20. **Fickett, J. W.,** Recognition of protein coding regions in DNA sequences, *Nucl. Acids Res.,* 10, 5303, 1982.
21. **Liquori, A. M., Ripamonti, A., Sadun, C., Ottani, S., and Braga, D.,** Pattern recognition of sequence similarities in globular proteins by Fourier analysis: a novel approach to molecular evolution, *J. Mol. Evol.,* 23, 80, 1986.
22. **Shulman, M. J., Steinberg, C. M., and Westmoreland, N.,** The coding function of nucleotide sequences can be discerned by statistical analysis, *J. Theor. Biol.,* 88, 409, 1981.
23. **Weir, B. S.,** Statistical analysis of molecular genetic data, *IMA J. Math. Appl. Med. Biol.,* 2, 1, 1985.
24. **Elton, R. A.,** Doublet frequencies in sequenced nucleic acids, *J. Mol. Evol.,* 4, 323, 1975.
25. **Nussinov, R.** Some rules in the ordering of nucleotides in the DNA, *Nucl. Acids Res.,* 8, 4545, 1980.
26. **Nussinov, R.,** The universal dinucleotide asymmetry rules in DNA and the amino acid codon choice, *J. Mol. Evol.,* 17, 237, 1981.
27. **Nussinov, R.,** Strong doublet preferences in nucleotide sequences and DNA geometry, *J. Mol. Evol.,* 20, 111, 1984.
28. **Nussinov, R.,** Doublet frequencies in evolutionary distinct groups, *Nucl. Acids Res.,* 12, 1749, 1984.
29. **Nussinsov, R.,** Strong adenine clustering in nucleotide sequences, *J. Theor. Biol.,* 85, 285, 1980.
30. **Nussinov, R.,** Compilation of eukaryotic sequences around transcription initiation sites, *J. Theor. Biol.,* 120, 479, 1986.
31. **Nussinov, R., Owens, J., and Maizel, J. V., Jr.,** Sequence signals in eukaryotic upstream regions, *Biochim. Biophys. Acta,* 866, 109, 1986.

32. **Duggleby, R. G.,** A paucity of palindromes in φX174, *J. Theor. Biol.,* 93, 143, 1981.

33. **Kullback, S., Kupperman, M., and Ku, H. H.,** Tests for contingency tables and Markov chains, *Technometrics,* 4, 573, 1962.

34. **Erickson, J. W. and Altman, G. G.,** A search for patterns in the nucleotide sequence of the MS2 genome, *J. Math. Biol.,* 7, 219, 1979.

35. **Rowe, G. W. and Trainor, L. E. H.,** On the informational content of viral DNA, *J. Theor. Biol.,* 101, 151, 1983.

36. **Lipman, D. J. and Maizel, J.,** Comparative analysis of nucleic acid sequences by their general constraints, *Nucl. Acids Res.,* 10, 2723, 1982.

37. **Lipman, D. J. and Wilbur, W. J.,** Contextual constraints on synonymous codon choice, *J. Mol. Biol.,* 163, 363, 1983.

38. **Konopka, A.,** Is the information content of DNA evolutionarily significant?, *J. Theor. Biol.,* 107, 697, 1984.

39. **Almagor, H.,** A Markov analysis of DNA sequences, *J. Theor. Biol.* 104, 633, 1983.

40. **Blaisdell, B. E.,** A prevalent persistent global nonrandomness that distinguishes coding and non-coding eucaryotic nuclear DNA sequences, *J. Mol. Evol.,* 19, 122, 1983.

41. **Blaisdell, B. E.,** Markov chain analysis finds a significant influence of neighboring bases on the occurrence of a base in eucaryotic nuclear DNA sequences both protein-coding and noncoding, *J. Mol. Evol.,* 21, 278, 1985.

42. **Garden, P. W.,** Markov analysis of viral DNA/RNA sequences, *J. Theor. Biol.* 82, 679, 1980.

43. **Chatfield, C.,** Statistical inference regarding Markov chain models, *Appl. Stat.,* 22, 7, 1973.

44. **Basawa, I. V. and Prakasa Rao, B. L. S.,** *Statistical Inference for Stochastic Processes,* Academic Press, New York, 1980.

45. **Katz, R. W.,** On some criteria for estimating the order of a Markov chain, *Technometrics,* 23, 243, 1981.

46. **Tong, H.,** Determination of the order of a Markov chain by Akaike's Information Criterion, *J. Appl. Probab.,* 12, 488, 1975.

47. **Raftery, A. E.,** A model for high-order Markov chains, *J. R. Stat. Soc. Ser. B,* 47, 528, 1985.

48. **Sanger, F., Coulson, A. R., Hong, G. F., Hill, D. F., and Petersen, G. B.,** Nucleotide sequence of bacteriophage Lambda DNA, *J. Mol. Biol.,* 162, 729, 1982.

49. **Weis, J. A., Word, C. J., Rimm, D., Der-Balan, G. P., Martinez, H. M., Tucker, P. W., and Blattner, F. R.,** Structural analysis of the murine IgG3 constant region gene, *EMBO J.,* 3, 2041, 1984.

50. **Trifonov, E. N. and Brendel, V.,** *GNOMIC. A Dictionary of Genetic Codes,* Balaban Publishers, 1986.

51. **Kubota, Y., Takahashi, S., Nishikawa, K., and Ooi, T.,** Homology in protein sequences expressed by correlation coefficients, *J. Theor. Biol.,* 91, 347, 1981.

52. **McLachlan, A. D. and Karn, J.,** Periodic features of the amino acid sequence of the nematode myosin rod, *J. Mol. Biol.,* 164, 605, 1983.

53. **Felsenstein, J., Sawyer, S., and Kochin, R.,** An efficient method for matching nucleic acid sequences, *Nucleic Acids Res.,* 10, 133, 1982.

54. **Silverman, B. D. and Linsker, R.,** A measure of DNA periodicity, *J. Theor. Biol.,* 118, 295, 1986.

55. **Trifonov, E. N. and Sussman, J. L.,** The pitch of chromatin DNA is reflected in its nucleotide sequence, *Proc. Natl. Acad. Sci. U.S.A.,* 77, 3816, 1980.

56. **Kennett, B. L. N.,** Introduction to the Finite Walsh Transform and the theory of the Fast Walsh Transform, in Proc. Conf. Theory and Application of Walsh Functions, Hatfield Polytechnic, London, 1971.

57. **Press, W. H., Flannery, B. P., Teukolsky, S. A., and Vetterling, W. T.,** *Numerical Recipes. The Art of Scientific Computing,* Cambridge University Press, London, 1986.

58. **Federoff, N. V. and Brown, D. D.,** The nucleotide sequence of oocyte S DNA in *Xenopus laevis.* I. The AT-rich spacer, *Cell,* 13, 701, 1978.

59. **Proudfoot, N. J., Gil, A., and Maniatis, T.,** The structure of the human zeta-globin gene and a closely linked, nearly identical pseudogene, *Cell,* 31, 553, 1982.

Chapter 6

PATTERNS IN DNA AND AMINO ACID SEQUENCES AND THEIR STATISTICAL SIGNIFICANCE

Samuel Karlin, Friedemann Ost, and B. Edwin Blaisdell

TABLE OF CONTENTS

I. INTRODUCTION

There are now more than 7000 DNA sequences totaling more than 15 million bases in the GenBank and EMBL data bases. About 5000 of these sequences contain coding regions that can be translated into amino acid sequences and supplement the approximately 2500 directly determined protein sequences in the Protein Identification Resources (PIR) data base.

DNA sequences that are well conserved over multiple species may indicate regions important to biological functions maintained by virtue of selective forces or they may correspond to nonfunctional evolutionary remnants of ancestral DNA fragments. Eukaryotic DNA sequences are typically different from random letter sequences as described by independence or Markov models.[1] However, the nonrandomness displays patterns that are conserved in some sets of genes or in limited subsequences of them. For example, the longest statistically significant word (defined here as a succession of contiguous letters) common to the human, mouse, rabbit, and chicken genomic β-globin DNA sequences (each about 2000 bp long) is 17 bp in length covering the interface between the second exon and its following intron. The second longest common word is 14 bp which covers the interface between the first exon and its following intron.[2,3] It appears that accuracy in RNA splicing requires conservation of definite sequences bounding the splice junctions for the same gene in similar species.

Among the objectives of nucleic acid and protein sequence analysis is discovering significant patterns and interpreting them in relation to the course of DNA processing, polypeptide folding, protein biochemical function, and evolutionary development at each of these levels. Similarities and differences among sequences can aid in phylogenetic classifications,[4-6] in assessing facets of analogy vs. homology,[7] and in gaining insights into the kinds and processes of substitutions, insertions, deletions, and recombination events.[8,9]

Specific word relationships (e.g., dyad symmetries) can be biologically meaningful. Relative to sequence composition, word relationships can be characterized with reference to spacings, proximity to natural biological sites, unusual lengths, clustering attributes, substantial iterations of certain letter types and count distributions of certain words. The specification of and examples demonstrating the utility of such concepts is the first main objective of this review (Section III).

II. ASSESSING STATISTICAL SIGNIFICANCE

Distinguishing significant features from features arising by chance is important in sequence comparisons. Means for assessing statistical significance of sequence patterns can be based on theoretical models and on permutations of the observed data. A description of useful theoretical formulas and their interpretation on molecular sequence data is the second main objective of this review article (Section IV).

A. Theoretical Sequence Models

We use a "random" model appropriate to the data as a standard in order to ascertain the distributional properties of the various data statistics. The independence random model provides a reasonable benchmark by which to assess statistical significance of various sequence patterns. In this model, the original sequences are generated in the manner that the successive letters of the vth sequence are sampled independently having the letter A_i occur with probability $p_i^{(v)}$ (in the case of DNA, the $p_i^{(v)}$ are usually specified as the actual A, T, C, and G frequencies in the observed sequences).

A standard based on a random model that incorporates first order neighbor dependencies can be constructed as follows. In the vth sequence, let $p_{ij}^{(v)}$ be the conditional probability of sampling letter A_j following letter A_i. The realization of successive letters of the vth sequence is accordingly governed by the transition probability matrix $\|p_{ij}^{(v)}\|$. $p_{ij}^{(v)}$ would correspond to the dinucleotide frequencies in the case of DNA and to diresidue frequencies for protein sequences. We refer to this sequence model as the first order Markov dependent random model. More complex random models would accommodate higher order Markov dependence or more elaborate long-range neighbor dependence.[10-12] For these models, theoretical results (limit distributional properties) have been obtained on (1) the length $K_{r,s}$ of the longest common word present in at least r out of s sequences; (2) on the numbers of moderate to long common words in these sequences; (3) on the longest run length of certain letter types; and (4) on the length of the longest word satisfying a prescribed relationship. We review some of these results in Section IV. Some similar results pertaining to matching words for the independence model have been given.[13,14] Waterman[15] has given a review of methods of comparing sequences that contains several examples of estimation of significance.

B. Data Shuffling Methods

These methods are widely practiced in many areas of data analysis.[16-18] The idea is to compare the observed sequences against a collection of independent restructured sequences each obtained by repeatedly randomizing or shuffling the data. Usually a data statistic evaluated on the original sequence is compared with its values determined from the randomly reconstructed data sets. For protein sequences, permutation methods have been used by Dayhoff,[5] and have been reviewed in Doolittle,[19] among others.

We use a spectrum of shuffling (permutation) procedures that selectively shuffle the sequence letters. This process alters certain alphabet relationships while keeping others intact. We identify each permutation model by the class of letters to be permuted; for example, purine-only shufflings permute randomly all the A + G positions while all C and T letters are left in their original positions.

Sequence statistics are computed for 100 to 500 permutations of the data to assess the variability of the statistics under each permutation class. The value of the original statistic relative to the collection of values of the statistic for the permutations of the data provides an opportunity to assess the special (nonrandom) characteristics of the original data. If the original statistic is more extreme than most (95 or 99%) of the values of this statistic when evaluated over the permuted data sets, then the original statistic is considered to be significant.

Insights into the data can also be gained by comparisons between different classes of permutations. Comparing between the permutation models of shuffled purines only and that of shuffled pyrimidines only affords a way to assess the relative preservation of purines vs. pyrimidines. Table 1 gives a listing of several useful permutation classes.

III. SEQUENCE STATISTICS AND CONCEPTS

Table 2 gives examples of sequence patterns and Table 3 gives appropriate statistics computable for them. These patterns and statistics are instrumental for classifying and

Table 1
EXAMPLES OF PERMUTATION CLASSES

1. Complete shuffling of a DNA or amino acid sequence
2. Complete shuffling of a set of sequences: each sequence independently
3. Complete shuffling of letters in a set of domains (exons, introns, flanks), each domain independently
4. Complete shuffling of a pooled set of sequences
5. a. Shuffle only purines
    b. Shuffle only pyrimidines
    c. Shuffle purines among themselves and pyrimidines among themselves
6. Shuffle among letters of the same alphabet classification
7. Shuffling of codons
8. Shuffle only sites 3 of codons

Table 2
EXAMPLES OF WORD RELATIONS (IN ANY ALPHABET)

1. Matching (aligned or close or in unrestricted locations)
2. Matching with a prescribed number or percentage of errors
3. Matching with systematically located errors in aligned sequences (e.g., errors in codon site 3)
4. Dyad words (exact or with some errors)
5. Inverted words (block inverted words)
6. Complementary words (relabeled words)
7. Matching structure independent of content
8. Change of alphabet

Table 3
EXAMPLES OF SEQUENCE STATISTICS (IN ANY ALPHABET)

1. Length of longest (second longest, etc.) repeats (without and with errors)
2. Counts of long repeats
3. Spacing between repeats
4. Close repeats
5. Periodic repeats
6. Repeats of special composition or structure
7. Any of the above for various word relationships (e.g., dyad symmetry combinations, charge complementary words in the charge alphabet)
8. Long common words among many sequences
9. Long runs of certain letter types
10. Long patterned runs
11. Counts of long runs
12. Count occurrence distributions of words in a defined relationship (one and multidimensional)

interpreting sequence attributes and for suggesting useful functions for them. We shall illustrate the ideas mostly in terms of two sequence functionals: count occurrence distributions and certain maximal length word relationships.

A useful concept applicable for all sequence statistics is the grouping of letters in one alphabet to form natural new alphabets. Many possible alphabets can be imagined and those that are tried are generally suggested by a correlation of sequence pattern with reasonable physiochemical properties. Thus, it is meaningful to group the nucleotides to form the two-letter purine vs. pyrimidine classification, characterized by chemical type and size, $R = \{A,G\}$, $Y = \{C,G\}$, or to form the two-letter alphabet of strong vs. weak hydrogen bonding bases, $W = \{A,T\}$ and $S = \{C,G\}$. Amino acids can be classified according to structural, chemical, charge, functional, and hydrophobicity properties. Other possible criteria in grouping amino acids could be based on physical endowments (e.g., molecular weight, shape), kinetic properties (e.g., turnover rates), associations with secondary structure (e.g., α he-

Table 4
EXAMPLES OF ALPHABETS

I. Two letter DNA alphabets
    1. Purines vs. pyrimidines {R, Y}
    2. Strong vs. weak hydrogen bonding {S, W}
    3. Two letter alphabet of less physiochemical significance: keto, K = {T, G} vs. amino, M = {A, C}
II. Amino acid alphabets
    4. The 3-letter structural alphabet:[28] ambivalent (Ala, Cys, Gly, Pro, Ser, Thr, Trp, Tyr); external (Arg, Asn, Asp, Gln, Glu, His, Lys); internal (Ile, Leu, Met, Phe, Val)
    5. The 8-letter chemical alphabet:[29] acidic (Asp, Glu); aliphatic (Ala, Gly, Ile, Leu, Val); amide (Asn, Gln); aromatic (Phe, Trp, Tyr); basic (Arg, His, Lys); hydroxyl (Ser, Thr): imino (Pro); sulfur (Cys, Met)
    6. The 4-letter functional alphabet:[26] acidic and basic (same as in chemical alphabet): hydrophobic nonpolar (Ala, Ile, Leu, Met, Phe, Pro, Trp, Val); polar uncharged (Asn, Cys, Gln, Gly, Ser, Thr, Tyr)
    7. The 3-letter charge alphabet: acidic and basic (as above in chemical alphabet); neutral (all the other amino acids)
    8. The 2-letter hydrophobic alphabet: hydrophobic (Ala, Ile, Leu, Met, Phe, Pro, Trp, Val); hydrophilic (Arg, Asn, Asp, Cys, Gln, Glu, Gly, His, Lys, Ser, Thr, Tyr)
III. Other alphabets
    9. Statistical (empirical) substitutability alphabet[5,22]
    10. Random partition of 20 amino acids into k classes
    11. Optimal partition of 20 amino acids into k classes that maximizes a similarity measure between sequences

lixes, β-sheets, turns). Classifications of amino acids into various alphabets different from those that we employ have been based on chemical categorizations and minimal base differences between codons.[20-24] Dayhoff[5] studied groups of closely related proteins from more than 70 evolutionary trees for various superfamilies of proteins and constructed a statistical substitutability alphabet.

We have also employed random alphabets of a prescribed size as controls[25] and constructed optimal amino acid groupings (alphabets) for particular sequence comparisons. Table 4 highlights various DNA and amino acid alphabets.[25-29]

The use of different alphabets can contribute in several ways. Finding significant identities at the same position in many alphabets underscores their possible significance (it should be recognized that the alphabet size and the sequence composition influence the determination of significance; see Section IV). Multiple alphabet comparisons can expose significant regions that are conserved in some, but not in other alphabets. These results may suggest contrasting functional or structural properties for different regions of the sequence.

Consider a sequence of letters drawn from an m-letter alphabet $A = (A_1, A_2, \ldots, A_m)$ (e.g., m = 4 for DNA sequences, m = 20 for amino acid sequences, and m = 8 for the "chemical" classification of amino acids). The following definition is convenient. A k-word is a set of k consecutive letters of the sequence. As we traverse each position, for a linear (circular) sequence of length N there are, not necessarily distinct, N − k + 1 (N) k-words.

A. Repeats and Associated Functionals within a Single Sequence

For a given sequence S of total length N based on the alphabet A a υ-fold repeat of length k is a k-word appearing exactly υ times in S.

1. Frequency Distributions of Word Occurrences

Relative to S for each given word length k we define the frequency distribution, $f_k(\upsilon)$, $\upsilon = 0,1,2, \ldots$ as the count of k-words occurring υ times. The number of distinct k-words

Table 5
REPEAT-OCCURRENCE DISTRIBUTION OF OLIGONUCLEOTIDES (WORDS) OF LENGTH 6 AND 8

							$f_6(\nu)$								
ν	1	2	3	4	5	6	7	8	9	10	11	12	13	14	18
BKV-Dun	898	628	361	175	87	57	30	14	7	1	0	0	2	0	1
SV-40	943	627	363	183	90	47	29	11	7	5	1	3	1	2	0
Polyoma	1174	740	421	198	78	22	5	2	1	0	0	0	0	0	0
Random polyoma	1391	899	423	132	42	11	3	1	0	0	0	0	0	0	0

			$f_8(\nu)$			
ν	1	2	3	4	5	6
BKV-Dun	4158	383	57	12	2	0
SV-40	4198	434	46	7	1	1
Polyoma	4709	269	11	3	0	0

Note: The entries indicate the number of distinct k-words that occurred exactly ν-times for the specified sequence. The row labeled random is obtained from the pointwise minimum of the cumulative distribution derived from 10 random permutations of the polyoma sequence.

is $N^* = \sum_{\nu \geq 1} f_k(\nu)$. There are various summary statistics associated with the word occurrence frequency distribution $f_k(\nu)$ including mean, variance, range, measures of skewness, etc.

In Table 5, we present the count occurrence distributions of 6- and 8-words for the three papovavirus genomes, Simian virus-40 (SV-40; N = 5243 bp), polyoma (N = 5293), and human BKV Dunlop strain (N = 5153).

The distributions of SV-40 and BKV are very close indicating that the genomes are similar. Polyoma is distinguished from both SV-40 and BKV by the lower number of highly repeated lengthy words. This comparison holds for all repeat occurrence distributions $f_k(\nu)$, $4 \leq k \leq 15$. These observations suggest a greater degree of duplication or homogenization events, a more recent divergence, or a lesser mutation rate during the evolution of SV-40 and BKV when compared to the polyoma virus. The occurrence distributions in all the papovaviruses, even polyoma, show an excess of long repeated words when compared to the occurrence distributions of the same sequences with the letters randomly permuted.

In contrast, the amino acid sequences of the VPI and VP2 capsid proteins of polyoma (data not shown) have dipeptide counts with significantly fewer repeats than for corresponding random sequences. Thus, in the VP1 gene, more unique dipeptides have been selected for, possibly suggesting that assembly of the icosohedral nucleocapsid is facilitated by providing more distinct components for each face.

2. Long Repeat Words

For a sequence S of length N we define L_r as the length of the longest word appearing at least r times. Equivalently,

$$L_r = \max\left\{k \quad \text{such that} \quad \sum_{\nu=r}^{\infty} f_k(\nu) \geq 1\right\}$$

This functional will also be referred to as the maximal r-fold repeat length. For random

Table 6
COUNTS OF
NONEMBEDDABLE
REPEATS ≥ 12 BP
LENGTH AND ≥ 10 BP
LENGTH FOR THE
PAPOVAVIRUSES

Sequence	No. of repeat of length	
	≥12	≥10
SV-40	6*	38
BKV-Dun	8*	30
Polyoma	1	13

Note: The count of 6 distinct repeats of length ≥ 12 is highly significant; see Section IV.G.

sequence models it is possible to derive the asymptotic distributional properties of L_r for N large (see Section IV.D). A long repeat (L_2 value) is said to be statistically significant if the probability of observing a repeat of this length or more for the random model is at most 0.01.

Significant long direct repeats provide a dramatic contrast between two *Escherichia coli* phages, λ and T7.[30] T7 shows an impressive set of long repeats linking a number of its known promoter elements while λ phage shows no significant long repeats. These contrasts might be attributed to the differences in the transcription mechanism of λ phage vs. T7. In this context, all long repeats of T7 are related to promoters of late genes. The requirements on these promoter sites are quite stringent as attested to by conservation of the long repeat unit. On the other hand, there are no significant repeats in the region of the early genes that rely on a variety of bacterial enzymes for transcription. The λ phage uses a multiplicity of host enzymes for transcription of all its genes.

3. Numbers of Long Repeats
The number of r-fold repeats exceeding length k* is

$$Z_{r,k^*} = \sum_{k \geq k^*} \sum_{\nu \geq r} f_k(\nu)$$

It is natural to prescribe k* of the order of the expected maximal r-fold repeat length. The asymptotical distributional properties of Z_{r,k^*} for appropriate random models are described in Section IV.G.

Excess counts of very long nonembeddable repeats of words of length k for SV-40 and BKV compared with polyoma are shown in Table 6 (a repeat is said to be nonembeddable if the corresponding matching oligonucleotides cannot be extended to a longer matching length). Can this excess be a reflection of a greater mutation rate in the mouse species and its viral inhabitants than in the primates[31,32] with consequent disruption of longer repeats?

4. Conditional Repeat Structures
It is of interest to consider the statistics described heretofore subject to a variety of conditions. For example, the occurrence distributions $f_k(\upsilon|d)$ which counts only k-word

repeats restricted to distances between copies $\leq$ d. The d-restricted analog of the L functional is the maximal repeat length satisfying the condition of distance $\leq$ d letters between successive copies.

One expects that, over a given random sequence, long repeats be spaced out at approximately equal intervals. However, in the papovaviruses all the statistically significant long repeats (there are four such repeats $\geq$ 14 bp length) occur in close proximity. These repeats include the familiar enhancer and promoter elements. All significantly long repeats in the Epstein-Barr virus (there are about 30 distinct sets) are also strikingly close (many comprise tandem iterates and most occur in coding regions or open reading frames, which is unusual). One set includes four copies of a long (about 540 bp) terminal tandem direct repeat.[33] By contrast, the herpes simplex virus I and the varicella zoster virus of the same general virus family exhibit two pairs of long, inverted complementary repeats, the two members of each pair widely separated.[34] These two viruses have notably fewer significant repeats elsewhere.

Other conditionings on the repeat structure could reflect on the content of the words. For example, we might focus on the repeat occurrence distribution of k-words with high G + C content or emphasize the presence of a specific word structure as almost periodic alternations of certain nucleotide types.[30]

B. Repeats and Other Similarity Functions for Multiple Sequences

For s sequences, $S = \{S_1, S_2, \ldots, S_s\}$, of lengths $N = \{N_1, N_2, \ldots, N_s\}$, respectively, all from the alphabet A, an r-of-s word identity of length k is a k-word appearing, at least once, in each of at least r of the s sequences. The number of representatives of a specific k-word across the various sequences is described by the vector $\boldsymbol{v} = (v_1, v_2, \ldots, v_s)$, where v_i is the number of times the k-word appears in the sequence S_i.

1. Multi-Sequence Frequency Distribution of Word Occurrences

This is the s-dimensional analog of the frequency distribution of word occurrences. We define $f_k(v_1, v_2, \ldots, v_s) = f_k(v) = n_v$ as the number of k-words that are represented across the sequences according to the vector v. Table 7 gives an example (for a different presentation of similar data, see Reference 3). Note at coordinate (1,1) human and mouse share more common words in this immunoglobulin genomic sequence than do human and rabbit or mouse and rabbit (33, 19, and 12 words, respectively), perhaps reflecting the fact that human and mouse, by sharing the same domicile, also share the same pathogens.

2. Long Common Words

Maximal r-of-s common words: for the s sequences S we define the quantity $K_{r,s}$ as the maximal length of a word occurring in at least r out of the s sequences. The asymptotic distributional properties of $K_{r,s}$ for large N have been developed for a collection of random sequence models (Section IV.B). On the basis of these formulas, the statistical significance of a long r-of-s shared word can be assessed.

We compared the family of human β-like globin genomic sequences (β,δ,γ,ε) in terms of both the standard DNA alphabet and the R-Y alphabet. Table 8 displays the significant (0.01) long common words in three of four or in four of four of the sequences.

The longest conserved oligonucleotides common to all four human globin genes of chromosome 11 (β,δ,γ,ε) are 20 and 19 bp in perfect alignment, starting, 181 5' in E2 (i.e., the 181st bp from the 5' end of exon 2) and 202 5' in E2, respectively. These may be concatenated to produce a 40-bp sequence with a single mismatch between the (β,δ) and (γ,ε) pairs of genes. This matching region expands to the longest word identity (58 bp) between β and δ covering the second exon 3' splice junction (overlapping the second intron by 7 bp) and to a 48-bp block identity between γ and ε (overlapping the second intron by 6 bp). The other three significant word identities common to the four genes (lengths 11,

Table 7
COMMON 4-WORD COUNT
OCCURRENCE DISTRIBUTION
IN THE CHEMICAL AMINO
ACID ALPHABET WITH
RESPECT TO THE HUMAN,
MOUSE, AND RABBIT
IMMUNOGLOBULIN-κ-C-
DOMAIN

Human Ig-κ-C

		0	1	3	>3
	0	3931	65	0	0
Mouse	1	63	33	1	0
Ig-κ-C	2	2	0	0	1
	>3	0	0	0	0

Human Ig-κ-C

		0	1	3	>3
	0	3929	77	0	0
Rabbit	1	64	19	0	0
Ig-κ-C	2	3	1	0	0
	>3	0	1	1	1

Mouse Ig-κ-C

		0	1	3	>3
	0	3923	81	2	0
Rabbit	1	71	12	0	0
Ig-κ-C	2	1	3	0	0
	>3	1	1	1	1

Note: The (i,j) entries of the first subtable give the counts of the 4-words occurring i times in the mouse sequence and j times in the human sequence.

10, and 11 bp) retain perfect alignment and are located, respectively, at 19 bp 5′ into E2, 74 bp 5′ into E2, and 97 bp 5′ into E2.

Most three-sequence significant word identities are extensions of the four-sequence significant word identities. For example, the longest distinct common oligonucleotide of the β-δ-γ genes extends to 20 bp the 11-bp identity at 19 bp 5′ into E2. The longest distinct β-δ-ε word identity extends to 29 bp, the 20 bp identities at 181 5′ in E2. The longest δ-γ-ε extends to 17 bp, the 11 bp at 97 bp 5′ into E2. The combination, β-γ-ε, shows a significant 12 bp common oligonucleotide starting 4 bp before E3, the longest three-sequence identity covering the 5′ E3 splice junction.

In the cases of DNA conservation across all 4 genes (segments of lengths 11, 10, 11, and 40 specifying a total of 24 codons), these segments code for 8 of the 18 amino acids in contact with the heme. They also code for 7 of the 12 amino acids engaged in those contacts between α and β globins that are involved in the change of conformation between the oxygenated and deoxygenated states. These two classes of amino acid contacts in globins

Table 8
SIGNIFICANT COMMON WORDS IN FOUR β-LIKE HUMAN GENES[a]

Base sequence	Genes β δ γ ε	{R,Y} sequence	Base sequence
42 to 53 5' in E1	X X X	42 to 65 5' in E1	CCT GTG GGG CAA
17 to 27 5' in E2	X X X		CTG AGG AGA AG
19 to 38 5' in E2	X X X	10 to 38 5' in E2	TGG ACC CAG AGG TTC TTT GA
19 to 29 5' in E2	X X X X	19 to 38 5' in E2	TGG ACC CAG AG
73 to 83 5' in E2	X X X	66 to 89 5' in E2	ATG GGC AAC CC
74 to 83 5' in E2	X X X X X	74 to 89 5' in E2	TG GGC AAC CC
	X X X	91 to 113 5' in E2	
97 to 113 5' in E2	X X X X	97 to 113 5' in E2	CAT GGC AAG AAG GTG CT
97 to 107 5' in E2	X X X X X		CAT GGC AAG AA
143 to 156 5' in E2	X X X		TGG ACA ACC TCA AG
151 to 161 5' in E2	X X X	139 to 165 5' in E2	C TCA AGG GCA C
172 to 200 5' in E2	X X X		CTG AGT GAG CTG CAC TGT GAC AAG CTG CA
	X X X	170 to 223 5' in E2[b]	
181 to 200 5' in E2	X X X X X		CTG CAC TGT GAG AAG CTG CA
202 to 220 5' in E2	X X X X X	171 to 231 5' in E2[c]	GTG GAT CCT GAG AAC TTC A
−4 to 8 5' in E3[d]	X X X		ACA GCT CCT GGG
49 to 59 5' in E3	X X X	36 to 59 5' in E3	GAA TTC ACC CC
38 to 59 5' in E3	X X X X	38 to 59 5' in E3	
65 to 76 5' in E3	X X X	105 to 130 5' in E3	TGC AGG CTG CCT
	X X X		

[a] Significant ($p = 0.01$) common words are given for 3 of 4 and 4 of 4 sequences. Results are given for two alphabets: base = {T,C,A,G} and {R,Y}, R = {A,G}, Y = {T,C}. For these alphabets (and these sequences) the $p = 0.01$ significant lengths are respectively, 9 and 17 for 4 of 4 and 11 and 21 for 3 of 4. Common words are located relative to the 5' end of the nearest exon. For example, 42 to 53 5' in E1 means the cited common word occupies positions 42 to 53 of exon 1, placing the 5' base of the exon at position 1.

[b] Extends 11 bp into following intron 2.

[c] Extends 9 bp into following intron 2.

[d] Extends 4 bp into preceding intron 2.

generally comprise the most highly conserved amino acids in globins across several species (data not shown). These facts support the suggestion that tertiary and quartenary structures and possibly preferential codon usage in these regions are important.

The cumulative significant DNA word identities of β with δ is 419, mostly in the coding region but with some segments in the 5' flank and the first intron. A pairwise word identity is significant, provided it exceeds 14 bp. This includes a 43-bp word identity perfectly aligned in the first intron 57 bp 3' to E1. The pronounced similarity of β and δ is attributed to gene conversion events of the region from the first through the second exon.[35] However, the significant word identities traverse all coding domains including all the splice boundaries. The extent of the cumulative pairwise conserved segments among the four genes is consistent with their order in the chromosome and the distances separating them.

When the α and β human globin families (α,ζ,ψ_α; β, δ, γ, ε) DNA sequences are compared, the length of the significant common word is 7 bp for 7/7 or 6/7. No 7/7 is observed in reasonable alignment. The heptamer TGCTGGT occurs in 6/7, at 17 5' in E2 for α, ζ, ψ_α, and at 14 5' in E2 for β, δ, γ. In ε, this location is occupied by TGATGGT with one mismatch (underlined) that changes leucine into methionine, both very hydrophobic amino acids. The heptamer TGGACCC occurs in 7/7 but in different locations for the α and β families: at 185, 165, and 185 5' in E2 for α, ψ_α, and ζ, respectively, of the α family and at 19 5' in E2 for the β family. This supports the proposition that the α- and β-globin genes are ancient and have complementary roles in hemoglobin function.

The human β-,δ-,γ-, and ε-globin gene regions with respect to the R-Y alphabet reveal a remarkable extent of similarity. DNA (R-Y) preservation around the splice junctions plus the 5' and 3' ends of the genes are emphasized. The longest R-Y word identity common to all four sequences is 61 bp starting at 171 bp 5' in E2, and extending 9 bp into the following intron. This segment is embedded in a 64-bp R-Y word identity of δ,ε, and γ, that is in turn embedded in a 77-bp identity between δ and γ extending 21 bp beyond the splice junction. The sequences β and δ contain a 76-bp R-Y word identity starting 19 bp 5' to exon 2.

The extent of R-Y word identities both in coding and noncoding regions suggests that DNA mutations tolerate transitions more than transversions. Since synonymous codon replacements for the degeneracy-two amino acids must be transitions, coding regions subject to functional constraints are expected to show a bias toward transitions. Furthermore, transitions conserve the size of the nucleotides.

We also investigated the nature of the identities in the two-letter S-W alphabet. Excluding long stretches of exact DNA identities, no other significant S-W identity blocks were observed. The absence of significant S-W block identities both in coding and noncoding regions suggests that exact DNA hydrogen bonding configuration plays a relatively minor role in control or function at any level.

3. Conditional Similarity Structures

a. Repeat Occurrences Conditioned on Clustering

Analogous to Part A.4, we may define $f(\upsilon_1,\upsilon_2, \ldots ,\upsilon_s|d)$ to be the number of clustered (intervening distance between neighbors ≤ d) k-words having the cluster size υ_i for sequence S_i, respectively; see Reference 36 for applications.

b. Repeat Occurrences Conditioned on Alignment.

Given a distinguished location $\ell_i{}^*$ in the sequence S_i, 1≤i≤s, we formalize the notion of an aligned k-word which in S_i occurs at location ℓ_i. A k-word w is said to be in an exact alignment occurrence if its location ℓ_i in S_i satisfies

$$\ell_i - \ell_i^* = \ell_j - \ell_j^* \quad \text{for all} \quad 1 \leq i, j \leq s$$

Thus, these instances of w are all in alignment with respect to the distinguished locations ℓ^*. An r out of s consensus would satisfy the requirements for at least r of the s sequences.

An approximate alignment occurrence with window d refers to a common k-word such that $|(\ell_i - \ell_i^*) - (\ell_j - \ell_j^*)| \leq d$ for all $1 \leq i, j \leq s$. Thus these instances of w are within d of being in exact alignment.

C. Word Relationships

The example of dyad symmetries (inverted complements) points up a further generalization of the repeat occurrence distribution to allow for related words. Let Δ be a one-to-one mapping of the alphabet A to itself. For instance, DNA base pairings possess a complementarity association on the four-letter alphabet {A,C,G,T} leading to the special mapping $\{\Delta^c: A \rightarrow T, T \rightarrow A, G \rightarrow C, G \rightarrow G\}$. Let $\pi = \{\pi_k\}$ be a family of permutations such that π_k rearranges the set of letters in a k-word. For example, for each given k, we designate $\pi_k^{(1)}$ as the inversion permutation, moving the ith letter to the $k + 1 - i^{th}$ position, e.g., $\pi_8^1(ATGCCGCT) = TCGCCGTA$. A relationship R of words is defined by combining a mapping Δ and a set of permutation $\{\pi_k\}$ operations. In particular, the composed mapping of Δ^c and $\pi^{(1)}$ defines the dyad relationship D, independent of the order of application of Δ^c and $\pi^{(1)}$. The two 5-words ATTCG and CGAAT, D(ATTCG) = CGAAT, are in dyad symmetry relation. A word is called a self-dyad (abbreviated self-D or palindrome) if it is invariant under the mapping D.

Other possible relationships among DNA words can involve simple inversion (i.e., applying only $\pi_k^{(1)}$ or word inversions. A speculative role of the existence of close inverted words is that they can furnish recognition sites for a DNA-interacting protein dimer whose individual peptides are oppositely oriented such that the separate units most effectively bind to inverted words.

For amino acid sequences represented in the charge alphabet (see Table 4), we define the mapping $\Delta^*: \{+ \rightarrow -, - \rightarrow +, 0 \leftrightarrow 0\}$. The composed mapping of Δ^* and $\pi^{(1)}$, called the charge complement relationship, inverts the order of the residues with subsequent complementation of their charge. Thus the 7-word "$0 + 0 - 0 0 0 -$" is in charge complementary relationship to the word "$+ 0 0 0 + 0 - 0$". Identifying such charge complementary words may help discern specific regions in a polypeptide where paired β-sheets are likely to form. The charge complementarity relationship specifically identifies antiparallel segments that exhibit aligned electrically attractive side chains. Alternatively, the complementary mapping Δ^* alone may identify β-sheets in parallel pairings.

1. Count Distribution of Occurrences of R-Related Pairs

The occurrence distribution of a word relationship within a single sequence is encompassed in the two-dimensional distribution $g_{R,k}(\upsilon,\mu)$, which enumerates for each length k the numbers of k-word pairs (w, w*) in relation R where w occurs υ times and its R-word, w*, occurs μ times in S. Table 9 presents as an example the bivariate distribution $g_{D,8}(\cdot,\cdot)$ of dyad symmetry pairs of length 8 for SV-40, polyoma, HPV, and BPV (human and bovine papilloma viruses). The count distributions, $g_{D,8}$ for polyoma and SV-40, display the same differences observed for the repeat occurrence distributions of these two viruses. Polyoma shows a reduced number of D-related 8-words compared to SV-40.

Comparison to the $g_{D,8}$ permutation ranges (Table 9) indicates that for both viruses $g_{D,8}(1,1)$ and $g_{d,8}(1,2)$ of the original sequences exceeds the maximum from the shuffled sets. This excess is evident for all $g_{d,8}(i,j)$, i = 1, . . . ,3, j = 1, . . . ,6 in SV-40.[2,3] The HPV and BPV genome adjusted for genome size is comparable to SV-40 in counts of dyad symmetry combinations.

2. Long R-Pairs

Suppose R is defined for all lengths. This is clearly the case for the dyad symmetry

Table 9
COUNT OCCURRENCE DISTRIBUTION OF $g_{D,8}$ FOR SV-40, POLYOMA, HPV, AND BPV COMPARED WITH $g_{D,8}$ FOR CORRESPONDING PERMUTED SEQUENCES[a]

SV40

	1	2	3	4	5	6
1	276 (195,260)	68 (0,25)	9 (0,3)	3	0	1
2		15 (0,4)	9 (0,1)	1	0	0
3			0 (0,0)	0	0	0

Polyoma

	1	2	3
1	248 (192,229)	36 (0,16)	0 (0,3)
2		2 (0,2)	0 (0,0)
3			0 (0,0)

HPV

	1	2	3	4
1	478 (341,407)	114 (40,92)	11 (0,7)	1 (0,2)
2		12 (0,6)	1 (0,1)	0 (0,0)
3			2 (0,0)	0 (0,0)

BPV

	1	2	3	4	11
1	486 (327,418)	115 (43,101)	10 (0,8)	0 (0,1)	0
2		17 (0,8)	2 (0,1)	0 (0,0)	1
3			3 (0,0)	0 (0,0)	0

[a] The range of counts for 30 permutations are shown in parentheses for each (i,j).

relation. For a sequence S, we define K^S_R as the length of the longest word w appearing at least once in S with the property that $R(w) = w^*$ also occurs. We can similarly ascertain $K^S_R(v^*, \mu^*)$ as the longest R-pair with w occurring at least v^* times and its R-related word $R(w) = w^*$ occurring at least μ^* times.

The asymptotic distributional properties of K^S_D are available (see Section IV.F). This knowledge can be used to assess statistical significance of long dyad pairs.

3. Conditional R-Relationship Structures

As is the case with repeat patterns, functionals of R-related words can be examined under various conditions. Of particular interest are *close* D-related words (i.e., close dyad symmetry pairs). Other conditions on R-related words can emphasize DNA content. Dyad symmetry pairs containing a preponderance of G + C nucleotides are known to make more stable stem-loop structures. The possible importance of such close dyad structures in DNA-protein interaction and enhancer activity are discussed in Reference 36.

4. Multiple Sequence R-Related Occurrence Distributions

Consider s letter sequences $\{S_1, S_2 \ldots, S_s\}$ and r word relations $R_1, R_2, \ldots, R_r$ each determined by mapping Δ_i among the alphabet letters and a family of permutations π^i applied to the positions of each k-word. Let the relations divide into groups

$$\{R_1, R_2, \ldots, R_{\alpha 1}\}\{R_{\alpha_1 + 1}, \ldots, R_{\alpha 2}\}, \ldots, \{R_{\alpha_{s-1}+1}, \ldots, R_{\alpha_s}\}$$

where $\{R_{\alpha_{i-1}+1}, \ldots, R_{\alpha_i}\}$ are relevant to sequence S_i. Here $\Sigma_{i=1}^s \alpha_i = r$. Some of the α_i may be zero and some of the R_i may invoke identity mappings. We define $f_k(\upsilon_1, \upsilon_2, \ldots \upsilon_r | R_1, \ldots, R_r)$ as the number of k-words w such that there exist υ_i, words R_i-related to w in sequence S_i. In terms of the distribution we can tabulate words and their R-related words of high frequency occurrence, the maximal length of a word fulfilling all the relations $\{R_1, \ldots, R_r\}$ and other statistics. For applications of this concept, see Reference 3.

5. Consensus Patterns Between and Among Sequences

A useful generalization of the notion of consensus words and word relationships is the concept of a consensus pattern. Instead of specifying that a single k-word be repeated within a window d relative to a distinguished alignment of the sequences $S_1, \ldots, S_s$, we suggest two extensions.

First, consider a relation R_i (or a set of relations) associated with the sequence S_i. In this context a consensus pattern involves the occurrence of a set of R_i-related words separated within a window d. A consensus pattern might accommodate limited variation within a category (for example, purine-rich words) or different word relations between sequences in alignment. When each R_i signifies a close dyad symmetry pair, then the consensus pattern identifies close dyad symmetry pairs of generally different stem content in approximate alignment with respect to special positions for each sequence.

6. Mismatches, Inexact Repeats, and Inexact Consensus Sequences

By allowing one, two, or any constant number of mismatches within a repeated word, it may be possible to detect nearly conserved biological sequences. The extension to inexact repeat occurrence distributions within a sequence or between multiple sequences is straightforward (Section IV.E).

Table 10 shows, for the hepatitis B virus of human (3182 bp) and ground squirrel (3311 bp), significant matching segments allowing errors. The 225 bp sequence displayed lies near the middle of a long open reading frame (ORF) that occupies bases 1050 to 2345 in squirrel, and is in turn embedded in a much longer ORF of different phase that occupies bases 380 to 3139. Matching segments in this case are defined as aggregates of exactly matching words of length at least 5, interrupted in one or both aggregates by blocks of contiguous bases, of lengths not greater than 3, that are not exactly matched. Such blocks may be caused by substitutions, insertions, or deletions. The numbers of total exact matches required for $p \leq 0.01$ significance for the given sequences are 14, 17, 20, 22, 25, 27 for 0, 1, 2, 3, 4, 5 interrupting nonmatch blocks, respectively, based on Section IV.E.

Table 10

SIGNIFICANT MATCHES, EXACT AND WITH ERRORS, OF HUMAN AND GROUND SQUIRREL HEPATITIS B VIRUS[a]

```
1649 GAT TGG GGA CCC TGc gct gaa cat gga gaa cat caC ATC AGG ATT CCT AGG ACc cct tct cgt gtt aca ggc ggg
     GAT TGG GGA CCC TGt act ttc gac gga gat gtc aCC ATC AGG TCT CCT AGG ACt cct cgt cgc att aca ggt ggt

1723 gtt TTT CTT GTT GAC AAG AAT ACC GCA GAG TCT AGA CTC GTG GAC TTC TCT CAA TTT TCT AGG
     ata TTT CTT GTG GAC AAA AAT CCT TCA GAG TCT AGA CTG GTG GAC TTC TCT CAG TTT TCC AGG
     GGG gac tac cgt tct gca AAA TTC GCA GTc ccc aac ctc caa tca ctc aCC AAC CTC TTG TCC AAC

1798 GGG GGG cat tcc cga gtg cac TGG CCA AAA TTT GCA GTt cca aac ctg caa aca ctt gCC AAC CTC TTG TCC ACC AAC 1873
```

[a] Significantly matched bases without or with errors are in upper case; other bases are in lower case. Nonmatched bases are underlined.

The tabulated sequence begins with a significant exact word match of length 14 bp at squirrel positions 1649 to 1662 and has another such 14 bp exact match near the end at positions 1854 to 1867 that extends to a significant segment of 19 exact matches with one internal mismatch from 1848 to 1873. There is another significant exact match of length 17 bp at 1772 to 1788 that extends from 1727 to 1801 to a significant segment of 66 exact matches with 7 mismatch interruptions. There are nearly significant segments, not extensions of significant exact matches, of 16 exact matches and an internal block of 2 nonmatches from 1684 to 1701, and of 16 exact matches and 1 internal nonmatch from 1817 to 1833. All of the cited subsequences are upper case in Table 10 with mismatches underlined.

There are two significant matching sequences in all three of the viruses of human, ground squirrel, and duck (data not shown). One is an exact match of length 12 at 2245 to 2256 in the squirrel virus which extends in human and squirrel to 2221 to 2257 with 33 exact matches interrupted by two blocks of 1 and 3 nonmatches. The other consists of 21 exact matches interrupted by two blocks of 1 and 2 nonmatches at 1764 to 1788, thus lying within the long 75 base significant sequences shown in Table 10. A more detailed analysis of these hepatitis B virus sequences was published elsewhere.[37]

7. Periodic Word Structures

Another level of generality may be introduced by allowing variant forms of k-words. Where previously a k-word was formed by k consecutive letters, we might substitute letters chosen periodically or by some other rule. Such notions might be germane in amino acid comparison bearing on tertiary protein structure and protein-protein interactions.

D. Extended Concept of Word Relationship

It is useful to incorporate the concept of word relations into a more general framework. A binary relation $R(.,.)$ between two words is defined by a set A of ordered pairs $(\mathbf{a},\mathbf{b})$ of words for which the relation is said to hold. Words $\mathbf{a},\mathbf{b}$ are then called R-related. The relation does not hold or is violated for the rest of pairs, i.e.,

$$R(\mathbf{a},\mathbf{b}) = \begin{cases} 1 & \text{for } (\mathbf{a},\mathbf{b}) \in A \\ 0 & \text{for } (\mathbf{a},\mathbf{b}) \notin A \end{cases}$$

$A \subset \mathfrak{L}^* \times \mathfrak{L}^*$, where $\mathfrak{L}^*$ denotes the set of all k-words from $\mathfrak{L}$. Thus the identity relation R = Id is valid only when strings match perfectly (i.e., $Id(\mathbf{a},\mathbf{b}) = 1$ signifies $\mathbf{a} = \mathbf{b}$). Matching with at most e aligned mismatches, corresponds to the relation

$$R(\mathbf{a},\mathbf{b}) = 1 \quad \text{if and only if} \quad \mathbf{a} = (a_1, \ldots, a_k),$$

$$\mathbf{b} = (b_1, \ldots, b_k) \text{ for some length k,}$$

have

$$a_i = b_i \text{ for at least } k - e \text{ indexes}$$

Matching allowing insertions, deletions and a percentage of errors is also encompassed in this formulation. The dyad symmetry relation D = Dyd between two strings again constitutes a bijective (1-1) relation, such that for any word $\mathbf{a}$ there is exactly one dyad word $\mathbf{b}$ for which $Dyd(\mathbf{a},\mathbf{b})$ is true.

Further bijective relations include the inverse word relationship for words of length

$$Rev(\mathbf{a},\mathbf{b}) = 1 \quad \text{if and only if} \quad \mathbf{b} = (a_n, a_{n-j}, \ldots, a_1)$$

and a relabeling relationship

$$\text{Sym}(\mathbf{a},\mathbf{b}) = 1 \text{ if and only if } \mathbf{b} = (\overline{a_1},\overline{a_2}, ..., \overline{a_n})$$

induced by a 1:1 mapping $\mathbf{a} \to \overline{\mathbf{a}}$ of the letters in $\mathfrak{L}$. Many of these relations are accessible to probabalistic analyses with determination of corresponding asymptotic statistical distributions (see Section IV.F).

Nonbijective relations allow more scope between related words. In this context a single word is related to many words. Relations based on patterns of aligned mismatches are examples of nonbijective relations. Some cases of probability formulas for their occurrence are given by Karlin and Ost.[11,12] Generally, the calculations are prohibitive.

Another simple type of nonbijective relation is determined by coalescing different letters as with amino acid classifications. In this purview, two letters belonging to the same class are called equivalent. This elementary relationship of letters naturally extends to the word relation

$$R(\mathbf{a},\mathbf{b}) = 1 \text{ if and only if } a_i \, b_i \text{ belong to the same letter grouping } i = 1, ..., k$$

In the 61 letter codon alphabet two triplets of nucleotides are deemed equivalent if they translate to the same amino acid. Then the associated oligonucleotide identity will identify strings of codons yielding the same peptide. Observe that the sequence based on groups of states of a Markov chain is in general no longer a Markov sequence of any finite order. Although this complicates the theoretical development, the desired formulas are accessible.[11,12]

IV. DISTRIBUTIONAL PROPERTIES OF SIZES AND COUNTS OF LONG COMMON WORDS AND PATTERNS BETWEEN AND WITHIN SEQUENCES FOR RANDOM SEQUENCE MODELS

In this section we present a number of typical asymptotic formulas pertaining to the length of the longest exact word match between sequences and also with a prescribed pattern of errors, the length of the longest r-fold repeat in a single sequence, distributional properties on the extent of long runs of certain letter types, Poisson limit laws for the counts of moderate length repeat words, and assessments of significance for certain word relationships among random sequences.

A. Maximal Common Words, Two Sequences
1. Independence Model
Consider two independent letter sequences, the first sequence of length N_1 having m possible letters sampled independently with probabilities $p_1, ..., p_m$, the second sequence of length N_2 having letters sampled independently with probabilities, $q_1, ... q_m$. Provided the probability laws $\{p_i\}$ and $\{q_i\}$ are not substantially different (a sufficient condition to serve our purposes is given in Equation 6, see p. 151) the length K of the longest word shared by both sequences is of the order $\log(N_1N_2)/(-\log \lambda)$ where the parameter

$$\lambda = \sum_{i=1}^{m} p_i q_i$$

reflects the probability of a local match.

The asymptotic distribution of K is

$$\Pr\left\{ K \geq \frac{\log(N_1 N_2)}{-\log \lambda} + z \right\} - [1 - \exp(-(1 - \lambda)\lambda^{z + \rho(n,z)}\gamma)] \to 0 \qquad (1)$$

as N_1 and $N_2 \to \infty$ at about the same rate and $\rho(N,z)$, $0 \leq \rho(N,z) < 1$, is defined such that $\log(N_1 N_2)/(-\log \lambda) + z - \rho(N,z)$ is an integer. γ is 1 in the independence, but not in the Markoff model. Equation 1 affords the estimate of the probability that there exists a word match between the two sequences exceeding length $\log(N_1 N_2)/(-\log \lambda) + z$ being at most

$$1 - \exp\{-(1 - \lambda)\lambda^z\} \qquad (2)$$

In practice, we determine z so that this quantity is 0.01. For example if fractions of A, T, C and G are $1/4$ then $\lambda = 0.25$ and the z of Equation 2 yielding 0.01 is 3.11. Therefore, when $N_1 = N_2 = 400$, the criterion length is 11.75 and since K is an integer, $K \geq 12$ gives a significant word match. Quadrupling the lengths to N_1 and $N_2 = 1600$ increases the criterion length to 14. For the asymmetric frequencies 1/5, 1/5, 1/5, 2/5 and $N_1 = N_2 = 400$ the criterion length is $K \geq 12.77$, i.e., $K \geq 13$.

Asymptotic formulas for the first two moments of K up to an additive constant at most $1/2$ are

$$\text{Expected length of K} \approx \frac{\log(N_1 N_2)}{-\log \lambda} + \frac{0.5772 + \log(1 - \lambda)\lambda + \log \gamma}{-\log \lambda} + 0.5$$

$$\text{Variance of K} \approx \frac{\pi^2/6}{(-\log \lambda)^2} \qquad (3)$$

For the cited example the expected length of K is about 8.35 with standard deviation about 0.93. Notice that the variance is asymptotically independent of the lengths N_1 and N_2

2. Markov Sequence Models

A standard based on a random model that accommodates first order neighbor dependencies is constructed as follows. In the vth sequence a letter sequence of the vth process is governed by the transition probability matrix $\|p_{ij}^{(v)}\|$. More complex random models would take account of higher order Markov or more long-range dependencies.[10-12]

The formulas corresponding to Equation 1 for Markov dependent sequence models are available. We illustrate with the case of two Markov letter sequences governed by the transition probability matrices $P = \|p_{ij}\|$ and $Q = \|q_{ij}\|$, respectively. Provided the matrices P and Q are not substantially disparate (see Equation 7) Equations 1 and 2 apply where λ is replaced by the spectral radius ρ (largest positive eigenvalue)

$$\lambda = \rho(P \cdot Q) \text{ of the Schur product matrix } P \cdot Q = \|p_{ij}q_{ij}\| \qquad (4)$$

The parameter γ in Equation 1 is calculated from the principal eigenvectors of $P \cdot Q$, as follows

$$\gamma = \left(\sum_{i=1}^{m} \pi_i^{(P)} \pi_i^{(Q)} \varphi_i\right)\left(\sum_{i=1}^{m} \psi_i\right) \Big/ \lambda \qquad (5)$$

where π^P is the stationary frequency vector of P, i.e., the coordinates of π^P are determined as the solution of the linear system of equations

$$\pi_j^{(P)} = \sum_{i=1}^{m} \pi_i^{(P)} p_{ij}, \quad j = 1, \ldots, m, \quad \sum_{i=1}^{m} \pi_i^{(P)} = 1$$

and similarly

$$\pi_j^{(Q)} = \sum_{i=1}^{m} \pi_i^{(Q)} q_{ij}, \quad j = 1, \ldots, m, \quad \sum_{i=1}^{m} \pi_i^{(Q)} = 1$$

ϕ and ψ are right and left principal eigenvectors of $P \cdot Q$ associated with the eigenvalue λ normalized such that

$$\sum_{i=1}^{m} \phi_i \psi_i = 1$$

A caveat that the p_i and q_i be not too different was indicated concerning the validity of Equation 1. Arratia and Waterman[13] have shown that the order of magnitude log $N_1 N_2 /$ $(-\log\lambda)$ is not correct for the independence model when the sequences are generated by strongly deviant probability laws. However, the formula can be applied provided the sequences being compared come from probability laws that do not differ strongly.

For the independence model, a sufficient condition for the applicability of Equation 2 is the fulfillment of the inequality

$$\max_{1 \leq i \leq m} \{p_i, q_i\} < \sqrt{\sum_{i=1}^{m} p_i q_i} = \sqrt{\lambda} \qquad (6)$$

If all $p_i = q_i$, the above condition is always satisfied. If all $p_i = 1/m$, then the condition becomes

$$\max_i q_i < \sqrt{\frac{1}{m}}$$

Thus, for DNA sequences, if one sequence has about equal base frequencies, then Equation 6 is violated only if one of the q_i is greater than $1/2$ which has never been encountered for actual genomic sequences. The condition (Equation 6) is practically always verified when comparing similar genes between species in any alphabet.

In the case of Markov random models, a sufficient condition corresponding to Equation 6 comprises the inequalities

$$\lim_{r \to \infty} \rho(P^{[r]})^{1/r} < \sqrt{\lambda}$$

$$\lim_{r \to \infty} \rho(Q^{[r]})^{1/r} < \sqrt{\lambda} \qquad (7)$$

where $P^{[r]} = \|(p_{ij})^r\|$ is the rth Schur power matrix and similarly for $Q^{[r]}$, see Reference 11 for mathematical proofs.

B. Maximal Common Word, Multiple Random Sequences

For comparisons of multiple, random sequences (independence model) S_σ (length N_σ) $\sigma = 1, \ldots, s$ with letter probabilities $[p_i^\sigma]$ the order growth of the length of the longest common word K^* is

$$E^* = \frac{\log(N_1 N_2 \ldots N_s)}{-\log \lambda} \qquad (8)$$

depending on the local match probability parameter

$$\lambda = \sum_{i=1}^{m} \prod_{\sigma=1}^{s} p_i^\sigma$$

The analog of Equation 6 is the condition that

$$\max_{i,\sigma} (p_i^{(\sigma)}) < \lambda^{1/s} \tag{9}$$

for the multiple sequence random model. The asymptotic distribution of K* (compare to Equation 1) is

$$\text{Prob}\{K^* \geqslant E^* + z\} - (1 - \exp\{-(1-\lambda)\lambda^{z+\rho}\}) \to 0 \tag{10}$$

provided all $N_i \to \infty$ at about the same rate.

We illustrate the application of the significance procedures of Section IV to the case of 4 of 4 for the genomic β-globin family sequences. The lengths of β,δ,γ,ε are 2165, 1985, 1648, 3915, respectively, and their fractions of (T,C,A,G) are (0.327, 0.203, 0.261, 0.210), (0.318, 0.198, 0.275, 0.208), (0.264, 0.203, 0.263, 0.270) (0.274, 0.181, 0.307, 0.238). Therefore (see Equation 8) in this case $\lambda = 0.01760$ and E* = 7.662. We now use the criterion derived from Equation 10. Accordingly a common word in all four sequences is statistically significant at the level 0.01 provided its length is at least 9.

C. Maximal Repeats within Sequences, Two Occurrences

Let the fractions of letter A_i be p_i. Then for the independence model, the length of the longest word repeated at least twice in a single sequence, L_2^N has the asymptotic distribution

$$\Pr\left\{L_2 \geqslant \frac{\log\binom{N}{2}}{-\log \lambda_2} + z\right\} - [1 - \exp(-(1-\lambda_2)\lambda_2^{z+\rho(N,z)})] \to 0 \tag{11}$$

as $N \to \infty$ for any real number z where $\rho(N,z)$, $0 \leqslant \rho(N,z) < 1$, is defined such that

$$\frac{\log\binom{N}{2}}{-\log \lambda_2} + z - \rho(N,z) \text{ is an integer.} \quad \text{Here } \lambda_2 = \sum_{j=1}^{m} p_j^2.$$

In practice, we specify $\rho(N,z) = 0$ and z is chosen to make the second term in Equation 11 at most 0.01.

D. Maximal Repeats, r-Fold Occurrences

Given a sequence of N independent random letters with p_i the probability of sampling letter A_i, let L_r denote the length of the longest r-fold repeat (words occurring at least r times in the sequence). Then

$$\Pr\left\{L_r \geqslant \frac{\log\binom{N}{r}}{-\log \lambda} + z\right\} - (1 - \exp\{-(1-\lambda_r)\lambda_r^{z+\rho(N,z)}\gamma_r\}) \to 0 \tag{12}$$

as $N \to \infty$ for any real z where

$$\lambda_r = \sum_{i=1}^{m} p_i^r \tag{12a}$$

Therefore

Pr {There is an r-fold repeat of length at least L} $\leq 1 - \exp\{-(1-\lambda_r)\lambda_r^L\gamma_r\binom{N}{r}\}$ (13)

$\gamma_r = 1$ in the independence model. As an example, consider $N = 400$, each $p_i = 1/4$ for $r = 2, 3,$ and 4. The criteria of Equation 13 give $L = 11.25, 7.47,$ and 6.10, respectively.

In the case of a Markov sequence model with successive letters governed by the transition probability matrix $P = \|p_{ij}\|$ we take $\lambda_r = \rho(P^{(r)}) = $ the spectral radius of the $r - $ th Schur power $P^{(r)} = \|(p_{ij})^r\|$ and determine γ_r paraphrasing Equation 5. Unlike the case of the distribution of K or K* for comparison between sequences, the asymptotic formula for the distribution of L_r entails no restriction on P, the underlying transition probability matrix of the random sequence; compare to Equations 6 and 7.

E. Matching with Errors

The importance of allowing for scattered errors in assessing sequence matches is well recognized in molecular contexts. For example, the SV-40 ($N_1 = 5243$) and polyoma ($N_2 = 5148$) virus genomic sequences contain the following matching segments:

$$\begin{array}{c}
\text{G A T C C G A T C A A C T A G C C T C A A T G T A A C} \\
\text{|}\qquad\qquad\quad\text{| |}\qquad\qquad\text{|} \\
\text{G A T C C G C T C A A C T A G G T T C A A T C T A A C}
\end{array} \qquad (14)$$

with mismatches at the places of vertical bars. Does this convey a statistically significant event? None of the perfectly matching parts of lengths 6, 8, 5, and 4 are long enough to qualify for the 1% significance level on its own. The formula extending Equation 2, allowing for a pattern of dispersed errors within matching segments, is given in Equations 15 and 16.

Consider two independent random letter sequences of lengths N_1 and N_2 generated as independently identically distributed letter sequences governed by the probability laws $[p_i]_1^m$ and $[q_i]_1^m$, respectively. We assume the $[p_i]$ and $[q_i]$ are not too different such that Equation 6 is satisfied. Let $K(n) = (n_1, \ldots, n_e)$ denote the cumulative length of the longest aggregate of matches interrupted by at most n_1 singlet mismatch positions, at most n_2 doublets of mismatches, at most n_3 triplets of mismatches, . . . and at most n_e groups of e-length block mismatches. Then $K(n)$ is of the order of magnitude

$$\frac{\log(N_1N_2) + n^*(\log\log(N_1N_2) - \log(-\log\lambda))}{-\log\lambda} = k_0 \qquad (15)$$

where

$$n^* = \sum_{\mu=1}^{e} n_\mu \qquad (15a)$$

counts the number of mismatch interruptions by clusters. The probability that an extended match of length at least $k = k_0 + z$ allowing mismatches conforming to the pattern $n = (n_1, \ldots n_e)$ can be approximated by

$$\Pr\{K(n) \geq k_0 + z\} \approx 1 - \exp\left[-\frac{(1-\lambda)\lambda^{z+\rho(N,z)}}{n_1! \ldots n_e!}\left(\frac{1-\lambda}{\lambda}\right)^s\right] \qquad (16)$$

where $\rho(N,z)$ is the noninteger part in excess of $k_0 + z$. Here

$$s = \sum_{\mu=1}^{e} \mu n_\mu$$

is the maximal number of mismatches permitted subject to the pattern $\mathbf{n} = (n_1, n_2, \ldots, n_e)$. The parameter

$$\lambda = \sum_{i=1}^{m} p_i q_i$$

as previously is the probability of a local match. Results analogous to Equation 16 for the Markov case are also available.[11,12]

The sequences in Equation 14 include two singlet mismatches ($n_1 = 2$) and one doublet mismatch ($n_2 = 1$). The probability that Equation 14 would happen between random sequences of lengths 5243 and 5148 governed by the probability laws (0.30, 0.21, 0.19, 0.30) and (0.26, 0.24, 0.24, 0.26) is approximately 0.013.

F. Long Dyad Symmetries

The permutation Dy in the DNA alphabet refers to the complementarity relationship Dy(A) = T, Dy(T) = A, Dy(C) = G, Dy(G) = C. For a given independence (or Markov) random sequence of length N, we ask for the distribution of the length of the longest dyad pairing. This variable is denoted by D. We find for its order of magnitude

$$D \sim \frac{\log\binom{N}{2}}{-\log \lambda_D}$$

with parameter $\lambda_D = \sum_{i=i}^{m} p_i p_{Dy^{(i)}}$ for the independence model and λ_D

$$= \rho(P \cdot P_D)$$

for a Markov model with transition probability matrix P. The transition matrix P_D associated with a Markov probability matrix P for dyad symmetry pairings corresponds to the time reverse process of P transformed into dual letters.

The formula by which to assess significance rests on the asymptotic relationship

$$\Pr\{\text{Dyad symmetry of length at least } k\} \approx 1 - \exp\{-(1 - \lambda_D)\lambda_D^k \gamma_D \binom{N}{2}\} \tag{17}$$

Since $\lambda_D \le \lambda_2 = \sum p_i^2$ with generally strict inequality the significant length for a dyad pair is usually less than that for a direct repeat. Again $\gamma_D = 1$ for independently generated letters. For N = 400 and p(T) = 0.15, p(C) = 0.2, p(A) = 0.3, p(G) = 0.35, $\lambda_D = 0.23$ the criterion length of a significant dyad pairing is 10.63.

In the case of a Markov model, the parameter γ_D is defined paraphrasing Equation 5 based on the eigenvectors of $P \cdot P_D$. (See the corresponding theoretical results for a hierachy of word relationships in multiple random sequences.[11,12]).

G. Counts of Long Matching Words

Let Z* denote the number of matching words (each preceded by a mismatch) between two sequences of length exceeding $\log(N_1 N_2)/(-\log \lambda) + z$ where λ is the local match parameter. In the independence random model, Z* has a limiting Poisson distribution of parameter $\lambda^{z+1}(1 - \lambda)$. In the Markov random model the corresponding parameter is $\lambda^{z+1}(1 - \lambda)\gamma$ (γ defined in Equation 5). A measure of similarity can be based on counts of matching words of length $\ge$ the order of the expected longest matching word size. A statistically significant count would be a number in the 0.01 tail of the corresponding Poisson distribution.[12]

For the SV-40 example used above N = 5243, λ = 0.200 and log $\binom{5243}{2}$$/(-\log \lambda)$ = 12.201. So z = -0.201 and $\lambda^{z+1}(1 - \lambda)$ = 0.252, and by the Poisson distribution the probabilities of counts of repeats of length at least 12 equal to 2 or more is 0.0022. Obviously the count of 6 in Table 6 is accordingly highly significant.

H. Long Runs

When is a run of a letter type or of a cyclic pattern significantly long? We describe three results of this kind for the following patterns: a long run of a single letter type, an alternating run, and a run of period 3 suggested by a particular amino acid arrangement. For definiteness, the random sequence under consideration is that of the independence model.

The probabilty of observing a succession (run) of a particular letter of length exceeding log $N/(-\log\lambda)$ + z (N is the sequence length and λ is the probability of sampling the prescribed letter) is bounded between

$$P_+ = 1 - \exp\{-(1 - \lambda)\lambda^z\} \quad \text{and} \quad P_- = 1 - \exp\{-(1 - \lambda)\lambda^{z+1}\} \quad (18)$$

For the former example N = 400, p_i = 1/4, log $N/(-\log\lambda)$ = 4.322. For $1 - \exp[-(1-\lambda)\lambda^z]$ = 0.01, z = 3.111 as in Equation 1 and L = 7.433. This suggests L = 8. Thus, a run of the same base of length $\geqslant 8$ is significant at confidence level <0.005.

In the context of independent identically distributed Bernoulli trials (probability λ of success) Erdös and Révész[38] provide strong laws and theorems of iterated logarithm type for the growth of the longest success run when λ = 1/2 allowing up to k (fixed) interspersed failure events. Guibas and Odlyzko[39] extend these results to include more general repetitive patterns of successes and failures. These authors concentrated on sequences of i.i.d. (independent, identically distributed) two-valued variables. The papers by Zubkov and Mikhailov[40] and by Samarova[41] are also relevant. The investigation of these problems for Markov or more general stationary generated letter sequences is discussed in Karlin and Ost.[11,12]

Consider a sequence composed from three letters A, B, and C occurring with probabilities α, β, and γ, respectively, ($\alpha + \beta + \gamma = 1$). Next, we assess the length of the longest run of either of the alternating forms {ABAB . . . } or {BABA . . . } in a sequence of length N. In this situation set $\lambda = \sqrt{\alpha\beta}$. Then an alternating run as prescribed of length exceeding log $N/(-\log \lambda)$ + z has asymptotic probability bounded between the distribution functions

$$1 - \exp\{-\sqrt{\alpha\beta}(2 - \alpha - \beta)\lambda^z\} \quad \text{and} \quad 1 - \exp\left\{-\left(\frac{\alpha + \beta - 2\alpha\beta}{\sqrt{\alpha\beta}}\right)\lambda^z\right\} \quad (19)$$

As another illustration of a periodic letter pattern for an i.i.d. sequence of two letters A and B generated with probabilities α and β, respectively, ($\alpha + \beta = 1$) we consider the longest run of the unit BAA or ABA or AAB. In this case set $\lambda = (\alpha^2\beta)^{1/3}$ and let

$$\rho_+ = \frac{(1 - \beta\alpha^2)\alpha\beta(\alpha^2 + 2\beta^2)}{(\alpha^3 + \beta\alpha + \beta)} \quad \text{and} \quad \rho_- = \frac{(1 - \beta\alpha^2)\alpha^2\beta(\alpha^2 + \beta)}{(\alpha^3 + \beta\alpha + \beta)\lambda^2}$$

then a periodic run of the unit BAA of length exceeding $\dfrac{\log N}{-\log \lambda}$ + z has asymptotic probability in the range

$$1 - \exp\{-\rho_+\lambda^z\} \quad \text{and} \quad 1 - \exp\{-\rho_-\lambda^z\} \quad (20)$$

Formulas are also available allowing for Markov dependence and some errors within the run.[42]

Examples of cases in the three paragraphs above occur in the Epstein-Barr virus (EBV) genomic sequence of the human herpesvirus family. The entire approximately 172 kbp EBV genome of one strain (B95-8) has been sequenced by Baer et al.[33] Viral proteins found in the nucleus during latent existence include the EBV-encoded antigens EBNA 1 (BKRF 1, coordinates 107950 to 109872), EBNA 2 (BYRF 1, 48429 to 49964), EBNA 3 (BERF 1, 92646 to 95162) and LYDMA (BNLF 1, encoded on the complementary strand, 169474 to 167001). Autonomous replication of the EBV episomes or maintenance of recombinant plasmids in latently infected cells requires the presence of EBNA 1 protein molecules. The latent genes all show long runs of alternating charged and uncharged amino acids of the form $(+,0)_n$ or $(+,0,0)_n$ or $(0,-,-)_n$, where $+(-)$ designates a positively (negatively) charged amino acid and 0 an uncharged amino acid. We observed in the EBNA 1 gene the iteration $(+,0)_{15}$ and $(0,-,-)_7$, each with a few errors, which are both statistically significant meaning that the probability is ≤ 0.01 of observing a run of the indicated length or longer for the corresponding independence model. The $(+,0)_{15}$ run contains an exact $(arg,gly)_4$ run. The EBNA1 open reading frame contains a long 237 bp sequence exclusively *gly* and *ala* and this has been removed in the following calculations because of its biasing the *gly* concentration. For the remainder of $N = 404$ residues, the fractions *arg* and *gly* are 0.124 and 0.243 so that $\lambda = 0.174$ and $-\log(400)/\log(\lambda) = 3.432$. The observed length of the run is 8, so that $z = 4.568$. Then by (19) the lower bound is 0.0000964 and the upper bound is 0.000598. Thus $(arg, gly)_4$ is significant to <0.001. For a further discussion of these examples, see Blaisdell and Karlin.[43]

ACKNOWLEDGMENTS

This work was supported in part by National Institutes of Health Grants GM10452-22, GM36056-02, and 1RO-1HL-30856 and National Science Foundation Grant MCS892-15131.

REFERENCES

1. **Blaisdell, B. E.,** Markov chain analysis finds a significant influence of neighboring bases on the occurrence of a base in eucaryotic nuclear DNA sequences both protein coding and noncoding, *J. Mol. Evol.,* 21, 278, 1985.
2. **Karlin, S. and Ghandour, G.,** Comparative statistics for DNA and protein sequences: multiple sequence analysis, *Proc. Natl. Acad. Sci. U.S.A.,* 82, 6186, 1985.
3. **Karlin, S.,** Comparative analysis of structural relationships in DNA and protein sequences, in *Evolutionary Processes and Theory,* Karlin, S. and Nevo, E., Eds., Academic Press, Orlando, Fla., 1986, 329.
4. **Zuckerkandl, E. and Pauling, L.,** Evolutionary divergence and convergence in proteins, in *Evolving Genes and Proteins,* Bryson, V. and Vogel, H., Eds., Academic Press, New York, 1965, 97.
5. **Dayhoff, M. O.,** *Atlas of Protein Sequence and Structure,* Vol. 5, Suppl. 3, National Biomedical Research Foundation, Washington, D. C., 1978.
6. **Blaisdell, B. E.,** A measure of the similarity of sets of sequences not requiring sequence alignment, *Proc. Natl. Acad. Sci. U.S.A.,* 83, 5155, 1986.
7. **Stebbins, G. L.,** *Darwin to DNA,* W. H. Freeman, San Francisco, 1982, 124.
8. **Efstradiadis, A., Posakony, J. W., Maniatis, T., Lawn, R. M., O'Connell, C., Spritz, R. A., DeRiel, J. K., Forget, B. G., Weissman, S. M., Slightom, J. L., Blechl, A. E., Smithites, O., Baralle, F. E., Shoulders, C. C., and Proudfoot, N. J.,** The structure and evolution of the human β-globin gene family, *Cell,* 21, 653, 1980.
9. **Olsen, G. J., Pace, N. R., Nuell, M., Kaine, B. P., Gupta, R., and Woese, C. R.,** Sequence of the 16S RNA gene from thermoacidophilic archaebacterium sulfolobus solfataricus and its evolutionary implications, *J. Mol. Evol.,* 22, 301, 1985.

10. **Karlin, S. and Ost, F.,** Maximal segmental match length among random sequences from a finite alphabet, in *Proceedings of the Berkeley Conference in Honor of Jerzy Neyman and Jack Kiefer,* Vol. 1, LeCam, L. M. and Olshen, R. A., Eds., Wadsworth, Belmont, Wash., 1985.

11. **Karlin, S. and Ost, F.,** Maximal length of common words among random letter sequences, *Ann. Prob.,* 16, 535, 1988.

12. **Karlin, S. and Ost, F.,** Counts of long aligned word matches among random letter sequences, *Adv. Appl. Prob.,* 19, 293, 1987.

13. **Arratia, R. and Waterman, M.,** Critical phenomena in sequence matching, *Ann. Prob.,* 13, 1236, 1985.

14. **Arratia, R. and Waterman, M. S.,** An Erdös-Renyi law with shifts, *Adv. Math.,* 55, 13, 1985.

15. **Waterman, M. S.,** General methods of sequence comparison, *Bull. Math. Biol.,* 46, 473, 1984.

16. **Edgington, E. S.,** *Randomization Tests,* Marcel Dekker, New York, 1980.

17. **Pratt, J. W.,** *Concepts of Nonparametric Theory,* Springer-Verlag, New York, 1981.

18. **Karlin, S. and Williams, P. T.,** Permutation methods for the structural exploratory data analysis (SEDA) of familial trait values, *Am. J. Hum. Genet.,* 36, 873, 1984.

19. **Doolittle, R. F.,** Similar amino acid sequences: chance or common ancestry, *Science,* 214, 149, 1981.

20. **Kyte, J. and Doolittle, R. F.,** A simple method for displaying the hydropathic character of a protein, *J. Mol. Biol.,* 157, 105, 1982.

21. **Fitch, W. M.,** An improved method of testing for evolutionary homology, *J. Mol. Biol.,* 16, 9, 1966.

22. **McLachlan, A. D.,** Repeating sequences and gene duplication in proteins, *J. Mol. Biol.,* 64, 417, 1972.

23. **Grantham, R.,** Amino acid difference formula to help explain protein evolution, *Science,* 185, 862, 1974.

24. **Goodman, M. and Moore, G. W.,** Use of Chou-Fasman amino acid conformational parameters to analyze the organization of the genetic code and to construct protein genealogies, *J. Mol. Evol.,* 10, 7, 1977.

25. **Karlin, S. and Ghandour, G.,** Multiple alphabet amino acid sequence comparisons of the immunoglobulin κ-chain constant domain, *Proc. Natl. Acad. Sci. U.S.A.,* 82, 8597, 1985.

26. **Karlin, S. and Ghandour, G.,** The use of multiple alphabets in kappa-gene immunoglobulin DNA sequence comparisons, *EMBO J.,* 4, 1217, 1985.

27. **Karlin, S., Ghandour, G., Foulser, D. E., and Korn, L. J.,** Comparative analysis of human and bovine papilloma viruses, *Mol. Biol. Evol.,* 1, 357, 1984.

28. **Dickerson, R. E. and Geis, I.,** *Hemoglobin Structure, Function, Evolution and Pathology,* Benjamin Cummings, Menlo Park, Calif., 1983.

29. **Mahler, H. R. and Cordes, E. H.,** *Biological Chemistry,* Harper & Row, New York, 1966.

30. **Karlin, S. and Ghandour, G.,** Comparative statistics for DNA and protein sequences: single sequence analysis, *Proc. Natl. Acad. Sci. U.S.A.,* 82, 5800, 1985.

31. **Fitch, W. M. and Atchley, W. R.,** Evolution in inbred strains of mice appears rapid, *Science,* 228, 1169, 1985.

32. **Wu, C. I. and Li, W. H.,** Evidence for higher rates of nucleotide substitution in rodents than in man, *Proc. Natl. Acad. Sci. U.S.A.,* 82, 1741, 1985.

33. **Baer, R., Bankier, A. T., Biggin, M. D., Deininger, P. L., Farrell, P. J., Gibson, T. J., Hatfull, G., Hudson, G. S., Satchwell, S. C., Seguin, C., Tuffnell, P. S. and Barrell, B. G.,** DNA sequence and expression of the B95-8 Epstein-Barr virus genome, *Nature (London),* 310, 207, 1984.

34. **Davison, A. J. and Scott, J. E.,** The complete DNA sequence of Varicella-Zoster virus, *J. Gen. Virol.,* 67, 1759, 1986.

35. **Slightom, J. L., Blechl, A. E., and Smithies, O.,** Human fetal G_γ and A_γ globin genes: complete nucleotide sequences suggest that DNA can be exchanged between these duplicated genes, *Cell,* 21, 627, 1980.

36. **Karlin, S. and Ghandour, G.,** DNA sequence patterns in human, mouse and rabbit immunoglobulin kappa-genes, *J. Mol. Evol.,* 22, 195, 1985.

37. **Karlin, S., Morris, M., Ghandour, G., and Leung, M.-Y.,** Efficient algorithms for molecular sequence analysis, *Proc. Natl. Acad. Sci. U.S.A.,* 85, 841, 1988.

38. **Erdös, P. and Revesz, P.,** On the length of the longest head run, *Colloq. Math. Soc. J. Bolyai,* 16, 219, 1975.

39. **Guibas, L. J. and Odlyzko, A. M.,** Long repetitive patterns in random sequences, *Z. Wahrscheinlichkeitstheorie Verw. Geb.,* 53, 241, 1980.

40. **Zubkov, A. M. and Mikhailov, V. G.,** Repetitions of s-tuples in a sequence of random trials, *Theor. Prob. Appl.,* 24, 269, 1979.

41. **Samarova, S. S.,** On the length of the longest head run for a Markov chain with two states, *Theor. Prob. Appl.,* 26, 498, 1981.

42. **Foulser, D. and Karlin, S.,** Maximal success runs for semi-Markov processes, *Stochastic Proc. Appl.,* 24, 203, 1987.

43. **Blaisdell, B. E. and Karlin, S.,** Distinctive charge configurations in proteins of the Epstein-Barr virus and possible functions, *Proc. Natl. Acad. Sci. U.S.A.,* in press.

Chapter 7

THE USE OF DYNAMIC PROGRAMMING ALGORITHMS IN RNA SECONDARY STRUCTURE PREDICTION

M. Zuker

TABLE OF CONTENTS

I. INTRODUCTION

An RNA (ribonucleic acid) molecule is made up of ribonucleosides linked together in a chain by covalent bonds. Each ribonucleoside, or nucleoside, comprises one of four different bases attached to a common element called a riboside. These bases are either adenine (A), cytosine (C), guanine (G), or uracil (U). The nucleosides are linked one to another by a phosphate backbone and are called nucleotides once the phosphate groups are attached. An RNA molecule is uniquely determined by the sequence of bases along the chain. There is a definite orientation to the molecule. The ith nucleotide has a phosphate group attached to the 3' position on the riboside. This is bonded to a phosphate group attached to the 5' position on the riboside of the next nucleotide. For this reason, we refer to the first nucleotide or base at the 5' end of the molecule and the last nucleotide or base as the 3' end.

The linear structure of RNA just described gives a very incomplete picture of the molecule. In the cell, or in vitro, the molecule is folded up in a complicated way like a ball of string. It is this three-dimensional or tertiary structure which determines the activity of the molecule. There are numerous reasons why researchers wish to determine such structures. To understand how ribosomes function, biochemists study the structure of ribosomal RNA (rRNA). The structure of messenger RNA (mRNA) might give clues about control mechanisms affecting processing and translation. Unfortunately, a precise determination of tertiary structure is only possible using X-ray diffraction methods on crystallized RNA. At best, these data are difficult to analyze and are usually not available at all. Biochemical probes yield structural information, but not nearly enough to determine complete conformations. Many structures which regulate transcription or translation are very short-lived and so direct measurement is impossible. Thus, in the absence of biochemical and other methods, there is a pressing need for mathematical tools to predict RNA structure.

The tertiary structure of an RNA molecule is held together principally by hydrogen bonds which form between pairs of complementary bases. These bonds are called base pairs and can form between G and C and between A and U. A rather weak bond is also possible between G and U. There are also electrostatic forces, solvent effects, and stereochemical constraints at work. The situation is even more complicated when ribosomes or other molecules are bound to the RNA. A natural approach would be to set up a molecular dynamics model of the RNA. At a low resolution, the nucleotides could be represented as hard balls joined to each other by flexible sticks. By assigning energy functions to describe tortional potential energies associated with each stick (the backbone phosphodiester bond) and all pairwise hydrogen bond and electrostatic interactions, a mathematician could formulate a simplified model of the RNA which could be solved by computing the conformation which would minimize the sum of all the energies built into the model. This sort of approach has been tried with protein molecules and has met with little success, except for small peptides. Mathematically, the problem is one of nonlinear optimization by adjusting a large number of continuous variables. Such problems require vast amounts of computer time and usually bog down in suboptimal solutions.

It should come as no surprise, then, that past and present algorithms to predict RNA structure have dealt with an even simpler model. This model looks only at which base pairs form and is called a secondary structure model. The name is appropriate because secondary structures of RNA molecules admit a pleasing two-dimensional representation. Apart from the tertiary structure of yeast phenylalanine transfer RNA,[1] determined using X-ray methods, all published conformational models for RNA have been secondary structures.

This article is devoted to a class of recursive algorithms for predicting RNA secondary structure. They are called dynamic programming algorithms and were first used about 30 years ago by people in operations research. They date back roughly to the days of the first digital computers. This is no coincidence, for without fairly powerful computers, these algorithms are useless. If the energy rules are not too complicated, such algorithms are efficient and unerring in finding minimum energy secondary structures. They can be readily adapted to take into account biochemical data and to predict structures compatible with these data. More recent improvements allow dynamic programming algorithms to predict an assortment of different structures close to the minimum energy. Used in conjunction with biochemical and phylogenetic data, they are a powerful tool in aiding the biochemist to predict RNA secondary structure.

II. FORMULATION OF THE SECONDARY STRUCTURE MODEL

Let us write the sequence of bases in an RNA molecule as $R = r_1, r_2, r_3, \ldots, r_N$ where $r_i = A, C, G$, or U and stands for the ith base from the 5' end. Mathematically, the linear structure of the molecule is represented by a sequence of letters from a four-letter alphabet. The real situation is more complicated, because bases can be chemically modified, and this affects their base-pairing potential. Biochemists simply use more letters or modified letters. For example, C_m refers to a cytosine modified by a methyl group. If $1 \leq i \leq j \leq N$, the notation R_{ij} refers to the subsequence or fragment from the ith nucleotide to the jth inclusive.

The secondary structure of an RNA molecule is defined to be the collection of base pairs which are formed between pairs of complementary bases. In the mathematical model, a secondary structure on R is simply a collection, S, of pairs of integers written as $i \cdot j$. If $i \cdot j$ belongs to S, then r_i and r_j form a base pair, and vice versa. From this point on, we will not differentiate between the base pair which bonds r_i to r_j and the mathematical object $i \cdot j$. It is always assumed that $i < j$. The only restriction imposed initially is derived from the fact that a ribonucleotide can form a base pair with at most one other ribonucleotide. Thus if $i_1 \cdot j_1$ and $i_2 \cdot j_2$ both belong to S, then $i_1 = i_2$ if and only if $j_1 = j_2$. This is called the exclusivity condition. If S is a secondary structure on R, S_{ij} is defined to be the collection of base pairs (possibly empty) belonging to S whose nucleotides lie in the fragment R_{ij}. S_{ij} is a secondary structure on R_{ij} and is called a substructure of S. If r_i is not part of a base pair, then r_i is called single stranded.

What further constraints need to be imposed in the definition of secondary structure? An obvious candidate is the condition that if $i \cdot j$ is a base pair, then r_i and r_j should be complementary bases. In addition, stereochemical facts dictate than an RNA molecule cannot fold back too sharply on itself. Specifically, at least three intervening bases must occur between base-paired ribonucleotides. This is equivalent to saying that if $i \cdot j$ is a base pair, then $j - i > 3$. Adopting these two constraints is a natural way to make the secondary structure model more realistic, but is unnecessary. These constraints complicate the algorithms to be presented later, clouding their essential simplicity. Nevertheless, hypothetical secondary structures which bend back too sharply on themselves or contain base pairs between bases which are not complementary must ultimately be eliminated from consideration. The approach taken here is to assign such secondary structures large destabilizing energies so that they will not be selected by energy minimizing procedures.

Unfortunately, one unnatural constraint must be imposed to enable the use of a dynamic programming algorithm to predict secondary structures. This is the elimination of knots. A secondary structure is said to be knotted if it contains two base pairs $i_1 \cdot j_1$ and $i_2 \cdot j_2$ satisfying $i_1 < i_2 < j_1 < j_2$. In a structure without knots, every base pair $i \cdot j$ divides the secondary structure into two disjoint parts. All base pairs are either between nucleotides in the fragment R_{ij} or between nucleotides in the excluded regions: r_1 to r_{i-1} and r_{j+1} to r_N. This fact is crucial in the construction of recursive algorithms to predict structure, as will be seen later. However, it is known that real secondary structures contain knots. Transfer RNAs (tRNAs), for example, have knotted secondary structures. Sequence analysis of many 5S RNAs have revealed precisely two universal structures which can exist in all of these molecules, and

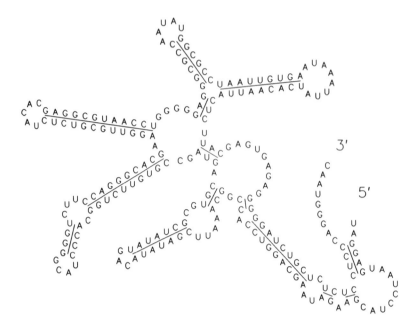

FIGURE 1.   A secondary structure of the last 231 bases from the bacteriophage Qβ. The solid lines are drawn between pairs of hydrogen-bonded bases.

one of them is knotted.[2] The strategy adopted here and by others is to predict unknotted structures and to relegate the prediction of knots to the study of tertiary structure. For example, once a secondary structure has been found, a computer search of single-stranded regions left over can reveal possible tertiary interactions which could result in knots. Purely mathematical considerations are not the only reason for eliminating knots. Once they are allowed, stereochemical considerations must be introduced to determine whether such structures are possible. Furthermore, no data are available on how knots affect the stability of structures. All in all, it seems reasonable to exclude knots. From this point on, a secondary structure will be assumed to be unknotted.

Secondary structures, which are also referred to as foldings of RNA molecules, can always be represented by a two-dimensional picture. The linear chain of bases can be folded back on itself so that base-paired nucleotides are in close proximity. This is illustrated in Figure 1.

III. ENERGY RULES

The two criteria which are used to select a best or a group of best secondary structures are free energy minimization and phylogeny. If the first is used, biochemical data must be available to assign free energies to hypothetical foldings. Use of phylogeny assumes at least two closely related RNA molecules and predicts common or similar foldings for the entire group. When one has a single sequence, energy minimization is the only path to follow. With the phylogenetic approach, energy considerations are a guide to how reasonable the predicted structures are.

There is an old story about a dairy that hired a systems analyst to advise them on how to improve milk production. After 6 months, the analyst walked into the seminar room at the dairy with a pile of graphs and computer printouts. He began his talk with the words: "Gentlemen, assume a perfectly spherical cow." This apocryphal story has a message to those engaged in RNA-folding prediction. If the energy rules are simple enough, an elegant and efficient folding algorithm is possible, but no biochemist is likely to trust it. On the other hand, as the energy rules become more and more complex, dynamic programming algorithms for folding prediction first become more intricate and slower to execute and finally break down altogether. It is natural for a biochemist to want energy assignment to be as realistic as possible, without regard to how difficult folding prediction becomes. However, secondary structure prediction is already a gross simplification of a more complicated three-dimensional process. It seems futile, therefore, to make the energy rules more complicated than this model warrants. Clearly, some sort of compromise is needed. Three basic levels of complexity for energy assignment are discussed here. Others are certainly possible, but these three have been chosen because they encompass all the work that has been done in this area.

The simplest method which has been used is to consider the hydrogen bonds in the secondary structure independently of all the others. A hydrogen bond potential energy is computed for each base pair, and the overall energy is the sum of the individual base pair energies. This can be written as:

$$E(S) = \sum_{i \cdot j \text{ in } S} e\,(i,\,j) \qquad (1)$$

where E is the total energy of the structure and e is the hydrogen bond potential energy for pairs of ribonucleotides. Note that if $e = -1$ when r_i and r_j are complementary and 0 otherwise, then $-E(S)$ simply counts the number of valid base pairs in the structure. In this case, an energy minimizing algorithm will find a structure with a maximum number of base pairs. Energy rules which assign values to individual base pairs and sum them to obtain a total energy can be called base pair dependent. In their earliest work on dynamic programming algorithms for RNA folding, Nussinov et al.[3] used such rules.

Base pair-dependent energy assignment is too crude to take into account biochemical data produced in the last 15 years. The next logical step in complexity is to assign energies to base pairs conditional on neighboring base pairs. This requires a formal definition of a new object. If $i \cdot j$ is a base pair in S, and if $i < h < j$, then h is called accessible from $i \cdot j$ if there is no base pair $k \cdot l$ in S such that $i < k < h < l < j$. The set of bases accessible from $i \cdot j$ is called a loop and is denoted by $L_{i \cdot j}$. The pair $i \cdot j$ is called the closing or exterior base pair of the loop, although it is not contained in the loop. The collection of bases which are not accessible from any base pair are called exterior bases. They form the exterior loop and can be denoted by L_{ext}. Then every secondary structure, S, on a sequence R decomposes R into disjoint loops. This follows from the definition of loop and the assumption that S is unknotted. The number of loops is the number of base pairs plus one for the exterior loop. The definitions given here are similar to those given for k-loops or k-cycles by Sankoff et al.[4] and by Zuker and Sankoff.[5] The reason for this decomposition is that loops rather than base pairs are now the primitive objects for assigning energy. An energy is computed for each loop, and the total energy is assumed to be the sum of these. Equation 1 becomes

$$E(S) = \sum_{i \cdot j \text{ in } S} e(L_{i \cdot j}) + e(L_{ext}) \qquad (2)$$

where e is now a function of loops. In this case, the energy rules can be called loop dependent.

Biochemists were referring to loops long before any abstract mathematical definition was given.[6] Let us define the loop size of a loop as the numer of single-stranded bases it contains. The index of a loop is defined to be the number of base pairs it contains. The no-knot assumption guarantees that if one base of a pair is in a loop, the other must also be in that loop. The base pairs contained in a loop are called the interior base pairs. In the following

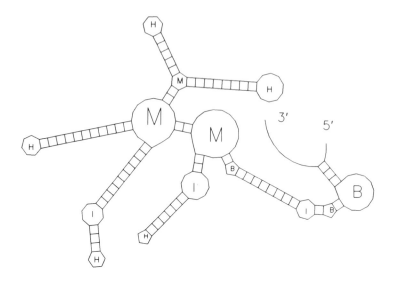

FIGURE 2.   A redrawing of Figure 1 showing only the linear backbone of the RNA molecule and the hydrogen bonds. All destabilizing loops are indicated according to the following code: B — bulge loop; H — hairpin loop; I — interior loop; and M — multiloop. The unmarked areas between consecutive hydrogen bonds are stacked pairs.

definitions, it is assumed that the loops discussed have a closing base pair. Loops of index 0 are called hairpin loops. Loops of index 1 are divided into three categories. If the loop size is 0, then it is called a stacked pair. Letting i·j and k·l denote the exterior and interior base pairs of the loop, it is clear that the loop size is $(k - i - 1) + (j - l - 1)$. If both the summands in brackets are > 0, then the loop is called an interior loop; if only one is >0, it is called a bulge loop. Loops of index 2 or greater are called multiloops. A stacking or helical region is a collection of stacked pairs: $L_{i \cdot j}$, $L_{i+1 \cdot j-1}$, $\ldots$, $L_{i+k-1 \cdot j-k+1}$, where k $\geqq 1$. Is is the stacking regions which stabilize the secondary structure, while the loops destablize it. Figure 2 illustrates the same folding as in Figure 1 redrawn to show only the backbone chain and the hydrogen bonds. All the various types of loops are shown. From this figure, it can be seen that loops correspond to planar regions between base pairs.

The energy rules which are in common use today are derived from melting experiments done on small RNA molecules or oligonucleotides.[7-13] They were summarized by Salser[14] and were modified by Tinoco,[15] although Salser's values are most often used. Each type of stacked pair is given its own negative (stabilizing) free energy, called the stacking energy, including those containing or closed by G-U base pairs. Hairpin loops are given positive (destabilizing) energies which depend only on the size of the loop and the closing base pair. Bulge and interior loops are assigned positive energies which depend upon the size of the loop, the interior base pair, and the exterior base pair. Stacking energies are also added to bulge loops, so that some small bulge loops can actually have a negative free energy. Multiloops are complicated, and there are no experimental data for assigning free energies. Sometimes they are ignored (given 0 energy), but most often they are treated as interior loops. Exterior bases are ignored altogether. Following Papanicolaou et al.,[16] we shall call this set of rules the "biophysical set" or BP set.

The loop destabilizing energies just mentioned are based on experimental data and are therefore arbitrary in some sense. However, apart from the dependence on interior and exterior base pairs, they depend only on loop size. For a given closing base pair and (possible) interior base pair, they increase with loop size. Thermodynamic considerations point to a logarithmic growth of loop-destabilizing energy as a function of loop size. Such computations have already been used by Steger et al.[17] who compute stacking and loop energies for folding at different temperatures. As we shall see, these energy rules are at the threshold of causing serious problems with energy-minimizing dynamic programming algorithms.

One could define a hierarchy of increasingly complex energy rules where energies are assigned to loops conditional on the kth nearest loop(s). We shall simply call all such rules arbitrary. Formally, energy rules which do not take the form in Equation 2 will be called arbitrary. Note that base pair-dependent rules are also loop dependent, since the loop closed by i·j can be given the energy e(i,j) and the exterior loop ignored. The BP set has been modified by Ninio[18] so that the well-known cloverleaf conformation would also be a minimum energy folding for transfer RNAs. This refinement was carried further by Papanicolaou et al.[16] to predict correct foldings for a group of 100 5S RNA sequences. They allow nonstandard base pairs, but their rules are still basically loop dependent. However, some of the special cases add correction energies to stacked pairs conditional on neighboring loops. It is likely that this trend to arbitrary energies will continue as researchers attempt to improve the rules still further. If this happens, then those who use such rules will have to abandon dynamic programming algorithms. Indeed, Gouy et al.[19] criticize the "physically unjustified" assumption that the energies of separate components of an RNA structure are strictly additive. They predict secondary structures by enumerating them.

IV. SOLUTION BY ENUMERATION

The obvious first approach to RNA-folding prediction is to use a computer to evaluate the energy of all possible structures and to choose the best or a group of the best. If this strategy is practical, there is no point trying a more sophisticated method. Unfortunately, the number of secondary structures grows exponentially with the size of the molecule. The first precise estimate of this number was obtained by Waterman[20] who showed that

$$T(N) \sim \sqrt{\frac{15 + 7\sqrt{5}}{8\pi}} \, N^{-3/2} \left(\frac{3 + \sqrt{5}}{2} \right)^{N} \tag{3}$$

where T(N) is the number of foldings on a molecule with N bases. For a modest 5S RNA molecule with 120 bases, this yields about 1.2×10^{47} different foldings! Of course, our definition of secondary structure is very broad, so this formula counts many biochemically invalid structures. If a probabilistic approach is taken and T'(N) is defined to be the expected number of valid structures in a molecule of size N, then it can be shown[5] that $T'(N) > 1.8^{N}$ for large N, where it is assumed that A, C, G, and U all occur randomly with equal likelihood. Thus, one is forced to admit that there will be an astronomical number of foldings to consider in molecules of interest.

Folding algorithms which enumerate structures have been around for some time[21] and are still in use.[19] They begin by compiling a list of all stacking regions and then proceed to piece them together in all possible ways. The total number of base pairs which can occur is the number of i, j pairs satisfying $1 \leq i < j \leq N$ and equals $N(N-1)/2$. If done efficiently, the computer time for constructing the list of regions will be proportional to $N^2/2$. A mathematician would say that the time is $O(N^2)$, that is, of the order N^2. This means that the ratio of the execution time to N^2 is bounded as N becomes large or that execution time grows at a rate that is proportional to N^2 as N grows. The constant factor is irrelevant. The list of regions is shortened by demanding that all regions contain at least k consecutive stacked pairs, where k is at least 2 and is frequently 3 or 4. If there are m regions, they can be sorted in order of increasing stability (energy) in time $O(m \log m)$.[22] Up to this point, there is no problem. However, the number of ways to piece them together to form structures is $O(2^m)$. Even allowing for the fact that the exclusivity and no-knot conditions eliminate many pairs of regions from occurring in the same structure, this number grows exponentially. The elegant tree search algorithm of Gouy et al.[19] is nothing more than an enumeration algorithm which takes into account the incompatibility of certain pairs of regions. It should come as no surprise that their algorithm is currently limited to folding molecules with no more than 200 nucleotides.

V. A DYNAMIC PROGRAMMING ALGORITHM FOR BASE PAIR-DEPENDENT ENERGY RULES

Although base pair-dependent rules are too simple for realistic energy assignment, it is instructive to examine how a dynamic programming algorithm can be used in this case. The method actually comprises two algorithms, called the fill algorithm and the traceback, and was first used by Nussinov et al.[3]

For $1 \leq i \leq j \leq N$, let $W(i,j)$ be the minimum possible energy for a secondary structure on R_{ij}. No secondary structure is possible on a single nucleotide, so $W(i,i)$ can be taken as 0. Now suppose that S_{ij} is a minimum energy structure on R_{ij}, where $i < j$. If j is not base paired, then S_{ij} must also be a minimum energy folding on R_{ij-1}, because any better structure on R_{ij-1} would also be a folding on R_{ij} with lower energy than $E(S_{ij})$. In this case, $W(i,j) = W(i,j-1)$. If j is base paired, then $k \cdot j$ is in S_{ij} for some k between i and $j-1$ inclusive. If $k = i$, then S_{ij} must be a minimum energy folding on $R_{i+1 \, j-1}$ plus the extra base pair $i \cdot j$, so $W(i,j) = W(i+1, j-1) + e(i,j)$. If $k > i$, then the no-knot condition ensures that all base pairs are either between nucleotides in R_{ik-1} or between nucleotides in R_{kj}. Thus, S_{ij} must be the union of a minimum energy folding on R_{ik-1} and a minimum energy folding on R_{kj}, so that $W(i,j) = W(i,k-1) + W(k,j)$ in this case. Putting together all the cases yields the formula:

$$W(i, j) = \min\{W(i, j-1), W(i+1, j-1) + e(i, j),$$
$$\min_{i<k<j}(W(i, k-1) + W(k, j)\}$$

(4)

When $j - i$ is small, $i + 1$ could be $> j - 1$. Rather than explicate special cases, it is better to adopt the convention that $W(i,j) = 0$ whenever $i > j$. Note that $W(i,j-1) = W(i,k-1) + W(k,j)$ when $k = j$, so that Equation 4 can be simplified to:

$$W(i, j) = \min\{W(i+1, j-1) + e(i, j),$$
$$\min_{i<k\leq j} [W(i, k-1) + W(k, j)]\}$$

(5)

The reason for deriving a formula such as Equation 5 is that it can be used recursively. Note that the left-hand side of Equation 5 is the energy of a subsequence containing $j - i + 1$ bases. The right-hand side uses the best folding energies of fragments at most $j - i$ long. Thus the minimum folding energy for fragments of length d can be computed using Equation 5 as long as minimum folding energies are known for all shorter fragments. If the number $W(i,j)$ is placed in the ith row and jth column of a triangular half-matrix, we say that the matrix is "filled" as these numbers are computed and stored. This can be done in several different ways.

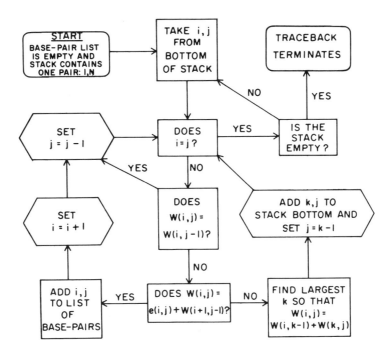

FIGURE 3. A traceback flow chart for the simple folding algorithm in Section V. It succeeds as long as W(i,j) is defined acording to Equation 5. The list of base pairs contains an optimal secondary structure upon completion.

Once the fill algorithm described above has been completed, the number W(1,N), the minimum folding energy for the entire RNA sequence, is known. However, a folding corresponding to this energy is still unknown. It is the traceback algorithm which actually identifies the base pairs. As with the fill algorithm, the traceback algorithm uses Equation 5, but in reverse. A minimum energy structure on R_{ij} either contains the base pair i·j if W(i,j) = W(i + 1, j − 1) + e(i,j) or else splits into a folding on R_{ik-1} and a folding on R_{kj} for some k between i + 1 and j inclusive. The recursion proceeds from longer fragments to shorter ones, and is described in detail in Figure 3.

The fill algorithm executes in time $O(N^3)$. To see this, it suffices to examine the computation in Equation 5. A total of j − i + 1 different sums are checked for each i,j pair satisfying $1 \leqq i < j \leqq N$. The total number of sums checked is

$$\sum_{j=1}^{N} \sum_{i=1}^{j-1} (j - i + 1)$$

which equals N(N + 1) (N + 2)/6. This is far more satisfactory than an exponentially increasing time. The traceback algorithm is very swift and executes in time O(N). Very often, computer memory is the limiting factor in a computation rather than execution time. The biggest demand for memory in the fill algorithm is the requirement to store the N(N + 1)/2 numbers W(i,j). We say that the computer storage or memory requirement of the algorithm is $O(N^2)$.

One of the drawbacks of the traceback algorithm just described is that it yields a single solution, even if two or more foldings of minimum energy exist. With some difficulty, the algorithm can be modified to predict a family of solutions within a certain range of the minimum energy. This is discussed later. One of the positive aspects of using dynamic

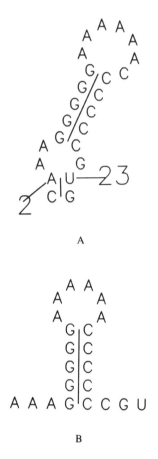

A

B

FIGURE 4.   (A) A minimum energy folding (-15.0 kcal/mol) of a small RNA molecule containing 24 bases. Both $S_{2,23}$ and $S_{3,22}$ are suboptimal substructures. (B) The minimum energy folding on $R_{2,23}$ (-14.9 kcal/mol) contains completely different base pairs from the folding in A.

programming for folding prediction is that the traceback algorithm can be used on any fragment R_{ij}, so that once the fill algorithm is completed, a minimum energy structure can be computed for any subsequence of the original RNA molecule in a very short time. This is useful, for example, to simulate the structures that might form as the molecule grows nucleotide by nucleotide from the 5' end.

VI. ALGORITHMS FOR LOOP-DEPENDENT ENERGY RULES

As soon as loop-dependent energy rules are introduced, the simple algorithm given in the previous section breaks down. With base pair-dependent rules, the energy contributions of each base pair are independent of one another, so that if S is a minimum energy folding on R, then S_{ij} is always a minimum energy folding on R_{ij}. This is what makes Equation 5 work. When energy assignment is loop dependent, S_{ij} is no longer a minimum energy folding on R_{ij} when i·j is a base pair of S which closes a destabilizing loop. Figure 4A illustrates a minimum energy folding of a small RNA sequence using the BP set of energy rules. The substructure on bases 2 to 23 is suboptimal. The minimum energy folding for this fragment, shown in Figure 4B, is totally different. The point is that the stacked pair $L_{1·24}$ (Figure 4A) more than makes up for the destabilizing energy incurred by creating the interior loop $L_{2·23}$.

A dynamic programming algorithm is still possible, but execution time is increased and storage requirements double. For each pair i,j satisfying $1 \leqq i \leqq j \leqq N$, we must now keep track of two quantities. $W(i,j)$ is redefined to be the minimum possible energy of a secondary structure on R_{ij} which contains at least 1 bp. Since no folding is possible on a single nucleotide, $W(i,i)$ is taken to be ∞. When a stable folding is possible on R_{ij}, then $W(i,j)$ has the same meaning as in the previous section. A new quantity $V(i,j)$ is defined to be the minimum possible energy of a folding on R_{ij} which contains the base pair i·j. Because the base pair i·j is forced, $V(i,j)$ is the energy of a structure on R_{ij} which may be suboptimal. Obviously, $V(i,j) \geqq W(i,j)$, and $V(i,i)$ can be set equal to ∞. Because these two quantities are stored for each i,j pair, computer memory requirements are doubled.

In defining the general algorithm, no assumptions are made on how energies are assigned to loops. The initial conditions are $W(i,i) = V(i,i) = \infty$. When $i < j$, we must examine all possible external loops for structures on R_{ij} when defining $W(i,j)$. The definition of $V(i,j)$ requires the examination of all possible loops closed by i·j. It is easily seen that

$$W(i, j) = \min_{\substack{i \leqq i_1 < j_1 < i_2 < j_2 < \ldots < i_k < j_k \leqq j \\ k > 0}} \left\{ e(L_{ext}) + \sum_{l=1}^{k} V(i_l, j_l) \right\} \tag{6}$$

and that

$$V(i, j) = \min_{\substack{i < i_1 < j_1 < i_2 < j_2 < \ldots < i_k < j_k < j \\ k \geqq 0}} \left\{ e(L_{i \cdot j}) + \sum_{l=1}^{k} V(i_l, j_l) \right\} \tag{7}$$

For this completely general version of the folding algorithm, Equation 7 does not depend on Equation 6. Therefore, it suffices to compute and store only $V(i,j)$ for all $i < j$. $W(i,j)$ need only be computed for fragments R_{ij} for which a folding is desired, and these values need not be stored. Nevertheless, the computation in Equation 7 is not much faster than counting all possible structures. The number of k-tuples of pairs i_1, j_1; i_2, j_2; $\ldots$; i_k, j_k which must be examined is $O(2^{j-i})$, making overall execution time $O(2^N)$. Thus, even with loop-dependent energy rules, we end up with an impractical algorithm in the general case.

The first simplification is to assume that the exterior loop contributes nothing to the overall energy. Up to the present, this seems to have been a universal assumption in folding prediction since no data are available on the effect of external bases. However, some biochemists[36] feel that multiloops or external loops which contain 2 bp of the form i·k and k + 1·j should add the stacking energy of 1 bp over the other to the overall sum. If this idea were adopted, external loops would have to be assigned nonzero energies. Ignoring exterior bases greatly simplifies the computation of W. If S_{ij} is a minimum energy folding on R_{ij}, then either i is not base paired, j is not base paired, i is base paired with j, or i and j are both base paired, but not with each other. In the first case, the ith base can be dropped without affecting the energy, so $W(i,j) = W(i + 1,j)$. Similarly, the second case implies $W(i,j) = W(i,j-1.)$ For the third case, $W(i,j) = V(i,j)$. In the last case, i·k and k'·j are base paired for k and k' satisfying $i < k < k' < j$. Because the external bases contribute nothing to the overall energy, $W(i,j)$ splits into the sum of $W(i,l)$, and $W(l + 1,j)$ for any l satisfying $k \leqq l < k'$. Putting these cases together yields

$$W(i, j) = \min\{W(i + 1, j), W(i, j - 1), V(i, j)$$
$$\min_{i < k < j} (W(i, k) + W(k + 1, j))\} \tag{8}$$

Figure 5 illustrates how W and V can be stored in a single array.

Equation 8 is a great improvement over Equation 6. It now becomes necessary to compute and store $W(i,j)$ for all i,j pairs, but the computation of $W(i,j)$ for each pair now takes time

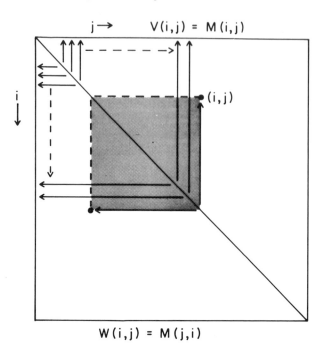

FIGURE 5.   Both W(i,j) and V(i,j) can be stored in a single square matrix, M, as shown. The solid arrows illustrate the order in which W and V can be computed. The broken arrows indicate the progression from one solid arrow to the next. Depending on which algorithm is used, the computation of V(i,j) will depend on some or all of the previously computed values in the shaded region above the diagonal. Computation of W(i,j) according to Equation 8 uses V(i,j) and the values stored in the jth row and ith column of M adjacent to the shaded region.

O(j − i), so the total computation time for W is $(O \sum_{1 \le i < j \le n} [j - i])$ which is equivalent to O(N³). Unfortunately, the computation time for V remains $O(2^n)$. What can be done about this?

The first step is to rewrite the formula for V. In Equation 7, k is the index of the loop closed by i·j. We separate the computation into three parts depending on whether k = 0, k = 1, or k > 1. Let VH(i,j) be the energy of the structure on R_{ij} containing the single base pair i·j. Let VBI(i,j) be the minimum energy of a folding on R_{ij} containing i·j and for which i·j closes a bulge or interior loop. Finally, let VM(i,j) be the minimum energy of a folding on R_{ij} containing i·j where i·j closes a multiloop. Then Equation 7 can be rewritten as

$$V(i, j) = \min\{VH(i, j), es(i, j) + V(i + 1, j - 1),$$
$$VBI(i, j), VM(i, j)\} \tag{9}$$

where es(i,j) is the energy of the stacked pair i·j over i + 1·j − 1. The way in which energy is assigned to destabilizing loops determines the computation time required for VH, VBI, and VM. The first point to recognize is that the energy of a loop can always be assumed to depend in part on the closing pair. This does not add to the computation time in Equation 9. An energy rule which looks at the size of the loop in addition to the nature of its paired and unpaired bases is called context dependent. An energy function which depends on the size of the loop is called size dependent. Finally, a size-dependent function which is a linear function of loop size is called linear.

When i·j closes a stacked pair, only a single computation is required in Equation 9 (second term). What this means is that the stacking energies can be arbitrarily complex without any problem. This is fortunate, because stacking energies have been studied the most[23] and certainly are known more accurately than other energies. The BP set considers GC, AU, and GU base pairs and assigns energies to all possible combinations of one over the other. The inclusion of GG, UU, CC, CA, AA, AG, and UC base pairs by Papanicolaou et al.[16] presents no problem to dynamic programming algorithms. What does cause problems are their special rules which look at neighboring loops.

A context-dependent energy rule for hairpin loops would require the examination of all $j - i - 1$ bases between r_i and r_j to compute VH(i,j). This would make the overall time $O(N^3)$ for VH. In fact, the BP set looks only at the closing base pair and the size of the loop. This requires a single calculation for each i,j pair, so total computation time for VH is $O(N^2)$. Tinoco modification of these rules[15] removes the dependence on the closing pair. Papanicolaou et al.[16] also use a size-dependent function. They have a special rule concerning the occurrence of Us, but this is only for loops of size three, so overall computation time remains $O(N^2)$.

The clash between realistic energy rules and an efficient algorithm begins with the consideration of bulge and interior loops. Let L(i,j,i′,j′) denote the bulge or interior loop closed by i·j and containing the interior pair i′·j′. Then using Equation 7 with k = 1 and ruling out the case of a stacked pair covered explicity in Equation 9, we obtain

$$VBI(i, j) = \min_{\substack{i<i'<j'<j \\ i'-i+j-j'>2}} \{e(L(i, j, i', j')) + V(i', j')\} \qquad (10)$$

For a truly context-dependent energy function, the computation of e in Equation 10 would take time $O(i' - i + j - j')$ for each pair of base pairs i·j and i′·j′. This sums to $O([j-i]^3)$ for each base pair i·j, and the overall time would then be $O(N^5)$. In fact, it is difficult to imagine an energy rule this complex. The BP set looks only at the size of bulge and interior loops as well as the closing base pairs. They are almost size dependent. The specialized rules of Papanicolaou et al.[16] are more involved since they look at the two numbers $i' - i - 1$ and $j - j' - 1$ separately. In both cases, computation of e(L[i,j,i′,j′]) takes time $O(1)$, so the overall computation time for bulge and interior loops becomes $O(N^4)$.

The rate of $O(N^4)$ derived above would seem to be the best possible, even for a strictly size-dependent rule. Nevertheless, Waterman and Smith[24] have recently shown that this can always be improved to $O(N^3)$ for size-dependent bulge and interior loop destabilizing energies. They make use of the fact that e(L[i,j,i′,j′]) is constant when $j' - i'$ is constant and $i' - i$ as well as $j - j'$ are > 1. The price they pay is the introduction of another triangular array which requires an additional $N^2/2$ storage locations, but this is not a severe constraint. It is easy to show that their result can be extended to cover the BP set of energy rules where the destabilizing energy also depends on the closing base pairs.

It turns out that a further improvement is possible if a pragmatic approach is taken. The algorithm described by Zuker and Stiegler[25] uses two methods to limit the search for a best bulge or interior loop. The first method is to define an absolute limit on the size of a bulge or interior loop. If MAXSIZE is this maximum size, then no matter how large $j - i$ becomes, there are at most (MAXSIZE + 1) (MAXSIZE + 2)/2 interior base pairs i′·j′ to examine. This number, although possibly large, is fixed, and the resulting bulge and interior loop search time becomes $O(N^2)$. For folding at room temperature using the BP set or even the rules of Papanicolaou et al.,[16] there is little risk of obtaining a suboptimal solution if MAXSIZE is 30 or so. This risk becomes unacceptable when folding is attempted at elevated temperatures using the energy rules of Steger et al.,[17] because large loops are expected in these circumstances. The second method employs an optimal stopping rule to limit the search. The program computes $V(i',j') + e(L[i,j,i',j'])$ for all loops of size s, for s = 1,2, and so on. For a particular s, VBEST is the minimum value obtained for loops of that size or smaller. The best energy possible for larger loops is certainly greater than or equal to

$$\min_{\substack{j'-i'=j-i-2-s \\ i<i'<j'<j}} W(i', j') + \min_{\substack{j'-i'=j-i-2-s \\ i<i'<j'<j}} e(L(i, j, i', j')) \tag{11}$$

This makes use only of the fact that destabilizing energies grow with loop size. When the number in Equation 11 is greater than or equal to VBEST, the algorithm gives up searching for larger loops. There is no sacrifice of rigor here, but there is also no way to predict how large s might become. In practice, s is bounded on the average. The net effect is to make the bulge and interior loop search time $O(N^2)$. Using the BP set, s was found to have an average value of 8 with a standard deviation of 5 in a folding of the MDV-1 RNA.[26] It is my conjecture that this stopping rule yields an $O(N^2)$ time for random RNA sequences.

Another way to arrive at a $O(N^2)$ time for bulge and interior loop searches is to employ a linear-destabilizing energy. This fact is contained in the review by Zuker and Sankoff[5] and has also been noted by Waterman and Smith.[24] Unfortunately, this is a "spherical cow" assumption and must be resisted no matter how appealing it might be to a mathematician. Destabilizing energies grow logarithmically, not linearly. However, Waterman and Smith[24] go on to conjecture that the $O(N^2)$ time remains possible for concave-destabilizing functions. This would cover logarithmic functions and would therefore cover all the energy rules in use today. All in all, a practical and realistic folding algorithm can compute Equation 10 in time $O(N^2)$ for all i,j.

The most difficult case to consider is when i·j closes a multiloop. The computation time for

$$VM(i, j) = \min_{\substack{i<i_1<j_1<i_2<j_2<...<i_k<j_k<j \\ k>1}} \{e(L_{i\cdot j}) + \sum_{l=1}^{k} V(i_l, j_l)\} \tag{12}$$

will be $O(2^N)$ unless some way can be found to reduce the computation. Very little is known about the destabilizing effects of multiloops. They are sometimes ignored altogether. Usually, they are treated as interior loops. It is certainly reasonable to assume a size-dependent energy rule, perhaps modified by the nature of the accessible base pairs. For a strictly size-dependent energy rule, Waterman and Smith[24] have reduced computation time to $O(N^4)$. Using our notation, they introduce the quantity WM'(i,j,s) which is defined to be the minimum folding energy of a structure on R_{ij} whose exterior loop is of size s. This exterior loop is given the multiloop energy. If em(s) is the destabilizing energy of a multiloop of size s, then

$$WM'(i, j, s) = \min\{em(s) - em(s-1) + WM'(i, j-1, s-1),$$
$$\min_{j'}(WM'(i, j',s) + V(j'+1, j))\} \tag{13}$$

The first term in the braces examines the case where r_j is not base paired, and the second examines all the possible base pairs between r_j and some $r_{j'}$ in the fragment R_{ij}. From here, it is clear that

$$VM(i+1, j-1) = \min_s WM'(i, j, s) \tag{14}$$

This will work as long as em(s) is greater than the energy given to bulge or interior loops of the same size. For fixed i,j,s, computation time for Equation 13 is O(j − 1). This makes computation time for Equation 14 O([j − i]²) for each i,j pair, so the overall time is O(N⁴). This is not bad, but unlike VH, VBI, and VM which do not have to be stored, WM′ appears on the right to Equation 13. This means that a three-dimensional array must be stored, bringing storage requirements up to O(N³). This is a heavy price to pay.

How can multiloop computation time be brought down to a reasonable level? One can limit the index of these loops to be no larger than some fixed number K. This is not a very good approach. Computation time becomes O(N²ᴷ) which is still too large even for K = 3, the index of the multiloop in the tRNA cloverleaf structure. The linear assumption is not so unpalatable in this case because of the lack of biochemical data and of a good alternative. Within the constraints of linearity, the multiloop destabilizing energy can be fairly general. It can depend arbitrarily on the closing base pair as well as the interior base pairs, as long as these contributions are additive. The form which the energy function can take is

$$\text{em}(L(i, j, i_1, j_1, \ldots i_k, j_k)) = \text{emc}(i, j) + a \times (\text{size of loop}) + \sum_{l=1}^{k} \text{emi}(i_l, j_l) \quad (15)$$

where emc and emi are the contributions of the closing base pair and the interior base pairs, respectively, and a is the constant. This allows the user, for example, to differentiate between GC, AU, and possibly GU base pairs. A new array W′(i,j) is introduced which must be computed and stored. It is the same as W(i,j) except that it includes a destabilizing energy for the exterior loop given by the last two summands in Equation 15, even if the index is 1. The recursions for VM and W′ are

$$\text{VM}(i, j) = \text{emc}(i, j) + \min_{i < h < j-1} \{W'(i + 1, h) + W'(h + 1, j - 1)\} \quad (16)$$

and

$$W'(i, j) = \min\{(V(i, j) + \text{emi}(i, j), W'(i + 1, j) + a, W'(i, j - 1) + a,$$

$$\min_{i < k < j} W'(i, k) + W'(k + 1, j)\} \quad (17)$$

The computation of Equation 17 is rate limiting, requiring time O(N³). Note that if one is prepared to penalize exterior bases according to Equation 15 (without the emc term), then one can dispense with the array W. Sankoff et al.[4] first introduced this algorithm with emc and emi both constant. It was later presented by Zuker and Sankoff[5] with emi constant. It can be generalized still further by allowing a to depend on individual bases in the sequence.

The method of Waterman and Smith discussed above is an important theoretical advance because it shows that exponential computing time can be avoided in a rigorous algorithm for size-dependent energy. If multiloops are to be treated as interior loops, then the use of a linear rule as an approximation will penalize larger multiloops more than the logarithmically increasing interior loop energies would. The compromise adopted by Zuker and Stiegler[25] is to break with rigor in the treatment of multiloops. Two auxiliary arrays, S(i,j) and S′(i,j), are introduced. S(i,j) is the number of exterior single-stranded bases in a best structure on R_{ij}, and S′(i,j) = 0, 1, or 2 depending on whether this best structure contains both AU and GC external base pairs, only AU base pairs, or only GC base pairs, respectively. In practice, S and S′ are encoded together so that only a single array need be stored. Interior loop energies from the BP set as summarized by Salser[14] are used. The form of this function is ei(loop size, type), where type is 0, 1, or 2 as described above, including the closing base pair. The recurrences for S and S′ are

$$S(i, j) = S(i + 1, j) + 1, S(i, j - 1) + 1, 0,$$

or

$$S(i, k) + S(k + 1, j) \tag{17a}$$

and

$$S'(i, j) = S'(i + 1, j), S'(i, j - 1), \text{type for } r_i \cdot r_j,$$

or $\tag{18}$

$$-(S'(i, k) + S'(k + 1, j))S'(i, k)S'(k + 1, j) \ (\text{mod } 3)$$

according to which case in Equation 8 yields the minimum value for $W(i,j)$. In this algorithm, $VM(i,j)$ is given by

$$VM(i, j) = \min_{i < k < j - 1} \{ei(S(i + 1, k) + S(k + 1, j - 1),$$

$$\text{type}(i, j, k)) + W(i + 1, k) + W(k + 1, j - 1)\} \tag{19}$$

where $\text{type}(i,j,k) = (-(x + y)xy + z) (x + y)xyz \ (\text{mod } 3)$, $x = S'(i + 1,k)$, $y = S'(k + 1, j - 1)$, and z is 1 or 2 if the closing base pair $i \cdot j$ is AU or GC, respectively. Execution time for the multiloop search is $O(N^3)$, making it the rate-limiting step in the algorithm because of the $O(N^2)$ method used to handle bulge and interior loops. The method of Zuker and Stiegler[25] is more effective than just using a best structure on $R_{i+1\,j-1}$ when closing a multiloop, but it still risks finding a suboptimal solution.

The many different methods discussed in this section are summarized in Table 1. The overall rate of an algorithm is the rate of its weakest link. It must be remembered that these rates are only rough guides. On molecules of fixed size, an $O(N^4)$ algorithm might execute faster than an $O(N^3)$ algorithm. The only certainty is that the latter will be faster for sufficiently large molecules. Algorithms which are slower but more realistic biochemically or more rigorous mathematically can still be very useful.

VII. CONSTRAINED OPTIMIZATION

The entire folding model with loop-dependent energy rules is not accurate enough to predict folding with any degree of reliability. Only about 25% of RNAs are predicted to have the cloverleaf conformation. This is probably because tRNAs have several modified bases which affect base pairing and because the cloverleaf structure is further stabilized by tertiary interactions. Nevertheless, the 359 bases of the potato spindle tuber viroid (PSTV) are correctly folded into a long rod-like secondary structure by the algorithm of Zuker and Stiegler;[25] so folding algorithms cannot be simply dismissed as nonsense. The modifications of the BP set by Ninio[18] and Papanicolaou et al.[16] have been successful for a limited class of molecules. It is not clear whether these rules can be extended to other molecules, and their methods are arbitrary rather than rooted in thermodynamics.

It is therefore desirable to be able to take into account other physical data which might be available for a particular molecule. Broadly speaking, the available data tell the scientist that certain parts of the RNA molecule are single stranded or base paired. How can this information be used? The answer lies in the nonthermodynamic use of the energy function. The energy assignment given by Equation 2 was made with the BP set or similar rules in mind. However, once the formula is written down, it becomes an abstract entity and need

Table 1
A SUMMARY OF DIFFERENT WAYS OF ASSIGNING ENERGIES TO LOOPS AND OF THE RESULTING COST IN EXECUTION TIME

Loop type	Energy rule	Execution time
Stacked pair	Arbitrary	$O(N^2)$
Hairpin	Content dependent	$O(N^3)$
	Size dependent	$O(N^2)$
Bulge/interior	Context dependent	$O(N^5)$
	Size dependent	$O(N^4)$
	Size dependent with auxiliary $N^2/2$ array (Waterman and Smith)	$O(N^3)$
	Linear	$O(N^2)$
	Loop size limitation	$O(N^2)$
	Stopping rule (Zuker and Stiegler)	$O(N^2)$
	Concave (Waterman and Smith conjecture)	$O(N^2)$
Multiloop	Context dependent	$O(2^N)$
	Size dependent (Waterman and Smith: auxiliary array requires N^3 storage)	$O(N^4)$
	Linear	$O(N^3)$
	Compromise of Zuker and Stiegler with auxiliary $N^2/2$ array	$O(N^3)$

not correspond to experimentally determined energies. This observation is the key to using dynamic programming algorithms for predicting foldings which agree with auxiliary information.

The first technique is to prohibit unwanted base pairs by assigning large destabilizing energies to loops which are closed by such base pairs. Recall that the definition of secondary structure in Section II allowed base pairs between arbitrary ribonucleotides and allowed r_i and r_j to base pair even if $j - i < 4$. This was for mathematical simplicity. In practice, a stacked pair closed by i·j is given a large destabilizing energy if r_i and r_j are not complementary bases. Similarly, a large penalty energy is given to a hairpin loop closed by i·j when $j - i < 4$. This alone is adequate to eliminate the prediction of biochemically invalid structures. However, there is no need to stop here. It is known that certain bases are sometimes chemically modified so they cannot base pair. These bases can be tagged by the folding algorithm and any stacked pair containing one of them is given a large penalty energy. Similarly, in some cases a protein (e.g., a ribosome) is known to bind to a region of an RNA molecule so that a number of consecutive bases are "protected" from base pairing. The folding technique is the same; these bases are all individually prevented from base pairing.

Another more subtle form of information on single-stranded regions is often available. Certain enzymes known as ribonucleases (RNases) cleave an RNA molecule by cutting the phosphodiesther bond linking two ribonucleotides. Some are very specific. For example, T1 RNase cuts only the 3' bond after a G. The most exposed bonds will be cut first. If a large amount of RNase is used, initial cuts will allow the molecule to rearrange and more cuts will follow, making it hard to interpret the data. However, under conditions of partial hydrolysis, the cuts which occur can be assumed to be in single-stranded regions. If the cut occurs between r_i and r_{i+1}, what sort of constraint should be used? The approach adopted by Zuker and Stiegler[25] and later used in Cech et al.[15] is a cautious one. Ribonucleotides r_i and r_{i+1} cannot both be base paired in a folding. This allows the bond linking them to be exposed or accessible to RNase attack. In the folding algorithm, one gives a large penalty energy to a stacked pair closed by r_i and r_j for $j > i$ or closed by r_k and r_{i+1} for $k < i$.

Biochemical data often yield information about double-stranded regions. Nuclease digestion data might reveal base pairing between distant regions in an RNA molecule, or it can show that two regions are not related by base pairing. For example, in the study of 16S rRNA from *Escherichia coli* by Stiegler et al.,[27] digestion data indicated that the first 560 bases out of 1541 did not base pair with the rest of the molecule. This simplified the folding prediction because it broke up the problem into two more easily handled parts. In fact, in this case, digestion data reduced the problem still further. A biochemical technique known as crosslinking can sometimes "cement" together double-stranded regions in an RNA molecule by creating a strong covalent bond between base-paired nucleotides. When possible, this can uncover specific base pairs, sometimes involving distant regions of the molecule. There is a RNase isolated from cobra venom which cleaves RNA in double-stranded regions. Vary and Vournakis[28] have reported a nonenzymatic chemical with a similar specificity. Depending on the data available, one might know that certain specific base pairs form, that a region from r_i to $r_{i'}$ somehow base pairs with another region from $r_{j'}$ to r_j, or that certain individual nucleotides are base paired with some unknown region.

Specific base pairs are most easily handled. If r_i and r_j are known to base pair, then any loop closed by r_i and r_j is given a bonus energy. The size of the bonus energy is not important as long as it forces the desired base pair to appear in a predicted folding. Something like 30 kcal/mol is more than enough in practice. This bonus energy must be in addition to the thermodynamic energy. The traceback algorithm can be modified to substract all the bonus energies used in order to arrive at the correct energy of the structure. When all that is known is that r_i is base paired, then all loops closed by r_i and r_k ($k > i$) or by $r_{k'}$ and r_i ($k' < i$) are given the bonus energy. The result is that r_i will be base paired in any predicted structure. The algorithm will select its "mate" in order to minimize the overall folding energy.

When specific base pairs are known to occur between distant regions in a large molecule, a folding problem which might otherwise be too large to handle on a given computer can be broken into two parts. If the base pair i·j is known to occur, the segment from r_i to r_j can be folded separately, forcing the ends to base pair with one another. Then the bases from r_{i+1} through r_{j-1} may be replaced by three "phantom" bases (the letter X may be used). This excised molecule can then be folded forcing r_i and r_j to base pair and giving no energy to the "pseudo hairpin loop" closed by i·j. The sum of the energies of these two foldings is then equal to the energy of a folding of the entire molecule constrained by the forced occurrence of i·j. The procedure used in the second folding can be called a closed excision. The important point is that r_i and r_j must be base paired. If the region between these nucleotides were simply excised and the ends spliced together, the folding energy would not come out correctly.

When all that is known is that two separated regions somehow base pair, it is best to excise all of the molecule except for the regions of interest. A folding of what is left might reveal some good double-stranded regions which can then be forced in a repeat folding of the entire molecule. If one is simply "fishing" for distant base pairing, the energy rules may be used to prohibit base pairs between bases which are less than K apart, where K might be several hundred, for example. Similarly, one can fold looking only for short-range interactions.

To summarize, folding prediction requires the use of whatever information is available to increase reliability. The simple use of bonus and penalty energies allows much information to be incorporated into folding algorithms. A mathematician would call this approach constrained optimization.

VIII. VARIATIONS ON FOLDING

Waterman[20] and Zuker and Sankoff[5] discuss different levels of complexity of secondary structures. It is the multiloops which cause structures to have a tree-like or branched ap-

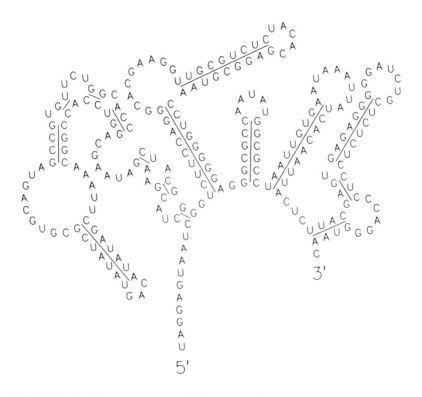

FIGURE 6. A minimum energy open folding (BP set of energy rules) of the 3′ Qβ fragment from Figure 1. The energy is −99.0 kcal/mol. The energy of the structure in Figure 1 is −106.9 kcal/mol (optimal).

pearance. A folding with no multiloops can be called an open folding. If it has k exterior base pairs: $i_1 \cdot j_1$, $i_2 \cdot j_2$, . . . $i_k \cdot j_k$, then each of the substructures on $R_{i_l j_l}$ is called a hairpin. A hairpin has a possibly twisted, rod-like appearance. Figure 6 shows an open folding of a molecule. Minimum energy open foldings can clearly be generated using the algorithms already discussed. All that needs to be done is to give a large penalty energy to multiloops. This is obviously inefficient, and it would be better to redesign these algorithms.

Letting W and V have the same meaning as in Section VI, the recursions are

$$W(i, j) = \min\{W(i + 1, j), W(i, j - 1), V(i, j),$$
$$\min_{i<k<j} (W(i, k) + W(k + 1, j))\} \tag{20}$$

and

$$V(i, j) = \min\{VH(i, j), es(i, j) + V(i + 1, j - 1), VBI(i, j)\} \tag{21}$$

Equation 20 is identical to Equation 8, and Equation 21 differs from Equation 9 only in the absence of VM(i,j) term which covers the case of i·j closing a multiloop. All the problems with multiloops vanish. If a practical approach is taken as discussed in Section VI, overall computation for Equation 21 will be $O(N^2)$. Almost all of this time will be for bulge and interior loop searches. The last term in Equation 20 makes its computation time $O(N^3)$, but this can be reduced to $O(N^2)$. The last term covers the case when i and j are both base paired, but not with each other. Thus Equation 20 can be rewritten as

$$W(i, j) = \min\{W(i + 1, j), W(i, j - 1), V(i, j), \min_{i<k<j} (W(i, k) + V(k + 1, j))\} \quad (22)$$

General folding algorithms using linear-destabilizing energies for multiloops or the compromise method for Zuker and Stiegler[25] both require $W(i,j)$ for arbitrary i and j in the computation of $VM(i,j)$, and hence $V(i,j)$. This is no longer true with open foldings. $W(i,j)$ can be redefined to be the minimum energy for a folding on $W(i,j)$ including the case where there is no structure, as was done in Section V. Thus, $W(i,i) = 0$ and the first term, $W(i + 1,j)$, in Equation 22 can be dropped. Setting $i = 1$ yields

$$W(1, j) = \min\{W(1, j - 1), V(1, j), \min_{1<k<j} (W(1, k) + V(k + 1, j))\} \quad (23)$$

Therefore, $W(i,j)$ need only be computed with $i = 1$. This means that the $N^2/2$ storage locations for W can be reduced to only N and the computation time for Equation 23 is reduced to $O(N^2)$. The optimal open folding of fragments can still be computed when the fragment includes the 5' end of the molecule.

Some RNA molecules have a circular rather than linear covalent structure. They can be visualized as the result of bonding the last ribonucleotide to the first in a linear molecule. In such a molecule, there are no 5' and 3' ends, so the "first" base is designated arbitrarily. An example is the PSTV which is a small virus.[29] The definition of secondary structure is the same as with a linear molecule, but the decomposition into loops changes slightly. The exterior loop is "closed off" and becomes just like a hairpin, bulge, interior, or multiloop, with the appropriate energy. The only difference is that this loop contains its closing base pair(s), but this is just a mathematical formality. The simplistic approach is to fold a circular RNA as if it were a linear molecule. If this is done, the exterior loop will not be given its correct energy, so the folding may well depend on the excision point chosen. This was found to be the case by Steger et al.[17] in folding viroids at high temperatures.

A proper treatment of circular RNA follows from the crucial observation that any base pair i·j divides the folding into two separate foldings on two linear sequences. The first sequence is the "included" fragment from r_i to r_j inclusive. The second is the "excluded" fragment from r_j through the origin to r_i inclusive. The base pair i·j is common to both foldings, but the loops are disjoint and so the energies sum with loop-dependent energy rules. The definitions of W and V given in Section VI can be extended so that $W(j,i)$ and $V(j,i)$ refer to the linear RNA from r_j through the origin to r_i ($i < j$). All the recursions from Section VI generalize. The differences are that a search over all k satisfying $i < k < j$ becomes $j < k \leq N$ and $1 \leq k < i$ and similarly for pairs i' and j' satisfying $i < i' < j' < j$. The minimum overall folding energy is given by

$$E_{min} = \min_{1 \leq i < j \leq N} \{V(i, j) + V(j, i)\} \quad (24)$$

as observed by Steger et al.[17] A best structure can be computed by finding an i,j pair satisfying $E_{min} = V(i,j) + V(j,i)$ and by performing tracebacks on the included and excluded fragments defined by these bases. Both storage requirements and computation time are doubled with respect to a linear RNA of the same size. Zuker and Sankoff[5] discuss a practical way of modifying this algorithm so that time and storage increase only slightly.

IX. MULTIPLE SOLUTIONS

There is an intrinsic biochemical reason to look at foldings close to the minimum energy. Thermal motion alone implies a mixture of conformations. Simplifying matters greatly, if

S_1 and S_2 are two foldings with energies E_1 and E_2, respectively, then the equilibrium constant, K, describing the ratio of the number of molecules in S_2 over the number S_1 is given by

$$K = e^{-\Delta G/RT} \tag{25}$$

$\Delta G = E_2 - E_1$ and is called the free energy difference between the foldings. T is the temperature in degrees Kelvin, and R, the gas constant per mole, has the value 1.986×10^{-3} kcal/K/mol. A scientist might have as little as 1 pmol of RNA molcules in vitro. This corresponds to 6×10^{11} molecules. An energy difference of 16 kcal/mol between two foldings would mean that only a single molecule could be expected to be in the alternate folding at room temperature. More realistically, finding 1% or 0.1% of molecules in alternate foldings would correspond to energy differences in 2.8 and 4.1 kcal/mol. This is quite small, considering that the stacking energy of a GC base pair over another contributes 4.8 kcal/mol to the overall stability of a molecule. In a living cell, an mRNA which codes for a protein sequence might have a copy number of only a few thousand. It would seem from simple thermodynamic considerations that all of these molecules would have to fold within a few kilocalories from the energy minimum.

The simplistic discussion above ignores other factors which might alter RNA folding. Most important of all, it does not take into account our ignorance in assigning energy. Let us be optimistic and assume that the energy rules are good to within 10%. What this means is that any structure within 10% of the computed minimum energy might be the best. In most cases, this greatly exceeds the 3 to 4 kcal demanded by thermal motion alone.

What are the possible alternate foldings within 10% or so of minimum energy? The breaking of only 3 bp can raise the energy by up to 15 kcal/mol. If this were the only sort of suboptimal folding, our problems would be over. The real situation is in some sense the worst possible. It turns out that completely different foldings are possible in some cases within even 5% of the minimum energy.[30] This is a property of the mathematical folding model and the energy rules. Whether it corresponds to biochemical reality is another matter. For RNA folding algorithms, it means that a search for the suboptimal becomes a necessity. To facilitate the following discussion, a P-suboptimal folding is defined to be a folding within P% of the minimum energy, where P is a positive number. A P-suboptimal base pair is a base pair which can be part of a P-suboptimal folding.

Algorithms which enumerate foldings have a built-in advantage. They automatically generate a list of structures which can be ranked in terms of energy. Dynamic programming algorithms usually arrive at a unique answer because the traceback algorithm takes a single path through the matrix of energies. Multiple foldings can be generated only by changing the constraints and executing the time-consuming fill algorithm over and over again. The traceback algorithm can be modified in theory using ideas from Waterman[31] and Waterman and Byers[32] so that all solutions within some percent of the minimum energy are found. Nevertheless, the practical problems are immense. In general, there may be millions of alternate structures within 10% of the computed energy minimum. How can these be filtered so that only a small collection which somehow represents all possibilities can be displayed? Despite these problems, Williams and Tinoco[33] have reported a dynamic programming algorithm for finding alternate foldings. The fill algorithm is used only once, and multiple tracebacks identify alternate structures. There is also a feature for doing interactive tracebacks. They use the estimated error in energy values to limit the number of alternate solutions. For example, if an interior loop in a best folding has an energy uncertainty of 2 kcal/mol, then they would allow alternate loops only within 2 kcal of this loop. Their algorithm has been used to derive a biologically interesting suboptimal folding of the intervening sequence of the rRNA from *Tetrahymena thermophila*.[15]

The problem with using alternate tracebacks to generate suboptimal foldings is that the number of solutions probably grows exponentially with the size of the molecule. This would certainly be the case if some small but fixed percent of all foldings were P-suboptimal. Another possibility is to search for all P-suboptimal base pairs. The total number of possible base pairs grows only as $O(N^2)$ so that at least a computer, if not a human, could examine them all. The naive or brute force method is to fold the molecule over and over again, forcing each base pair to occur one at a time. This is out of the question because it would take too much computer time. It is also totally unnecessary.

Loop-dependent dynamic programming algorithms discussed in Section VI compute the numbers $V(i,j)$ which are the minimum folding energies of the fragments R_{ij} containing the base pair i·j. This is half of what is needed. For each possible base pair i·j, the folding energy of the included fragment is known, but not the energy of the excluded fragments. Recall that with circular RNA, an extension of the dynamic programming algorithms discussed earlier, yielded the numbers $V(j,i)$, the minimum folding energy on the excluded fragment (j through the origin to i) containing i·j. Thus, for a circular RNA, the fill algorithm need only be executed once, and then an $O(N^2)$ search will find all base pairs i·j which are P-suboptimal. The criterion for acceptance is

$$V(i, j) + V(j, i) \leq (1 - P/100)E_{min} \qquad (26)$$

where E_{min} is the minimum folding energy. What is good for circular RNA should also be good for linear RNA. With a mathematical *tour de force*, any linear sequence can be circularized. A few dummy bases, denoted by X, can be inserted at the end to allow for base pairing between the first and last nucleotides which would otherwise be adjacent. The circular algorithm must then be modified slightly so that destabilizing loops which contain the origin are given zero energy. This corrects the energy to the case of folding linear RNA where the exterior loop has no energy.

The results of the above analysis can be displayed in two ways. A complete picture can be obtained by plotting a dot in the ith row and jth column of a triangular matrix for every base pair i·j which is P-suboptimal. Better still, if $0 = P_1 < P_2 < \ldots < P_m = P$, then the P_1-suboptimal base pairs corresponding to each energy increment can be displayed using different characters or colors. This is illustrated in Figure 7 using four different levels. The first level shows the optimal folding and more and more possibilities are revealed as the energy increment increases to 10% of the minimum.

Although a dot plot of P-suboptimal base pairs is packed with information, it is not a good way to visualize actual structures. These can be obtained by performing two tracebacks for each base pair i·j which satisfies Equation 26. Note that once a base pair has been included in some P-suboptimal structure, it need not be examined again. In other words, the number of pairs of tracebacks which must be performed will be far less than the number of P-suboptimal base pairs. The alternate structures may all contain some common feature such as a very stable helix, but they will all differ from one another in some way.

To reduce the output of alternate structures still further and to avoid finding pairs of trivially different foldings, it seems necessary to define a distance between secondary structures. If S_1 and S_2 are two secondary structures on the same sequence, define the distance between them, $d(S_1,S_2)$, to be max $\{d'(S_1,S_2), d'(S_2, S_1)\}$, where

$$d'(S_1, s_2) = \max_{i_1 \cdot j_1 \text{ in } S_1} \quad \min_{i_2 \cdot j_2 \text{ in } S_2} \quad \max\{|i_1 - i_2|, |j_1 - j_2|\} \qquad (27)$$

It can be shown that this distance is actually a metric in the strict mathematical sense. Heuristically, if the distance is small, then every base pair in the first folding will be close to some base pair in the second, and vice versa. If the two structures are plotted on the

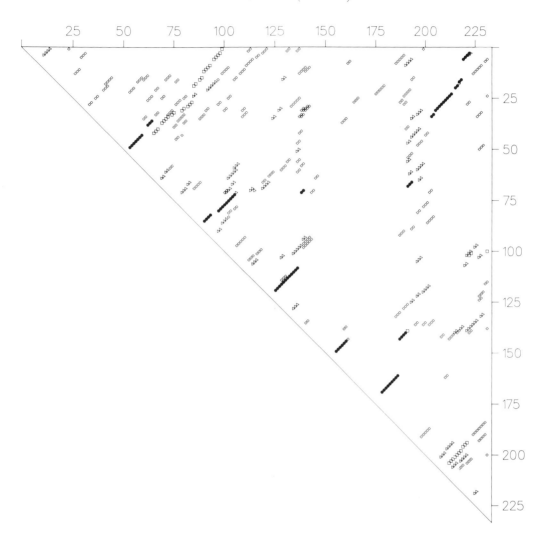

BACTERIOPHAGE QBETA (3' END)

FIGURE 7.   A dot plot of 10-suboptimal bp for the same Qβ fragment from Figure 1 . In this case, four levels are used. $P_1 = 0$, $P_2 = 3.3$, $P_3 = 6.7$, and $P_4 = 10$. On the plot, these correspond to the solid circles, the squares, the triangles, and the small diamonds, respectively. The solid circles are a dot plot of the structure in Figure 1. Not all 10-suboptimal bp are plotted. What is shown are the results of 235 tracebacks which generated suboptimal structures, no two of which are a distance of three or less from one another.

same dot plot using, for example, red dots for S_1 and blue dots for S_2, then a square of size 2d by 2d centered on each red dot will always contain a blue dot, and vice versa. In the multiple traceback algorithm, an auxiliary marker array can be used to keep track of which base pairs have already occurred in P-suboptimal foldings. A P-suboptimal base pair which is too close (say within d) to a base pair that has already appeared in an alternate folding will not be used to initiate a new pair of tracebacks. This will guarantee that all foldings generated will be a distance of at least $d + 1$ from one another. For example, setting $d = 1$ would eliminate one of the foldings in Figure 8. The dot plot in Figure 7 was generated using $d = 3$.

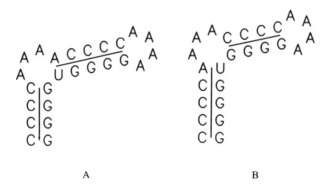

FIGURE 8.   Two minimum energy foldings of a small RNA molecule. The distance between them is 1. Multiple traceback algorithms should be designed to avoid displaying two such similar structures. The method described in the text will suppress one of these structures when d is set to 1.

X. CONCLUSIONS

When two or more closely related RNA sequences are expected to have similar secondary structures, it is very interesting to ask what sort of algorithm can simultaneously align and fold these sequences into a common structure. This procedure has been performed already by a number of biologists[34] without the use of labor saving algorithms. Although outside the scope of this article, Sankoff[35] has combined dynamic programming algorithms for alignment and folding into a single algorithm which requires time $O(N^6)$ and storage $O(N^4)$ for a pair of sequences of roughly equal length (N). This is too demanding of computer time and memory to be useful for practical problems, but it is still of theoretical interest, if only in that it forces one to define precisely what is meant by the term "common folding". One observation is that the energy rules become less important since it is the existence of common base pairs which will force the folding one way or another. Common secondary structures for the large and small subunits of rRNA were constructed without resorting to energy calculations at all.

The most important message of this chapter is that there is a tradeoff between biochemical realism and workable folding algorithms. Eliminating knots seems to be inescapable. The definition of loops breaks down when knots are allowed and even the simple algorithm in Section V fails. Currently accepted energy rules are on the verge of causing difficulties with dynamic programming folding algorithms. This is especially true in the treatment of multiloops.

The multiple traceback extension of dynamic programming algorithms may help to reconcile the conflict between the biochemist and the mathematician. The fill algorithm can be executed using the BP set of energy rules and by assigning linear destabilizing energies to multiloops. This can be done rigorously and efficiently in $O(N^3)$ time. The multiple traceback algorithm can then be executed to yield perhaps several hundred to several thousand alternate structures. This is far more than a human would want to examine, but it is nothing for a computer. The energies of each structure could then be recomputed using arbitrarily complicated revised energy rules designed by a biochemist, and the structures could be sorted according to the new energies. This last part is not a rigorous procedure, but if the more complicated energy rules do not differ radically from the BP set, there is reason to hope that a structure close to the minimum revised energy will be found.

ACKNOWLEDGMENTS

The secondary structure displays in Figures 1, 2, 4, 6, and 8 were produced using the DRAW program of Shapiro and Maizel. I wish to thank J. M. Ridgeway for creating the dot plot display program on short notice and for assistance in proofreading.

REFERENCES

1. **Kim, S. H., Suddath, F. L., Quigley, G. J., McPherson, A., Sussman, J. L., Wang, A. H. J., Seeman, N. C., and Rich, A.**, Three-dimensional tertiary structure of yeast phenylalanine transfer RNA, *Science,* 185, 435, 1974.

2. **Trifonov, E. N. and Bolshoi, G.,** Open and closed 5S ribosomal RNA, the only two universal structures encoded in the nucleotide sequences, *J. Mol. Biol.,* 169, 1, 1983.

3. **Nussinov, R., Pieczenik, G., Griggs, J. R., and Kleitman, D. J.,** Algorithms for loop matchings, *SIAM J. Appl. Math.,* 35, 68, 1978.

4. **Sankoff, D., Kruskal, J. B., and Mainville, S., and Cedergren, R. J.,** Fast algorithms to determine RNA secondary structures containing multiple loops, in *Time Warps, String Edits, and Macromolecules: The Theory and Practice of Sequence Comparison,* Sankoff, D. and Kruskal, J. B., Eds., Addison-Wesley, Reading, Mass., 1983, 93.

5. **Zuker, M. and Sankoff, D.,** RNA secondary structures and their prediction, *Bull. Math. Biol.,* 46, 591, 1984.

6. **Fresco, J. R., Alberts, B. M., and Doty, P.,** Some molecular details of the secondary structure of ribonucleic acid, *Nature (London),* 188, 98, 1960.

7. **Tinoco, I., Jr., Uhlenbeck, O. C., and Levine, M. D.,** Estimation of secondary structure in ribonucleic acids, *Nature (London),* 230, 362, 1971.

8. **Fink, T. R. and Crothers, D. M.,** Free energy of imperfect nucleic acid helices. I. The bulge defect, *J. Mol. Biol.,* 66, 1, 1972.

9. **Uhlenbeck, O. C., Borer, P. N., Dengler, B., and Tinoco, I.,** Stability of RNA hairpin loops: A_6-C_m-U_6, *J. Mol. Biol.,* 73, 483, 1973.

10. **Gralla, J. and Crothers, D. M.,** Free energy of imperfect nucleic acid helices. II. Small hairpin loops, *J. Mol. Biol.,* 73, 497, 1973.

11. **Gralla, J. and Crothers, D. M.,** Free energy of imperfect nucleic acid helices. III. Small internal loops resulting from mismatches, *J. Mol. Biol.,* 78, 301, 1973.

12. **Tinoco, I., Jr., Borer, P. N., Dengler, B., Levine, M. D., Uhlenbeck, O. C., Crothers, D. M., and Gralla, J.,** Improved estimation of secondary structure in ribonucleic acids, *Nature (London) New Biol.,* 246, 40, 1973.

13. **Borer, P. N., Dengler, B., Tinoco, I., Jr., and Uhlenbeck, O. C.,** Stability of ribonucleic acid double-stranded helices, *J. Mol. Biol.,* 86, 843, 1974.

14. **Salser, W.,** Globin messenger-RNA sequences — analysis of base-pairing and evolutionary implications, *Cold Spring Harbor Symp. Quant. Biol.,* 42, 985, 1977.

15. **Cech, T. R., Tanner, N. K., Tinoco, I., Jr., Weir, B. R., Zuker, M., and Perlman, P. S.,** Secondary structure of the tetrahymena ribosomal RNA intervening sequence: structural homology with fungal mito-chondrial intervening sequences, *Proc. Natl. Acad. Sci. U.S.A.,* 80, 3903, 1983.

16. **Papanicolaou, C., Gouy, M., and Ninio, J.,** An energy model that predicts the correct folding of both the tRNA and the 5S RNA molecules, *Nucl. Acids Res.,* 12, 31, 1984.

17. **Steger, C., Hofmann, H., Förtsch, B., Gross, H. J., Randles, J. W., Sänger, H. L., and Riesner, D.,** Conformational transitions in viroids and virusoids: comparison of results from energy minimization algorithm and from experimental data, *J. Biomol. Struct. Dyn.,* 2(3), 543, 1984.

18. **Ninio, J.,** Prediction of pairing schemes in RNA molecules — loop contributions and energy of wobble and non-wobble pairs, *Biochimie,* 61, 1133, 1979.

19. **Gouy, M., Marliere, P., Papanicolaou, C., and Ninio, J.,** Prédiction des structures secondaires dans les acides nucléiques: aspects algorithmiques et physiques, *Biochemie,* 67, 523, 1985.

20. **Waterman, M. S.,** Secondary structure of single-stranded nucleic acids, in *Studies in Foundations and Combinatorics, Advances in Mathematics Supplementary Studies,* Vol. 1, Academic Press, New York, 1978, 167.

21. **Pipas, J. M. and McMahon, J. E.,** Method for predicting RNA secondary structure, *Proc. Natl. Acad. Sci. U.S.A.,* 72, 2017, 1975.

22. **Tremblay, J.-P. and Sorenson, P. G.,** *An Introduction to Data Structures with Applications,* McGraw-Hill, New York, 1984.

23. **Ornstein, R. L. and Fresco, J. R.,** Correlation of T_m, sequence, and ΔH of complementary RNA helices and comparison with DNA helices, *Biopolymers,* 22, 2001, 1983.

24. **Waterman, M. S. and Smith, T. F.,** Rapid dynamic programming algorithms for RNA secondary structure, *Adv. Appl. Math.,* 7(4), 455, 1986.

25. **Zuker, M. and Stiegler, P.,** Optimal computer folding of large RNA sequences using thermodynamics and auxiliary information, *Nucl. Acids Res.,* 9, 133, 1981.

26. **Mills, D. R., Kramer, F. R., and Spiegelman, S.,** Complete nucleotide sequence of a replicating RNA molecule, *Science,* 180, 916, 1973.

27. **Stiegler, P., Carbon, P., Zuker, M., Ebel, J.-P., and Ehresmann, C.,** Structural organization of the 16S ribosomal RNA from *E. coli.* Topography and secondary structure, *Nucl. Acids Res.,* 9, 2153, 1981.

28. **Vary, C. P. H. and Vournakis, J. N.,** RNA structure analysis using methidiumpropyl-EDTA.Fe(II): a base-pair specific RNA structure probe, *Proc. Natl. Acad. Sci. U.S.A.,* 81(22), 6978, 1984.

29. **Riesner, D., Colpan, M., Goodman, T. C., Nagel, L., Schumacher, J., Steger, G., and Hofmann, H.,** Dynamics and interactions of viroids, *J. Biomol. Struct. Dyn.,* 1, 669, 1983.

30. **Zuker, M.,** RNA folding prediction: the continued need for interaction between biologists and mathematicians, *Lect. Math. Life Sci.,* 17, 1986.

31. **Waterman, M. S.,** Sequence alignments in the neighborhood of the optimum with general application to dynamic programming, *Proc. Natl. Acad. Sci. U.S.A.,* 80, 3123, 1983.

32. **Waterman, M. S. and Byers, T. H.,** A dynamic programming algorithm to find all solutions in a neighborhood of the optimum, *Math. Biosci.,* 77, 179, 1985.

33. **Williams, A. L., Jr. and Tinoco, I., Jr.,** A dynamic programming algorithm for finding alternative RNA secondary structures, *Nucl. Acids Res.,* 14(1), 299, 1986.

34. **Stiegler, P., Carbon, P., Ebel, J.-P., and Ehresmann, C.,** A general secondary structure model for procaryotic and eucaryotic RNAs of the small ribosomal subunits, *Eur. J. Biochem.,* 120, 487, 1981.

35. **Sankoff, D.,** Simultaneous solution of the RNA folding, alignment and protosequence problems, *SIAM J. Appl. Math.,* 45, 810, 1985.

36. **Turner, D. H.,** personal communication.

Chapter 8

CONSENSUS METHODS FOR FOLDING SINGLE-STRANDED NUCLEIC ACIDS

Michael S. Waterman

TABLE OF CONTENTS

I. INTRODUCTION

As the preceding chapter[1] has explained, the structure of single-stranded RNA macromolecules is crucial to the functioning of an organism. While it has recently become routine to directly read the primary structure of these molecules by sequencing techniques, the deduction of secondary and tertiary structure is much less straightforward. The secondary structure of DNA is well known: DNA is double-stranded according to the familiar Watson-Crick rules. Double-stranded DNA has alternate double helical structures. The classic B- and A-forms are both right-handed helixes while the Z-form is left-handed.[2,3] RNA has base-pairing rules corresponding to those for DNA; T in DNA is replaced by U so that base A pairs U (A*U) and base G pairs C (G*C). The pair G*U is usually added to this list. The fact that RNA occurs frequently as single-stranded often makes the secondary structure of RNA difficult to determine. Segments of the sequence will form base pairs between them, and the prediction of the resulting structure is a difficult task. Obviously the resulting structure — the folded molecule — is highly dependent on the specific linear sequence of the RNA.

It is quite surprising, to a mathematician at least, that biologists have been so successful at predicting some important secondary structures. In fact, the first primary (linear) sequence of a tRNA (transfer RNA) appeared in 1965[4] along with the cloverleaf form of secondary structure. This turned out to be the correct structure and has been verified by X-ray crystallography.[5] Other than by guessing or inspection, there seem to be two major techniques for prediction of secondary structure: the minimum energy method and the comparative method. The previous chapter gives an extensive treatment of the important minimum energy method, which utilizes dynamic programming. After briefly discussing the minimum energy approach we turn to the main topic of this chapter, comparative or consensus analysis of folding.

In an important paper Tinoco et al.[6] proposed assigning free energies to the components of secondary structure — the various base pairs, end loops, bulges, interior loops, and multibranch loops — and then finding the minimum free energy secondary structure. To accomplish this task they presented the base pairing matrix for an RNA, which is the analog of the dot matrix for sequence matching. One difficulty with fully implementing their proposal is the huge number of possible secondary structures. The number of configurations has been studied,[7] and it was found that for sequences of length 150, allowing end loops of two bases or more, there are 1.22×10^{54} possible secondary structures. Now this number counts all conceivable structures, and the base pairing of a given sequence reduces the number somewhat, but the point remains. There are too many candidate structures to simply consider them all and take the one with minimum free energy.

In 1978, two dynamic programming methods were proposed to solve this problem. Waterman[8] and Waterman and Smith[9] used general energy functions and, in an iterative fashion, built up the complexity of the optimal structures. Nussinov et al.[10] maximized the number of base pairs in a single pass algorithm. The advantages of both of these methods have been combined into a useful, efficient algorithm described in the preceding chapter.[1]

Some of the shortcomings of the minimum energy methods are (1) the lack of precise knowledge about the energy functions themselves, (2) the large amount of computer time required, and (3) the inability of the current algorithms to handle many sequences simultaneously. Item 3 is really a subcategory of 2, since computer time and storage is the main difficulty in 3. Sankoff[11] has an algorithm to simultaneously fold and align several sequences; three sequences seem to be an upper limit, but the ability to both fold and align several sequences is an important problem. To overcome these difficulties, it is instructive to take a careful look at some of the successful work of biologists who study these problems.

In a remarkable 1969 paper, Levitt[12] obtained a cloverleaf model that fit all the 14 tRNA sequences known at that time. He almost certainly obtained his consensus structure by

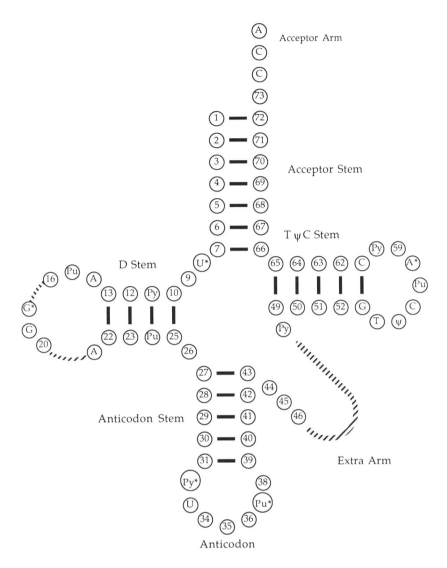

FIGURE 1. The cloverleaf structure of tRNA. The nucleotide positions are numbered, or whenever a position is conserved, the identity is indicated. Dashed lines indicate nucleotides that may or may not be present in any given molecule.

arranging the sequences by hand into an alignment in which helixes and homologies (identical bases) were represented. Later, the structure was largely confirmed by crystallography.[5] Essentially the same pattern of helix and homology is shown in Figure 1 where a so-called universal cloverleaf is shown.[13] The over 300 known tRNA sequences[14] fit this general structure, and we now discuss it in some detail.

The meaning of Figure 1 is that all known tRNA sequences can be arranged into an alignment with positions labeled as in the figure. The appearance of a base pair, between 1 and 72, for example, means that whatever the identity of the bases labeled 1 and 72, they form a base pair. The sequences end in CCA; this triplet has been conserved, independent of any base pairing. Actually the "universals" are in some positions violated by 5 to 10% of tRNA sequences. The variation in sequence length makes structure prediction and/or alignment a fascinating and difficult problem. The D arm varies in length by up to 4 bases, while the so-called extra arm varies in length by up to 18 bases. Therefore, the alignment is not simply given by shifts of the primary sequence, but must be found by inserting gaps into the sequences. Notice the large number of conserved bases in the interior of the sequence. Positions 53, 54, 55, and 56 are GUUC, the longest conserved sequence in the structure. In total, 14 of the bases of tRNA are conserved in the alphabet {A,U,G,C}, while 8 more are conserved in the Purine = Pu and Prymadine = Py alphabet, {Pu, Py}.

Let us take a brief look at the magnitude of the problem of sequence alignment, which we must solve to put the sequences into correspondence. The tRNA sequences can differ in length by as much as 20 bases. If there are R sequences and we want to look at them in all possible arrangements, not allowing gaps within the sequences, there are a minimum of $(20 + 1)^R$ possible arrangements. If R = 14, as was Levitt's situation, $(21)^{14} \approx 3.24 \times 10^{18}$. If R = 32, as in the example of this chapter, $(21)^{32} \approx 2.05 \times 10^{42}$. If R = 150, a reasonable number of tRNA sequences, $(21)^{150} \approx 2.15 \times 10^{198}$. In none of these cases is it possible to exhaustively consider all alignments on any modern computer. Allowing gaps from 1 to 20 letters only increases these numbers by many orders of magnitude. Even with no gaps and only R = 14 sequences, a direct approach to alignment is computationally hopeless. Clearly, the approach of considering all alignments individually is not feasible, even for the smallest cases of interest.

The approach of inferring structure by common (conserved) features, helixes, or homologous bases, has come to be known as the comparative or phylogenetic method. Features in rRNA (ribosomal RNA) essential to organisms must be conserved in evolution, and it is hoped that these features will be recognized as common in the sequences studied. For example, the CCA at the 5' end of tRNA is involved in the interaction between tRNA and the amino acids. By locating CCA in a tRNA sequence, we obtain valuable information about the location of the acceptor stem. Levitt's approach was based on these ideas.

After tRNA, the next RNA molecule for which this method was used was 5S rRNA, which is about 120 bases in length. Fox and Woese[15] and Nishikawa and Takemura[16] solved the structure after many attempts by investigators using other approaches. There is no crystallographic data for this molecule, but biochemical and physiochemical evidence support the structure. (See Waterman[17] for a consensus approach to folding 34 5S rRNA sequences on a computer.) The difficulties of unequal sequence lengths exist with 5S sequences also. A study of Trifonov and Bolshoi[18] studies 5S folding by a related method which has some drawbacks. First, the sequences must be aligned, a difficult problem in itself. Then the base pair matrix[6] for each sequence is obtained. The matrixes are summed and possible helixes appear as dark, antidiagonal regions. The methods presented in this chapter directly consider the helixes.

The next larger rRNA, 16S, and 16S-like molecules posed new difficulties for investigators, due in part to the greater sequence length of approximately 1540 bases. As in 5S sequences, bulge loops, interior loops, and noncanonical base pairs (those other than A*U or G*C) appear in 16S structures. As with 5S structure, 16S structure has been solved by the comparative method. The work was mainly done by three groups, and it is this work, notably that of Woese and Noller,[19,20] that provided the motivation and inspiration for this chapter (see also References 21, 22, and 23). The model of Woese and Noller and collaborators[24] for 16S rRNA of *Escherichia coli* is shown in Figure 2: These authors describe their approach[19] as progressing with alignment of 16S-like rRNA sequences in parallel with the development and testing of the secondary structure model. Preliminary alignments are then used to identify obvious primary and secondary structure features; these patterns are used as the basis for refinement of the sequence alignment. The procedure is then iterated, and new sequence information incorporated as it is obtained.

It is the goal of this chapter (1) to make some of the Noller-Woese procedures explicitly defined so that other groups can see exactly what the corresponding computer searches are, (2) to find efficient computer methods to perform the searches, and (3) to give some estimates

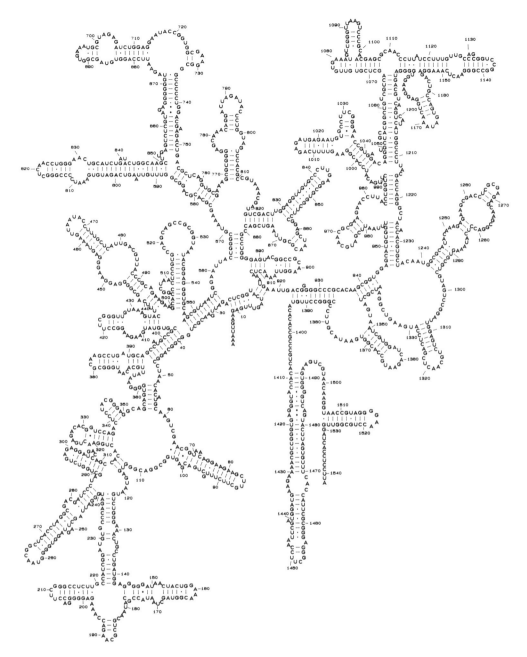

FIGURE 2. Secondary structure of *E. coli* 16S RNA. (Taken from Moazed, D., Stern, S., and Noller, H., *J. Mol. Biol.*, 187, 399, 1986. With permission.)

of statistical significance. The philosophy beneath the comparative method is that important features, such as specific bases or helixes, have been conserved over the course of RNA evolution and that these conserved features are still utilized by the organism. Our task is to make this approach into an algorithm.

For illustrative purposes we will study the set of 32 *E. coli* tRNA sequences whose names appear in Table 1. Since some of the sequences have the extra arm, the variation in length is from 74 to 93 bases. Several other interesting features arise. For example, the acceptor stem is shifted one base from the "universal" structure in the sequence of histidine tRNA. While tRNAs are the shortest RNA sequences we have discussed, they will serve well for

Table 1
THE 32 *E. COLI* tRNA SEQUENCE
NAMES WITH THE GenBank
ABBREVIATIONS

ala tRNA;	ECOTRA1A
ala tRNA;	ECOTRA1B
cys tRNA;	ECOTRC
asp tRNA;	ECOTRD1
glu tRNA;	ECOTRE1
glu tRNA;	ECOTRE2
phe tRNA;	ECOTRF
gly tRNA;	ECOTRG1
gly tRNA;	ECOTRG2
gly tRNA;	ECOTRG3
his tRNA;	ECOTRH1
ile tRNA;	ECOTRI1
ile tRNA;	ECOTRI2
lys tRNA;	ECOTRK
leu tRNA;	ECOTRL1
leu tRNA;	ECOTRL2
leu tRNA;	ECTORL5
initiator	ECOTRMF
met tRNA;	
met tRNA;	ECOTRM
asn tRNA;	ECOTRN
gln tRNA;	ECOTRQ1
gln tRNA;	ECOTRQ2
arg tRNA;	ECOTRR1
arg tRNA;	ECOTRR2
ser tRNA;	ECOTRS1
ser tRNA;	ECOTRS3
thr tRNA;	ECOTRTACU
val tRNA;	ECOTRV1
val tRNA;	ECOTRV2A
val tRNA;	ECOTRV2B
trp tRNA;	ECOTRW

illustration. Both 16S and 23S are too long with which to easily illustrate the algorithms, although even with their greater length they are still computationally feasible. 16S has about 1540 bases while 23S[25] has about 2500 bases. As will be seen, tRNAs are quite suitable for our purposes, being of manageable size and of sufficient difficulty of folding. Dynamic programming methods are reputed to fold approximately half of the tRNA sequences into a cloverleaf structure. Consensus methods, as will be seen, fold all *E. coli* tRNAs into the correct cloverleaf shape. In addition, tertiary structure can be studied by the same methods.

II. ALIGNMENT BY MATCHES

In earlier chapters on alignment by Karlin[26] and Waterman,[27] the authors discussed finding statistically significant matches between sequences. The motivation for that work is the hope that statistically significant matches between sequences will be biologically significant. In the setting of this chapter, there are several conserved (or "invariant" or "universal") sequences in tRNA. In Figure 1, we notice that the longest universal pattern is GTTC. In our data we will see that with a few exceptions this pattern is contained in a longer five letter pattern GGTTC, beginning at base 52 in the figure. The acceptor arm pattern of CCA is also present in all sequences. Several other one and two letter patterns can be seen on examining Figure 1.

There are several reasons for being interested in these invariant patterns. Their presence has been conserved over evolutionary time, and this gives us some reason to believe they are essential to the functioning of tRNA. Our basic reason for study of these data sets is to deduce structure, function, and evolution of the macromolecules. As an aid in deducing the structure, then, finding significant invariant patterns could be essential in deducing the correct alignment of the data set. While no shifting is necessary to find GGTTC if the sequences are already aligned on their right ends, such shifting into the correct alignment could allow us to locate other smaller patterns, as well as base pairing which might otherwise be undetectable. This turns out to be the case with 16S RNA.[20]

It is now time to ask some hard questions. What is the basis for concluding that such patterns are universal? The flaw in looking at a data set until a pattern is seen and then concluding it is significant has often led scientists to incorrect conclusions. Exactly what search is performed to find these patterns? Are other significant patterns missed in Figure 1? How is statistical significance to be estimated? These important questions are addressed in the remainder of this section.

A. Finding Matches

In the search for matches, our program simply finds all patterns of a specified length that occur at or above a present frequency in a specified section (column "a" to column "b") with the sequences arranged in some alignment. Even if a sequence, GTTC for instance, occurs several times within a single sequence, it is only counted once. For small data sets such as the tRNAs, to find k-letter (k-mer) repeats it is sufficient to make a table of all k-mers occurring in the sequence ($k \leq 9$) with their frequencies and then check to see which occur at the required frequency. The search for k-mer repeats can evidently be performed in time proportional to the number of letters (N say) in all sequences with storage bounded by $O(4^k)$. If the common sequences are longer, then the techniques of hashing allow the search to be done in NlogN time (see Martinez[28] for a useful algorithm to find repeats in molecular sequences by hashing). Thus it is seen that the search for common patterns is not computationally difficult in these problems. In these cases, we are interested in exact matches only.

B. Statistical Significance

1. The Log(n) Distribution

Estimates of statistical significance of matches are more difficult than finding the matches and were not well understood until recently. The model we study here is R sequences of length N that have iid (independent, identically distributed) letters. The event for which we calculate significance levels is that of finding a pattern of length k common to L of R sequences. First we present results for the case $N \to \infty$. In Chapter 3, the case of $R = L = 2$ is discussed with extensions to imperfect matchings, while in Chapter 6, extensions to larger R and L are given. We give the simplest of these extensions here. Let $p = P(X_1 = X_2 \ldots = X_L)$ where X_i, the letters in the sequences, are iid. If the alphabet has four equally likely letters, $p = 4(1/4)^L = (1/4)^{L-1}$. Let $M(R,L) =$ length of the longest pattern common to at least L of the R sequences. Then,

$$E(M(R, L)) \approx \log(\binom{R}{L}N^L) + \log(1 - p) + \gamma\log(e) - 1/2$$

and

$$Var(M(R, L)) = \sigma^2 \approx (\pi \log(e))^2/6 + 1/12$$

where

$$\log = \log_{1/p} \quad \text{and} \quad \gamma \approx .0577$$

For the R = 32 sequences of length $\approx 75 = N$, take L = 32 as well. If the letters are equally likely, $p = (1/4)^{31}$ and

$$E(M(32, 32)) \approx 3.1144 \ldots + 0.0134 \ldots - 0.5$$

$$= 2.6278 \ldots$$

and

$$\sigma^2 = 0.0842 \ldots$$

with

$$\sigma = 0.2902 \ldots$$

Therefore, $4 = k$ is almost 5 standard deviations above E(M), and this k is achieved in our sequences by the word GTTC.

2. The Binomial Distribution and Large Deviations

A glance at the locations of the pattern GTTC in the data set aligned as shown in Figure 5 brings up an interesting second question. The pattern occurs perfectly aligned in the figure as well as in some other locations. What is the significance of such a pattern of occurrence with little shifting? That is, in the case $N << \infty$. In Figure 5, we could take $k = W = 4$ and discover the pattern, where W is the width of the window in which the search is being performed.

For ease of exposition, take the case of equally likely letters of RNA. Then, if w is a k-letter sequence,

$$\alpha = P(w \text{ occurs in N letters})$$

$$= P\left(\bigcup_{i=1}^{W-k+1} \{w \text{ starts at } i\} \right) \leq (W - k + 1)(1/4)^4$$

The probability that w occurs in exactly L of R sequences is given by the binomial probability

$$\binom{R}{L}\alpha^L(1 - \alpha)^{R-L} \approx \binom{R}{L}(W - k + 1)^L(1/4)^{kL}(1 - (W - k + 1)(1/4)^k)^{R-L}$$

and, summing over all 4^k possible w, the desired probability is

$$\binom{R}{L}(W - k + 1)^L(1/4)^{k(L-1)}(1 - (W - k + 1)(1/4)^k)^{R-L}$$

For small R and L, this formula can be directly used to estimate significance. Otherwise we use the large deviations theory described next.

Now define $\beta = L/R$. If $\beta \leq \alpha$ and R is large, the strong law of large numbers assures us that we will have approximately $\alpha R \geq \beta R = L$ occurrences. Otherwise, when $\beta > \alpha$, a bound for the probability of a k-letter word common to at least L of R sequences is given by the large deviations estimate.[29-31]

The estimate is given by

Table 2
ESTIMATES OF STATISTICAL
SIGNIFICANCE FOR APPEARANCE OF SOME
k-LETTER WORD IN SOME WINDOW
POSITION AND IN AT LEAST L OF R = 32
SEQUENCES OF LENGTH N = 75

k	L	W	α	β	$H(\alpha,\beta)$	p
4	20	50	0.184	0.625	0.474	1.73×10^{-3}
4	24	75	0.281	0.75	0.472	7.14×10^{-5}
6	10	75	0.171	0.313	0.662	2.55×10^{-6}
7	7	75	0.004	0.188	0.547	4.17×10^{-4}

$$4^k \exp\{- RH(\alpha, \beta)\}$$

where $H(\alpha,\beta) = \beta\log\beta/\alpha + (1 - \beta)\log(1 - \beta)/(1 - \alpha)$. The factor of 4^k is to count the number of possible w. This quantity approximates the probability that some k-letter word is common to at least L of R sequences of length N. If a window of width W is placed in all $N - W + 1$ possible positions, then the estimate becomes

$$(N - W + 1)4^k \exp\{-RH(\alpha, \beta)\},$$

where $\alpha = P(w$ occurs in W letters).

Some sample estimates appear in Table 2. Finding some four letter word common to 24 of 32 sequences of length $N = 75$ will only happen with the probability of 7.15×10^{-5}. In our sequences, we find the word $w(=GTTC)$ in all 32 sequences perfectly aligned, a highly unlikely event!

III. ALIGNMENT BY BASE PAIRING

While alignment by matches common to many sequences is a very useful procedure, the striking feature of rRNA data sets is commonality of base pairing. The most conserved features in Figure 1 are not conserved letters, but conserved base pairs (bp) or helixes. The aminoacyl stem is a helix of 7 bp, while the TψC stem and the anticodon stem have 5 bp, and the D stem has 4 bp.

All of the invariant helixes are, in our data set, composed of differing sequences. The common feature is that a helix of the required length can be formed with a relatively small amount of shifting of individual sequences.

A. Finding Helixes

We have chosen the following implementation for our search for variant or consensus helixes. Position two nonoverlapping windows of width W on the data set, at a distance or separation of ℓ apart. Let k be the desired helix length where $k \leq W$. Then find the location of the best (if any) helix (or helixes if more than one exists) in each sequence within the specified windows. "Mismatches" correspond to interior loops, while the insertion/deletions of letters correspond to bulges. Usually we will simply search for helixes of some length with a specified amount of mispairing (mismatches). The score for a given window position is the sum of the scores for each sequence. We score a helix by the number of base pairs divided by helix length.

To do a full search of the data for length k helixes in windows of width W, we let ℓ, the separation between windows, vary from $\ell = 0$, where there are $N - 2W + 1$ window

Table 3
ESTIMATES OF STATISTICAL SIGNIFICANCE
p FOR APPEARANCE OF CONSENSUS BASE
PAIRING (k-LETTER HELICES) BETWEEN
TWO WINDOWS OF WIDTH W IN AT LEAST L
OF R = 32 SEQUENCES OF LENGTH N = 75

k	L	W	α	β	H(α,β)	p
4	16	8	0.010	0.500	0.521	1.29×10^{-4}
5	10	6	0.035	0.313	0.450	1.21×10^{-3}
6	16	25	0.010	0.500	0.521	7.23×10^{-5}
7	8	25	0.002	0.250	0.408	2.71×10^{-3}

positions, to $\ell = N - 2W$ where exactly one window position is possible. This causes any such search to take $O(N^2)$ time, where W and k are fixed.

B. Statistical Significance

Once again, it is natural to ask about the significance level of found base pairing patterns. Fortunately the work of the last section can easily be carried over.

The large deviation formulas for statistical significance go as follows. We have R sequences of length N, with a window width W and word size k. The probability α of finding a k letter helix in a given sequence with fixed window positions is

$$\alpha \cong (W - k + 1)^2 (1/4)^k$$

since there are $(W - k + 1)$ distinct ways to find the helix location in each window. As above, we want to find a helix at least L of the R sequences. If $\beta = L/R$ and $\beta > \alpha$, the estimate of statistical significance is

$$p = \frac{(N - W)(N - (W + 1))}{2} \exp\{ -RH(\alpha, \beta)\}$$

The coefficient of exp{ }, $\binom{N-W}{2}$, in the above equation counts window positions in sequences of length N. For our data set, Table 3 gives some relevant estimates.

Consensus alignment of many RNA sequences is, in principle, a simple straightforward procedure at this point. However, writing usable computer programs is a major problem and, in addition, there are many difficulties encountered in the analysis of actual sequences. Therefore, we illustrate this analysis by folding our set of tRNA sequences.

IV. FOLDING tRNAs

As emphasized in earlier sections, alignment and folding are interrelated problems. To fold a set of tRNAs, we need a strategy for approaching the problem. Not only are there dependencies between alignment and folding, but also dependencies within both operations of alignment and folding. In folding, for example, there are conflicts between different length helixes as well as quality (number of bulges and interior loops) of helixes. We approach these problems by first locating long (statistically significant) matches between the sequences. Then we locate common patterns of base pairing.

A. tRNA Alignment by Matches

We first explore alignment by matches. Recall from Section II that while a 4-mer is common to all 32 of our sequences (W = 75), the expected length of pattern common to

```
        80        70        60        50        40        30        20        10
8765432109876543210987654321098765432109876543210987654321098765432109876543210987654321
         GGGGGCATAGCTCAGCTGGGAGAGCGCCTGCTTTGCACGCAGGAGGTCTGCGgttcgaTCCCGCGCGCTCCCACCA
         GGGGCTATAGCTCAGCTGGGAGAGCGCCTGCTTTGCACGCAGGAGGTCTGCGgttcgaTCCCGCATAGCTCCACCA
          GGCGCGTTAACAAAGCGGTTATGTAGCGGATTGCAAATCCGTCTAGTCCGgttcgaCTCCGGAACGCGCCTCCA
        GGAGCGGTAGTTCAGTCGGTTAGAATACCTGCCTGTCACGCAGGGGGTCGCGGgttcgaGTCCCGTCCGTTCCGCCA
        GTCCCCTTCGTCTAGAGGCCCAGGACACCGCCCTTTCACGGCGGTAACAGGGgttcgaATCCCCTGGGGGACGCCA
        GTCCCCTTCGTCTAGAGGCCCAGGACACCGCCCTTTCACGGCGGTAACAGGGgttcgaATCCCCTAGGGGACGCCA
        GCCCGGATAGCTCAGTCGGTAGAGCAGGGGATTGAAAATCCCCGTGTCCTTGgttcgaTTCCGAGTCCGGGCACCA
         GCGGGCGTAGTTCAATGGTAGAACGAGAGCTTCCCAAGCTCTATACGAGGgttcgaTTCCCTTCGCCCGCTCCA
         GCGGGCATCGTATAATGGCTATTACCTCAGCCTTCCAAGCTGATGATGCGGgttcgaTTCCCGCTGCCCGCTCCA
        GCGGGAATAGCTCAGTTGGTAGAGCACGACCTTGCCAAGGTCGGGGTCGCGAgttcgaTCTCGTTTCCCGCTCCA
        GGTGGCTATAGCTCAGTTGGTAGAGCCCTGGATTGTGATTCCAGTTGTCGTGGgttcgaATCCCATTAGCCACCCCA
        AGGCTTGTAGCTCAGGTGGTTAGAGCGCACCCCTGATAAGGGTGAGGTCGGTGGTTCAAGTCCACTCAGGCCTACCA
        GGCCCCTTAGCTCAGTGGTTAGAGCAAGCGACTGATAATCGCTTGGTCGCTGGTTCAAGTCCAGCAGGGGCCACCA
        GGGTCGTTAGCTCAGTTGGTAGAGCAGTTGACTTTTAATCAATTGGTCGCAGgttcgaATCCTGCACGACCCACCA
  GCGAAGGTGGCGGAATTGGTAGACGCGCTAGCTTCAGGTGTTAGTGTCCTTACGGACGTGGGGGTTCAAGTCCCCCCTCGCACCA
  GCCGAGGTGGTGGAATTGGTAGACACGCTACCTTGAGGTGGTAGTGCCCAATAGGGCTTACGGGTTCAAGTCCCGTCCTCGGTACCA
  GCCCGGATGGTGGAATCGGTAGACACAAGGGATTAAAAATCCCTCGGCGTTCGCGCTGTGCGGGTTCAAGTCCCGCTCCGGGTACCA
         CGCGGGGTGGAGCAGCCTGGTAGCTCGTCGGGCTCATAACCCGAAGGTCGTCGGTTCAAATCCGGCCCCCGCAACCA
        GGCTACGTAGCTCAGTTGGTTAGAGCACATCACTCATAATGATGGGGTCACAGgttcgaATCCCGTCGTAGCCACCA
        TCCTCTGTAGTTCAGTCGGTAGAACGCGGGACTGTTAATCCGTATGTCACTGgttcgaGTCCAGTCAGAGGAGCCA
       TGGGGTATCGCCAAGCGGTAAGGCACCGGTTTTTGATACCGGCATTCCCTGgttcgaATCCAGGTACCCCAGCCA
       TGGGGTATCGCCAAGCGGTAAGGCACCGGATTCTGATTCCGGCATTCCGAGgttcgaATCCTCGTACCCCAGCCA
        GCATCCGTAGCTCAGCTGGTAGAGTACTCGGCTGCGAACCGAGCGGTCGGAGgttcgaATCCTCCCGGATGCACCA
        GCATCCGTAGCTCAGCTGGTAGAGTACTCGGCTGCGAACCGAGCGGTCGGAGgttcgaATCCTCCCGGATGCACCA
  GGAAGTGTGGCCGAGCGGTTGAAGGCACCGGTCTTGAAAACCGGCGACCCGAAAGGGTTCAGAgttcgaATCTCTGCGCTTCCGCCA
  GGTGGCCGAGAGGCTGAAGGCGCTCCCCTGCTAAGGGAGTATGCGGTCAAAAGCTGCATCCGGGgttcgaATCCCCGCCTCACCGCCA
        GCTGATATAGCTCAGTTGGTAGAGCGCACCCTTGGTAAGGGTGAGGTCGGCAgttcgaATCTGCCTATCAGCACCA
        GGGTGATTAGCTCAGCTGGGAGAGCACCTCCCTTACAAGGAGGGGGTCGGCGgttcgaTCCCGTCATCACCCACCA
        GCGTCCGTAGCTCAGTTGGTTAGAGCACCACCTTGACATGGTGGGGGTCGGTGgttcgaGTCCCATCGGACGCACCA
        GCGTTCATAGCTCAGTTGGTTAGAGCACCACCTTGACATGGTGGGGGTCGTTGgttcgaGTCCAATTGAACGCACCA
        AGGGGCGTAGTTCAATTGGTAGAACACCGGTCTCCAAAACCGGGTGTTGGGAgttcgaGTCTCTCCGCCCCTGCCA
        GGTGGGGTTCCCGAGCGGCCAAAGGGAGCAGACTGTAAATCTGCCGTCATCGACTTCGAAGgttcgaATCCTTCCCCCACCACCA
```
```

FIGURE 3.   The six letter pattern gttcga is common to 26 of 32 *E. coli* tRNA sequences. It is the most frequent six letter word.

all 32 was ≈ 2.6. Therefore, without decreasing the window size, we should not consider any pattern less than four letters long. What pattern length k should we begin with? Our approach is to start with larger k and work down to smaller k. The results for k = 6 appear in Figure 3 where gttcga appears in 26 of the 32 sequences. The sequences generally appear as upper case while the patterns we locate appear in lower case. The sequences are right justified in order to highlight these found matches, and the following results support such an alignment. With k = 5, the most common word is ggttc, which is found in 29 sequences and overlaps gttcga in every location where the latter sequence occurs (see Figure 4). Additionally ggttc occurs once upstream (5′ or left) of its "canonical" location. In Figure 5, the results for k = 4 are displayed and ggtc is found 32 times, perfectly aligned when the sequences are right justified. Even for k = 3, shown in Figure 6, the 3-mers which are common to all 32 sequences include only subpatterns of ggttcg and cca. Each of these patterns are included in the invariant "positions" of Figure 1, ggttcg(a) being in the TψC loop and cca being the acceptor arm pattern.

Of course, the positions in Figure 1 are the result of an alignment and provide a template for future investigators to fit tRNA sequences to. Here we have set ourselves the task of producing alignment and folding without a template with which to align or fold. Using matches we have now aligned the sequences on what is actually the known TψC loop. Now we turn to finding common folding patterns.

## B. tRNA Alignment by Base Pairing

In Section III, we gave a general description of the procedures to be employed in this section. Here we must present output from our program (fold), and we are required to be
```

```
      80        70        60        50        40        30        20        10
765432109876543210987654321098765432109876543210987654321098765432109876543210987654321

          GGGGGCATAGCTCAGCTGGGAGAGCGCCTGCTTTGCACGCAGGAGGTCTGCggttcGATCCCGCGCGCTCCCACCA
          GGGGCTATAGCTCAGCTGGGAGAGCGCCTGCTTTGCACGCAGGAGGTCTGCggttcGATCCCGCATAGCTCCACCA
          GGCGCGTTAACAAAGCGGTTATGTAGCGGATTGCAAATCCGTCTAGTCCggttcGACTCCGGAACGCGCCTCCA
          GGAGCGGTAGTTCAGTCGGTTAGAATACCTGCCTGTCACGCAGGGGGTCGCGggttcGAGTCCCGTCCGTTCCGCCA
          GTCCCCTTCGTCTAGAGGCCCAGGACACCGCCCTTTCACGGCGGTAACAGGggttcGAATCCCCTGGGGGACGCCA
          GTCCCCTTCGTCTAGAGGCCCAGGACACCGCCCTTTCACGGCGGTAACAGGgggttcGAATCCCCTAGGGGACGCCA
          GCCCGGATAGCTCAGTCGGTAGAGCAGGGGATTGAAAATCCCCGTGTCCTTggttcGATTCCGAGTCCGGGCACCA
          GCGGGCGTAGTTCAATGGTAGAACGAGAGCTTCCCAAGCTCTATACGAGggttcGATTCCCTTCGCCCGCTCCA
          GCGGGCATCGTATAATGGCTATTACCTCAGCCTTCCAAGCTGATGATGCGggttcGATTCCCGCTGCCCGCTCCA
          GCCGGAATAGCTCAGTTGGTAGAGCACGACCTTGCCAAGGTCGGGGTCGCGAGTTCGAGTCTCGTTTCCCGCTCCA
          GGTGGCTATAGCTCAGTTGGTAGAGCCCTGGATTGTGATTCCAGTTGTCGTGggttcGAATCCCATTAGCCACCCCA
          AGGCTTGTAGCTCAGGTGGTTAGAGCGCACCCCTGATAAGGGTGAGGTCGGTggttcAAGTCCACTCAGGCCTACCA
          GGCCCCTTAGCTCAGTGGTTAGAGCAAGCGACTGATAATCGCTTGGTCGCTggttcAAGTCCAGCAGGGGCCACCA
          GGGTCGTTAGCTCAGTTGGTAGAGCAGTTGACTTTTAATCAATTGGTCGCAggttcGAATCCTGCACGACCCACCA
  GCGAAGGTGGCGGAATTGGTAGACGCGCTAGCTTCAGGTGTTAGTGTCCTTACGGACGTGGGggttcAAGTCCCCCCCTCGCACCA
  GCCGAGGTGGTGGAATTGGTAGACACGCTACCTTGAGGTGGTAGTGCCCAATAGGGCTTACGggttcAAGTCCCGTCCTCGGTACCA
  GCCCGGATGGTGGAATCGGTAGACACAAGGGATTAAAAATCCCTCGGCGTTCGCGCTGTGCGggttcAAGTCCCGCTCCGGGTACCA
          CGCGGGGTGGAGCAGCCTGGTAGCTCGTCGGGCTCATAACCCGAAGGTCGTCggttcAAATCCGGCCCCCGCAACCA
          GGCTACGTAGCTCAGTTGGTTAGAGCACATCACTCATAATGATGGGGTCACAggttcGAATCCCGTCGTAGCCACCA
          TCCTCTGTAGTTCAGTCGGTAGAACGGCGGACTGTTAATCCGTATGTCACTggttcGAGTCCAGTCAGAGGAGCCA
          TGGGGTATCGCCAAGCGGTAAGGCACCGGTTTTTGATACCGGCATTCCCTggttcGAATCCAGGTACCCCAGCCA
          TGGGGTATCGCCAAGCGGTAAGGCACCGGATTCTGATTCCGGCATTCCGAggttcGAATCCTCGTACCCCAGCCA
          GCATCCGTAGCTCAGCTGGTAGAGTACTCGGCTGCGAACCGAGCGGTCGGAggttcGAATCCTCCCGGATGCACCA
          GCATCCGTAGCTCAGCTGGATAGAGTACTCGGCTGCGAACCGAGCGGTCGGAggttcGAATCCTCCCGGATGCACCA
  GGAAGTGTGGCCGAGCGGTTGAAGGCACCGGTCTTGAAAACCGGCGACCCGAAAGggttcCAGAGTTCGAATCTCTGCGCTTCCGCCA
  GGTGGCCGAGAGGCTGAAGGCGCTCCCCTGCTAAGGGAGTATGCGGTCAAAAGCTGCATCGGggttcGAATCCCGCCTCACCGCCA
          GCTGATATAGCTCAGTTGGTAGAGCGCACCCTTGGTAAGGGTGAGGTCGGCAGTTCGAATCTGCCTATCAGCACCA
          GGGTGATTAGCTCAGCTGGGAGAGCACCTCCCTTACAAGGAGGGGGTCGGCggttcGATCCCGTCATCACCCACCA
          GCGTCCGTAGCTCAGTTGGTTAGAGCACCACCTTGACATGGTGGGGGTCGGTggttcGAGTCCACTCGGACGCACCA
          GCGTTCATAGCTCAGTTGGTTAGAGCACCACCTTGACATGGTGGGGGTCGTTggttcGAGTCCAATTGAACGCACCA
          AGGGGCGTAGTTCAATTGGTAGAACACCGGTCTCCAAAACCGGGTGTTGGGAGTTCGAGTCTCTCCGCCCCTGCCA
  GGTGGGggttcCCGAGCGGCCAAAGGGAGCAGACTGTAAATCTGCCGTCATCGACTTCGAAGggttcGAATCCTTCCCCCACCACCA
```

FIGURE 4. The five letter pattern ggttc is common to 29 of 32 *E. coli* tRNA sequences. It is the most frequent five letter word.

specific about some details of our computer method. In particular we will first describe how we organize the (approximately) $N - 2W$ graphs of score vs. location of right-hand windows for the (approximately) $N - 2W$ separations of the windows. There are about $(N - 2W)^2/2$ window positions. Initial alignment of the sequences is also considered. Then we illustrate how base pairings found by the program are displayed along with their connections with the associated score graphs. Then we turn to our analysis of tRNA folding.

1. The Score Graphs

To make matters specific, take the window size, $W = 10$, and the helix length, $k = 5$, with the maximum number of allowed mispairs, $mm = 0$. There are approximately $(N - 2W)^2/2$ positions for the two windows. To organize ourselves, we take the horizontal axis to be the position of the rightmost base in the right window for a fixed separation of windows. The vertical axis is score. For the analysis in Figure 7, the sequences are left justified. Each separation is an individual graph. In Figure 7A, all $(N - 2W)$ graphs are superimposed, making a jumbled graph. Figure 7B gives a three-dimensional representation of the data. In Figure 7C, an individual graph is given for window separation 3. This peak corresponds to the anticodon stem and is further explored in Figure 9. To relate the single graph for a single separation to all separations, the data in Figure 7A is "redrawn" in Figure 7D keeping the separation = 3 graph solid and plotting all other separations in dotted lines. This procedure allows us to find our way among these complex data.

2. Sequence Alignments

Several sensible alignments of the sequence set are possible. We have already mentioned

```
         80        70        60        50        40        30        20        10
8765432109876543210987654321098765432109876543210987654321098765432109876543210987654321

         GGGGGCATAGCTCAGCTGGGAGAGCGCCTGCTTTGCACGCAGGAGGTCTGCGgttcGATCCCGCGCGCTCCCACCA
         GGGGCTATAGCTCAGCTGGGAGAGCGCCTGCTTTGCACGCAGGAGGTCTGCGgttcGATCCCGCATAGCTCCACCA
         GGCGCGTTAACAAAGCGGTTATGTAGCGGATTGCAAATCCGTCTAGTCCgttcGACTCCGGAACGCGCCTCCA
         GGAGCGGTAgttcAGTCGGTTAGAATACCTGCCTGTCACGCAGGGGGTCGCGGgttcGAGTCCCGTCCgttcCGCCA
         GTCCCCTTCGTCTAGAGGCCCAGGACACCGCCCTTTCACGGCGGTAACAGGGgttcGAATCCCCTGGGGGACGCCA
         GTCCCCTTCGTCTAGAGGCCCAGGACACCGCCCTTTCACGGCGGTAACAGGGgttcGAATCCCCTAGGGGACGCCA
         GCCCGGATAGCTCAGTCGGTAGAGCAGGGGATTGAAAATCCCCGTGTCCTTGgttcGATTCCGAGTCCGGGCACCA
         GCGGGCGTAgttcAATGGTAGAACGAGAGCTTCCCAAGCTCTATACGAGGgttcGATTCCCTTCGCCCGCTCCA
         GCGGGCATCGTATAATGGCTATTACCTCAGCCTTCCAAGCTGATGATGCGGgttcGATTCCCGCTGCCCGCTCCA
         GCGGGAATAGCTCAGTTGGTAGAGCACGACCTTGCCAAGGTCGGGGTCGCGAgttcGAGTCTCGTTTCCCGCTCCA
         GGTGGCTATAGCTCAGTTGGTAGAGCCCTGGATTGTGATTCCAGTTGTCGTGGgttcGAATCCCATTAGCCACCCA
         AGGCTTGTAGCTCAGGTGGTTAGAGCGCACCCCTGATAAGGGTGAGGTCGGTGgttcAAGTCCACTCAGGCCTACCA
         GGCCCCTTAGCTCAGTGGTTAGAGCAAGCGACTGATAATCGCTTGGTCGCTGgttcAAGTCCAGCAGGGGCCACCA
         GGGTCGTTAGCTCAGTTGGTAGAGCAGTTGACTTTTAATCAATTGGTCGCAGgttcGAATCCTGCACGACCCACCA
GCGAAGGTGGCGGAATTGGTAGACGCGCTAGCTTCAGGTGTTAGTGTCCTTACGGACGTGGGgttcAAGTCCCCCCCCTCGCACCA
GCCGAGGTGGTGGAATTGGTAGACACGCTACCTTGAGGTGGTAGTGCCCAATAGGGCTTACGGgttcAAGTCCCGTCCTCGGTACCA
GCCCGGATGGTGGAATCGGTAGACACAAGGGATTAAAAATCCCTCGGCgttcGCGCTGTGCGGgttcAAGTCCCGCTCCGGGTACCA
         CGCGGGGTGGAGCAGCCTGGTAGCTCGTCGGGCTCATAACCCGAAGGTCGTCGgttcAAATCCGGCCCCCGCAACCA
         GGCTACGTAGCTCAGTTGGTTAGAGCACATCACTCATAATGATGGGGTCACAGgttcGAATCCCGTCGTAGCCACCA
         TCCTCTGTAgttcAGTCGGTAGAACGGCGGACTGTTAATCCGTATGTCACTGgttcGCACGGTCCAGTCAGAGGAGCCA
         TGGGGTATCGCCAAGCGGTAAGGCACCGGTTTTTGATACCGGCATTCCCTGgttcGAATCCAGGTACCCCAGCCA
         TGGGGTATCGCCAAGCGGTAAGGCACCGGATTCTGATTCCGGCATTCCGAGgttcGAATCCTCGTACCCCAGCCA
         GCATCCGTAGCTCAGCTGGTAGAGTACTCGGCTGCGAACCGAGCGGTCGGAGgttcGAATCCTCCCGGATGCACCA
         GCATCCGTAGCTCAGCTGGATAGAGTACTCGGCTGCGAACCGAGCGGTCGGAGgttcGAATCCTCCCGGATGCACCA
GGAAGTGTGGCCGAGCGGTTGAAGGCACCGGTCTTGAAAACCGGCGACCCGAAAGGgttcCAGAgttcGAATCTCTGCGCTTCCGCCA
GGTGGCCGAGAGGCTGAAGGCGCTCCCCTGCTAAGGGAGTATGCGGTCAAAAGCTGCATCCGGGgttcGAATCCCCGCCTCACCGCCA
         GCTGATATAGCTCAGTTGGTAGAGCGCACCCTTGGTAAGGGTGAGGTCGGCAgttcGAATCTGCCTATCAGCACCA
         GGGTGATTAGCTCAGCTGGGAGAGCACCTCCCTTACAAGGAGGGGGTCGGCGgttcGATCCCGTCATCACCCACCA
         GCGTCCGTAGCTCAGTTGGTTAGAGCACCACCTTGACATGGTGGGGGTCGGTGgttcGAGTCCACTCGGACGCACCA
         GCgttcATAGCTCAGTTGGTTAGAGCACCACCTTGACATGGTGGGGGTCGTTGgttcGAGTCCAATTGAACGCACCA
         AGGGGCGTAgttcAATTGGTAGAACACCGGTCTCCAAAACCGGGTGTTGGGAgttcGAGTCTCTCCGCCCCTGCCA
       GGTGGGgttcCCGAGCGGCCAAAGGGAGCAGACTGTAAATCTGCCGTCATCGACTTCGAAGgttcGAATCCTTCCCCCACCACCA
```

FIGURE 5. The pattern gttc is found in all 32 *E. coli* tRNA sequences. It occurs perfectly aligned as well as some other locations.

right justification, which locates the TψC loop. The left justification of Figure 7 locates the anticodon stem. *A priori,* without the probability calculations justifying alignment on TψC, they are equally reasonable alignments. To see that the data analysis differs for left- and right-justified alignments, the superimposed graphs are given for right-justified sequences in Figure 8A and left-justified sequences in Figure 8B.

In all of Figure 8, W = 10, word size = 5, and the amount of mispairing is mm = 0. There is another reasonable possibility for initial alignment; the sequences can be aligned on *both* ends. This simply means that variable loop sizes will result. The superimposed graphs for such a search is presented in Figure 8C.

3. Presentation of Helixes

It is clearly possible, by moving the dotted vertical line, to move about in a graph of a single separation. To move from separation to separation, we move the relative positions of windows on the screen where the sequence set is displayed. To illustrate, Figure 9A is the graph for separation 3, where the sequences are aligned left and W = 10, k = 5, and mm = 0. Corresponding to the horizontal location of the dotted line are the window locations and displayed found pattern of Figure 9B. In summary: (1) moving the right window about in Figure 9B moves the dotted line in Figure 9A and, when separation between windows is changed, moves to another separation graph; and (2) moving the dotted line in Figure 9A moves the window positions in Figure 9B, while maintaining window separation.

Because the TψC loop matches we found above align perfectly when the sequences are right justified, we right justify and scan with W = 10, k = 7, and mm = 0. A highly significant 13 helixes are found in the 32 sequences. In examining this pattern, it is discovered

```
        80        70        60        50        40        30        20        10
4321098765432109876543210987654321098765432109876543210987654321098765432109876543210987654321

         GGGGGCATAGCTCAGCTGGGAGAGCGCCTGCTTTGCACGCAGGAggtCTGCggttcgATCCCGCGCGCTCccacca
         GGGGCTATAGCTCAGCTGGGAGAGCGCCTGCTTTGCACGCAGGAggtCTGCggttcgATCCCGCATAGCTccacca
         GGCGCgttAACAAAGCggttATGTAGCGGATTGCAAATCCGTCTAGTCCggttcgACTCCGGAACGCGCCTcca
         GGAGCggtAgttcAGtcggttAGAATACCTGCCTGTCACGCAGGGggtcgCGggttcgAGTCCCGTCCgttcCGcca
         GTCCCCttcgTCTAGAGGCccaGGACACCGCCCTTttcACGGCggtAACAGGgggttcgAATCCCCTGGGGGACGcca
         GTCCCCttcgTCTAGAGGCccaGGACACCGCCCTTttcACGGCggtAACAGGgggttcgAATCCCCTAGGGGACGcca
         GCCCGGATAGCTCAGtcggtAGAGCAGGGGATTGAAAATCCCCGTGTCCTTggttcgAttcCGAGTCCGGGCAcca
         GCGGGCGTAgttcAATggtAGAACGAGAGCttcccaAGCTCTATACGAGggttcgAttcCCttcgCCCGCTcca
         GCGGGCAtcgTATAATGGCTATTACCTCAGCCttccaAGCTGATGATGCGggttcgAttcCCGCTGCCCGCTcca
         GCGGGAATAGCTCAgttggtAGAGCACGACCTTGccaAggtcgGggtcgCGAgttcgAGTCtcgtttcCCGCTcca
         ggtGGCTATAGCTCAgttggtAGAGCCCTGGATTGTGAttccagttGtcgTGggttcgAATCccaTTAGccaCCcca
         AGGCTTGTAGCTCAggtggttAGAGCGCACCCCTGATAAGggtGAggtcggtggttcAAGTccaCTCAGGCCTAcca
         GGCCCCTTAGCTCAGTggttAGAGCAAGCGACTGATAAtcgCTTggtcgCTggttcAAGTccaGCAGGGGccacca
         GggtcgttAGCTCAgttggtAGAGCAgttGACTTTTAATCAATTggtcgCAggttcgAATCCTGCACGACccacca
GCGAAggtGGCGGAATTggtAGAGCGCGCTAGCttcAggtgttAGTGTCCTTACGGACGTGGGggttcAAGTCCCCCCCCCtcgCAcca
GCCCGAggtggtGGAATTggtAGAGCACGCTACCTTGAggtggtAGTGCccaATAGGGCTTACGggttcAAGTCCCGTCCtcggtAcca
GCCCGGATggtGGAAtcggtAGAGACACAAGGGATTAAAAATCCCtcgGCgttcgCGCTGTGCGggttcAAGTCCCGCTCCGggtAcca
         CGCGGggtGGAGCAGCCTGgtAGCtcgtcgGGCTCATAACCCGAAggtcgtcggttcAAATCCGGCCCCCGCAAcca
         GGCTACGTAGCTCAgttggtAGAGCACATCACTCATAATGATGGggtCACAggttcgAATCCCGtcgTAGccacca
         TCCTCTGTAgttcAGtcggtAGAACGCGGACTgttAATCCGTATGTCACTggttcgAGTccaGTCAGAGGAGcca
          TGGGgtAtcgccaAGCGgtAAGGCACCggttTTTGATACCGGCAttcCCTggttcgAATccaggtACCccaGcca
          TGGGgtAtcgccaAGCGgtAAGGCACCGGGAttcTGAttcCGGCAttcCGAggttcgAATCCtcgTACCccaGcca
         GCATCCGTAGCTCAGCTGgtAGAGTACtcgGCTGCGAACCGAGCggtcgGAggttcgAATCCTCCCGGATGCAcca
         GCATCCGTAGCTCAGCTGGATAGAGTACtcgGCTGCGAACCGAGCggtcgGAggttcgAATCCTCCCGGATGCAcca
GGAAGTGTGGCCGAGCggttGAAGGCACCggtCTTGAAAACCGGCGACCCGAAAGggttccaGAggttcgAATCTCTGCGCttcCGcca
ggtGGCCGAGAGGCTGAAGGCGCTCCCCTGCTAAGGGAGTATGCggtCAAAAGCTGCATCCGGggttcgAATCCCCGCCTCACCGcca
         GCTGATATAGCTCAgttggtAGAGCGCACCCTTggtAAGggtGAggtcgGCAgttcgAATCTGCCTATCAGCAcca
         GggtGATTAGCTCAGCTGGGAGAGCACCTCCCTTACAAGGAGGGggtcgGCgggtcgATCCCGTCATCACcacca
         GCGTCCGTAGCTCAgttggtAGAGCAccaCCTTGACATggtGGGggtcggtggttcgAGTccaCtcgGACGCAcca
         GCgttcATAGCTCAgttggtAGAGCAccaCCTTGACATggtGGGggtcgttggttcgAGTccaATTGAACGCAcca
         AGGGGCGTAgttcAATTggtAGAACACCggtCTccaAAAACCGggtgttGGGAgttcgAGTCTCTCCGCCCCTGcca
ggtGGggttcCCGAGCGGccaAAGGGAGCAGACTGTAAATCTGCCGTCAtcgACttcgAAggttcgAATCCttcCCccaccacca
```

FIGURE 6.   Several three letter patterns occur in 32 of 32 *E. coli* tRNA sequences. They are ggt, gtt, ttc, tcg, and cca.

that both right and left justification produces seven letter base pairing in all but three of the sequences! See Figure 10A for a display of this pattern. Notice that in several (seven) places there are actually eight letter base pairings. How is this abundance of base pairings to be handled? If the letters adjacent to the helix are random, then the helix is expected to extend in $1/4 \times 32 = 8$ cases. Therefore we decide not to extend the consensus helix to 8 bp.

Our idea to resolve these difficulties is that of consensus: locate the common features. This removes the ambiguity in all but one sequence, the 11th, which has patterns

ggtggcta ——————————————— tagccacc.

In this case if

ggtggct ——————————————— agccacc

is chosen, there is consensus of the left-hand pattern with the other left-hand patterns, but not consensus of the right-hand pattern with the other right-hand patterns. Similarly with gtggcta ——————— tagccac, some additional examination is required. If ggtggct ——————— agccacc is chosen, this will be the only sequence without a T in the column just 3′ right of the left-hand pattern and, as we will see, the TψC stem will be spoiled. Thus, we resolve the difficulty as in Figure 10B. Allowing one mispairing (mm = 1), we add the three other sequences to the consensus and align on the base pairing in Figure 10C.

The helix located in Figure 10C is, of course, the acceptor stem, involving areas of sequence at the 5′ and 3′ ends. The method of representing helixes by parentheses will allow us to unambiguously present secondary structure. The cloverleaf of Figure 1 has the symbolic form

$$5' (( ) ( ) ( )) 3'.$$

In our sequences "(. . .]" and [. . .)" are used to show helix size and location. This scheme, of course, does not work if we do not have secondary structure.

There is no significant pairing with k = 6 when we scan the area between the base-paired regions with W = 10 and mm = 0. Moving to k = 5, we show in Figure 11A the scan with separation 1. The rightmost slender peak corresponds to the TψC stem and is shown (mm = 1) in Figure 11B. The leftmost peak is refined by left justifying the remaining sequences. The consensus pairing pattern is shown in Figure 11C. We, of course, have located the anticodon stem.

Finally, we restrict attention to the segments of sequence between the left-hand k = 7 pattern and the anticodon stem. (Observe the position of the carets, ">" and "<", in Figure 12B). This scan has W = 5, k = 4, and mm = 0. Figure 12A shows one separation (of 7) in dark while the remaining separations are plotted lighter. The pattern corresponding to the peak of the dark line is shown in Figure 12B, and the consensus pattern (mm = 1) is shown in Figure 12C.

This is the complete study of secondary structure for this set of tRNAs, agreeing in detail with that published.[14] Figure 12C is our consensus folding of these tRNA sequences. This is the first time such a task has been accomplished in a mathematically rigorous fashion.

V. TERTIARY INTERACTIONS

The hydrogen bonding involved in the tRNA cloverleaf is known as secondary structure. See Chapter 7 for a mathematical definition of secondary structure.[1] Viewing the cloverleaf bonds as fixed, additional hydrogen bonds are formed between bases unpaired in the cloverleaf. These additional bonds form what is known as tertiary structure. Figure 13 is a diagram of secondary and tertiary interactions in yeast phe tRNA.[13] The tertiary bonds further fold tRNA into the familiar L-structure found by Kim et al.[5]

Recall that the tertiary interactions are frequently simply additional base pairings and that no changes in pairing rules need to be made for the search. Real difficulty, however, comes with these pattern searches. The sequences are locked into a fairly rigid alignment (see Figure 12C), but no longer is a helix of k ≧ 4 the object of interest. Instead, Figure 13 shows pairing between *single* letters. Due to the amount of conserved positions, there is a good deal of potential tertiary interaction. The good news is that such searches are possible; the bad news is that, unlike secondary structure, many conflicting possibilities exist.

Our goal is not to produce a complete analysis of tertiary interactions in tRNA, but to show what is possible with the program and methodology we have presented in this chapter.

Figure 12C shows the cloverleaf produced by our methods. We will now search this alignment for potential tertiary interactions. The D loop and the extra arm are of variable length, and the windows are set (for these runs) to have left and right justification. This should make clear just what alignment is used when the windows are in specified positions.

The first quite naive search is for windows of width 4 and helix size 4 and mm = 1. Thus, no shifting is allowed, even in the variable length regions. Figure 14A shows the full scan, with all separations superimposed. The four collections of peaks which reach maximum value correspond, obviously, to the four helixes of the cloverleaf. Figure 14B shows three of the peaks for a separation of 9 bases. To show some additional results, the medium height set of peaks of Figure 14A, adjacent to the TψC stem peaks, result from possible "pairing" between the left half of the TψC stem (positions 29 to 32) and positions 70 to 73 of the

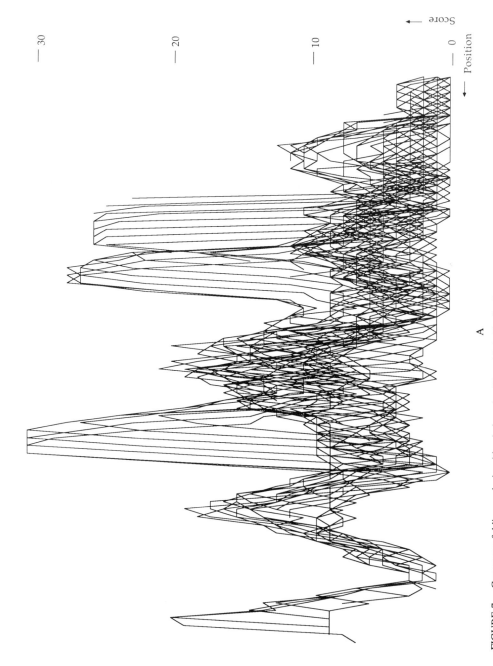

A

FIGURE 7.   Consensus folding analysis with window size W = 10, helix size k = 5, and no mispairs allowed. The sequences are right justified. (A) All separation graphs are superimposed, while in (B), an additional dimension makes a three-dimensional graph. (C) The graph for separation 3 appears alone, and in D, the remainder of the graphs appear with dotted lines.

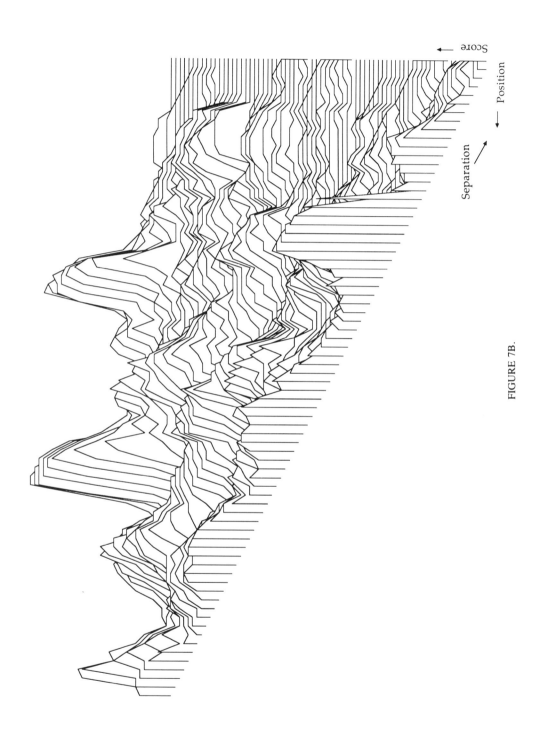

FIGURE 7B.

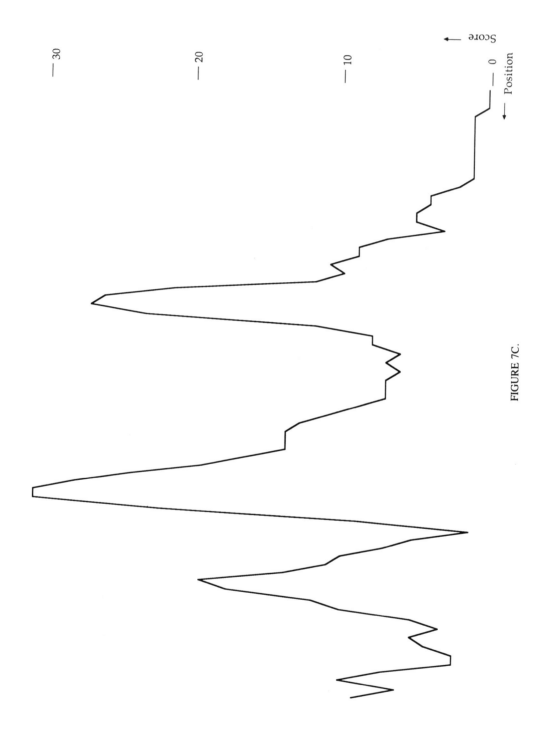

FIGURE 7C.

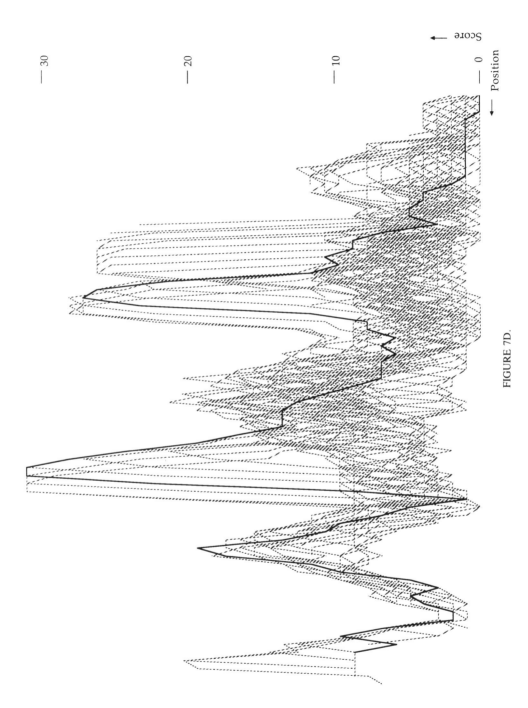

FIGURE 7D.

Score

Position

— 30

— 20

— 10

— 0

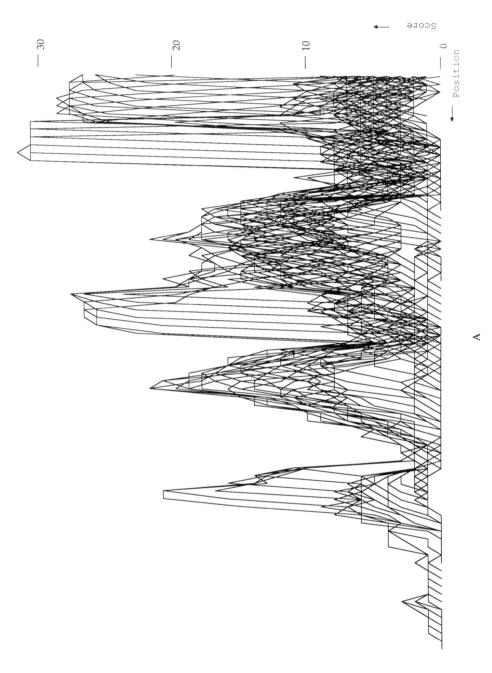

FIGURE 8.   Consensus folding analysis with window size = 10, helix size k = 5, and no mispairs allowed. (A) The sequences are left justified; (B) the sequences are right justified; and (C) the sequences are aligned on both ends.

205

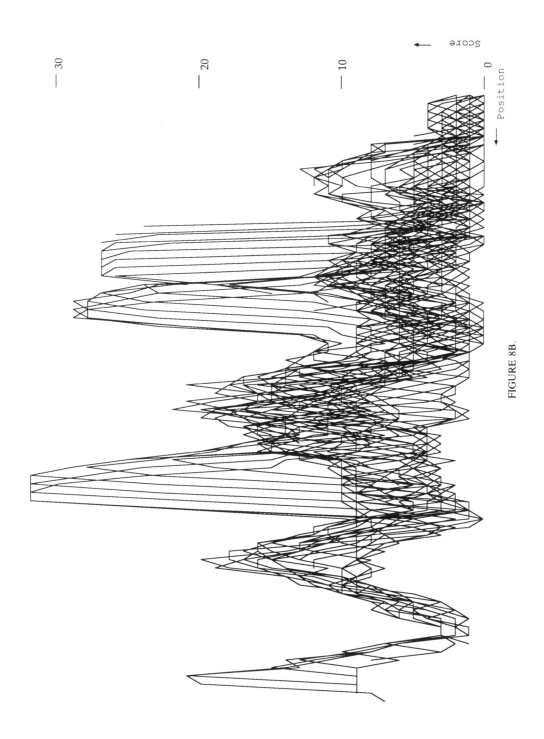

FIGURE 8B.

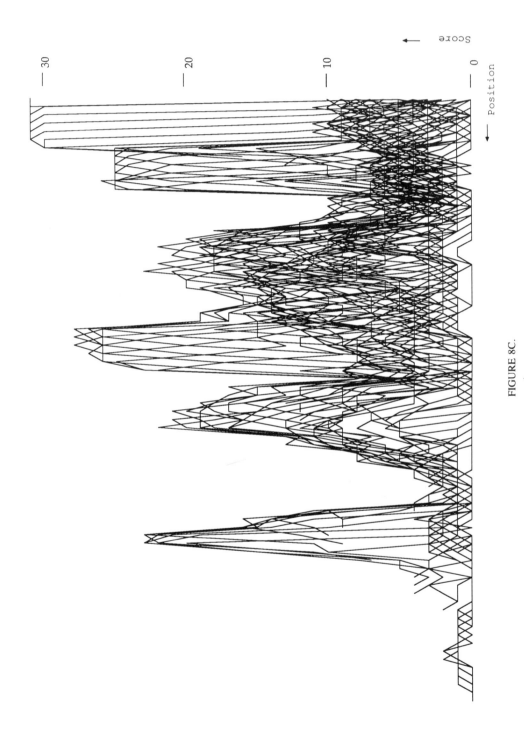

FIGURE 8C.

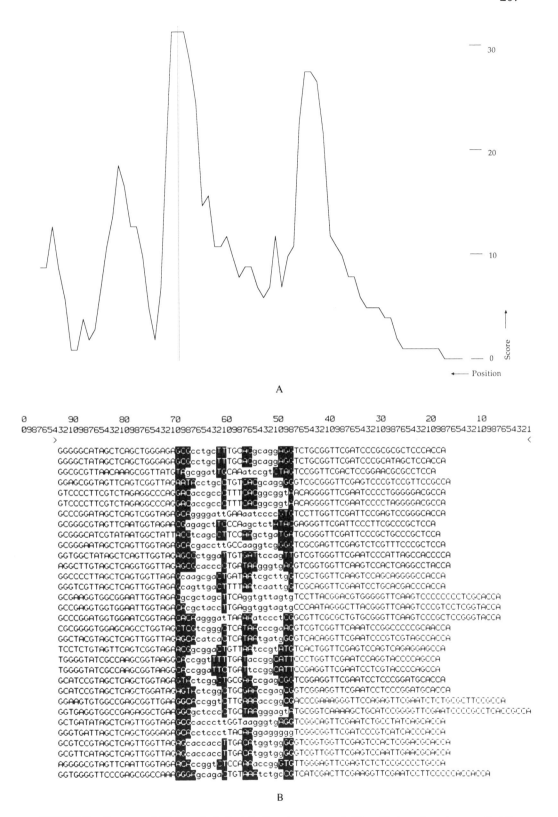

FIGURE 9. Consensus folding analysis for left-aligned sequences th W = 10, k = 5, and mm = 0. (A) The graph is for separation 3. The base pairing patterns producing the peak at the dotted line are shown in (B).

```
100        90        80        70        60        50        40        30        20        10
54321098765432109876543210987654321098765432109876543210987654321098765432109876543210987654321

GGGGGCCATA CTCAGCTGGGAGCGCCTGCTTTGCACGCAGGAGGTCTGCGGTTCGATCCGC                                  GGGGTCCGACTACA
ggggctgtACCTCAGCTGGGAGCGCGCTGCTTTGCACGCAGGAGGTCTGCGGTTCGATCCGC                                  atagctccGACCA
ggcgcgttACCAAAGCCGTTATGTAGCGGATTGCAAATCCGTCTAGTCCGGTTCGACTCCGG                                  aacgcgccTCGACCA
ggagcgggTACTTCAGTCGGTTAGAATACCTGCCTGTCACGCAGGGGGTCGCGGTTCGAGTCCCG                                tccgttccAGGGCA
gtccccctTCCTCTAGAGCCCGAAGCACCGGTCTTTCACGGCGGTAACAGGGGTTCGAATCCCC                                tggggacGACGCA
gtccccctTCCTCTAGAGCCCGAGACACCGCCCTTTCACGGCGGTAACAGGGGTTCGAATCCCC                                tagggacGGCA
gcccggaTACCTCAGTCGGTAGAGCAGGGGATTGAAAATCCCCGTGTCCTTGGTTCGATTCCGA                                gtccgggCGCCA
gcgggcgTACTTCAATGTAGAACGAGAGCTTCCCAGCTCTATACGAGGGTTCGATTCCCT                                     ctgcccgcTCGCCA
gcgggcaTCCTATATGGCTATTACCTCAGCCTTCCAAGCTGATGATGCGGTTCGATTCCCG                                    gtgcccgcTCGACCA
gcgggacTACCTCAGTCGGTAGCACAACCTTGCCAAGGTCGGGGTCGCGAGTTCGATCTCG                                    gttcccgcTCGACCA
ggtggctaTACGCTCAGTTGGTAGAGCCCCTGGATTGTGATTCCAGTTGTCGTGGGTTCGAATCCCA                              ttagcaccTCGACCA
aggcttgTACTCTCAGTCGGTTAGAGCACCGGACTGATAATCGCTTGCGCTTCGAGTCCAG                                    tcaggcctTCGACCA
ggccccctTACCTCAGTCGGTTAGAGCAGTTGACTTTTAATCAATTGGTCGCAGGTTCGAATCCTG                              taggggccACGACCA
gggGCAAGCTGCCGGAATTGGTAGAGCGGTTAGTGTCCTTACGGACGTGGGGTTCAAGTCCCC                                  GGCGGGTTTGACTACA
ggcgaggTGCTGGAATTGGTAGACACGGTACCTTGAGGTGGTAGTGCCCAATAGGGCTTACGGGTTCAAGTCCCG                      cgtagccAGGACA
gccggaTGCCTGAATCGGTAGACACAGGGGATTAAAATCCCTGGCGGTTCGCGCTGTCGCAGGTTCAAGTCCCG                       tcaggggaTCGACCA
DGCAAGGCTGCCAGCACCTGGTACCTCGTCGGGCTCATAACCCAAGGTCGTCGGTTCAAATCCGG                                DGCCCGGAGTTCGACTACA
ggctacgTACCTCAGTTGGTTAGAGCATCACTCATATAATGATGGGGCTCACAGGTTCGAATCCCG                               tgtagccCGCGACCA
tcctctgTACTTTCAGTCGGTTAGAGACGCGGACTGTTTTGATTACCCGCATTCCTGGTTCCGTCAGTCCAG                         tcagggaccaCGCGACCA
tggggtatTCCCAAGCGGTAAGGCACCGGGTTTTGATTACCCGCATTCCTGGCGAGGTTCGAATCCTC                             gtacccgaTCGACCA
tggggtatTCCCAAGGCGTAAGGCACCGGATTCTGATTCTCGGCCTCGGAACCGGCCGGGAGGTTCGAATCCTC                       gtacccccCTCGACCA
gcatccgTACCTCAGCTGAGTAGCTACCTCGGCCTGCGAACCAGCCGGTCGGAGGTTCGAATCCTC                               tcggatgcGCGACCA
gcatccgTACCTCAGCTGGATAGAGTACTCGGCCTGCGAACCAGCCGGTCGGGAGGTTCGAGTTCGAATCCTC                        tcggatgcCCGACCA
ggaagtgtTCCGAGCGGTTGAAGCAAGCCGGCCTCCCGTCTTGAAAACCCGGACGCCCGGAGCGGTTCGAGAGTTCGAATCTCT            gcgcttccCTCGACCA
ggtgaggtTCCCAGAGGCTGAAGCCTGAAAGCCGCTCCCTGCTAAGGGAGTATGCGGTCAAAAGCTGCATCCCGGGGTTCGAATCCCGcctcaccCCCA
gctgatgTTCCTCAGTTGGTAGAGCGCACCCTCCCTTACAAGGAGGGGGTCGGCAGTTCGAATCTGC                              tatcagcTCGCCA
gggtgatTACCTCAGCTGGGAGAGCACACCTCCCTTGACAAGGAGGGGGTCGGCGGTTCGATCCGT                               atcaccgCGCCA
gcgtccgTACCTCAGTTGGTAGAGCACAACCTTGACATGCGGTCGGTGGTTCGAGTCCAC                                     tcggagcGCGCCA
gcgttcctTACCTCAGTTGGTTAGAGCACACCTTGACATCGGGGTCGGGGTCGTTGGTTCGAGTCCAA                             ttgaacgcGCGCCA
aggggcgTACCTCAGTTGGTTAGAGACCGCGTCTCCAAAACCGGTGTTGGGGTCATCGCACTTCGAAGGTTCGAATCCTT               cgccccctGCGCCCA
ggtggggTTCCGGAGCGGCCAAAGGGGCGAGACTGTAAATCTCGCCATCCGCACTTCGAAGGTTCGAATCCTT                       ccccaccGCGCCH
```

A

FIGURE 10. Consensus folding patterns with W = 10, k = 7, and mm = 0. A shows ambiguity in eight sequences. These are removed in B. Allowing 1 mm gives the patterns in C.

FIGURE 10B.

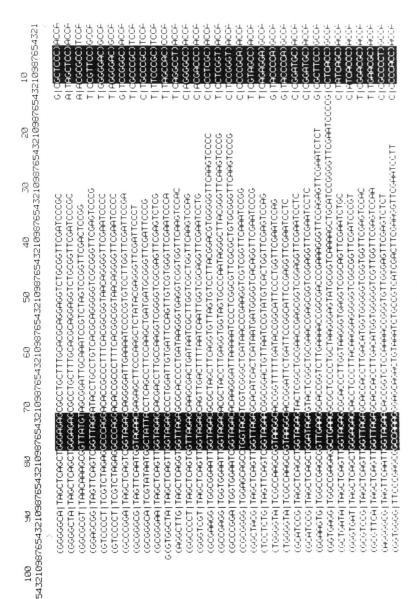

FIGURE 10C.

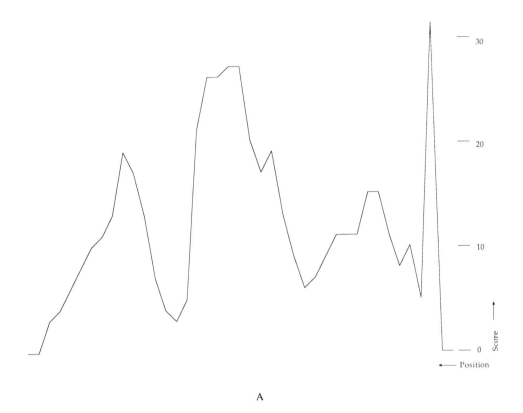

A

FIGURE 11. Analysis of the configuration of Figure 10C with W = 10, k = 5, and mm = 0. The graph with separation 1 is shown in A and the pattern of the rightmost peak shown in B. The leftmost peak can be refined to the pattern of C. In C, three consensus helixes are represented.

anticodon loop (see Figure 14C for illustration). Now this is not a real interaction, but one which the program easily locates.

We continue our study by showing graphs in Figure 15 of all separations superimposed for two letter (Figure 15A) and one letter (Figure 15B) interactions with no shifting. The strong two letter potential interactions are located as follows:

Peak	Locations
A_1:	D stem
A_2:	95-96 and 70-71
A_3:	Anticodon
A_4:	72-73 and 29-30
A_5:	29-30 and 26-27
	95-96 and 26-27
A_6:	26-27 and 23-24
A_7:	TψC stem
A_8:	Acceptor stem

Figure 15B contains most of the actual tertiary interactions. Obviously there is a good deal of data, and both computation and biology are needed to sort out such a situation if the answer is not already understood. It is our hope that computation can prove truly useful in a similar situation where the structure is not known.

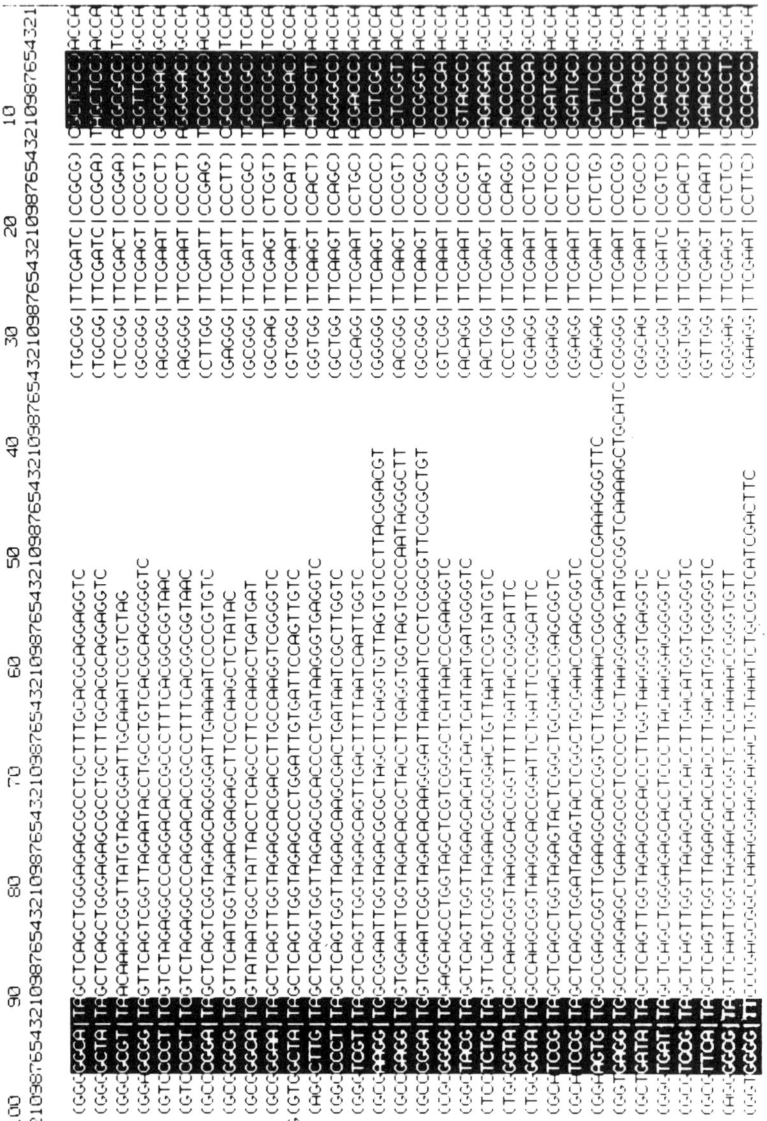

FIGURE 11B.

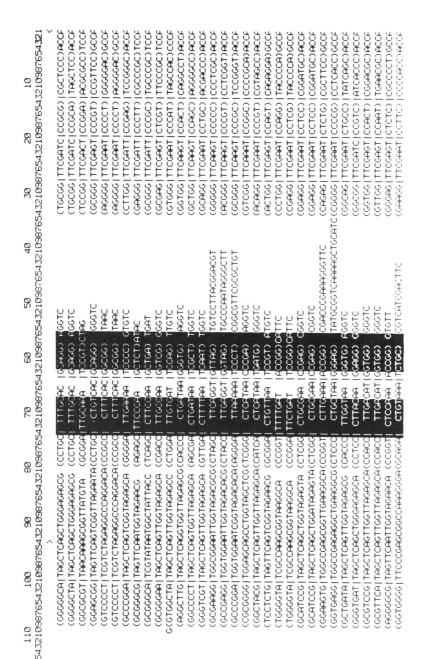

FIGURE 11C.

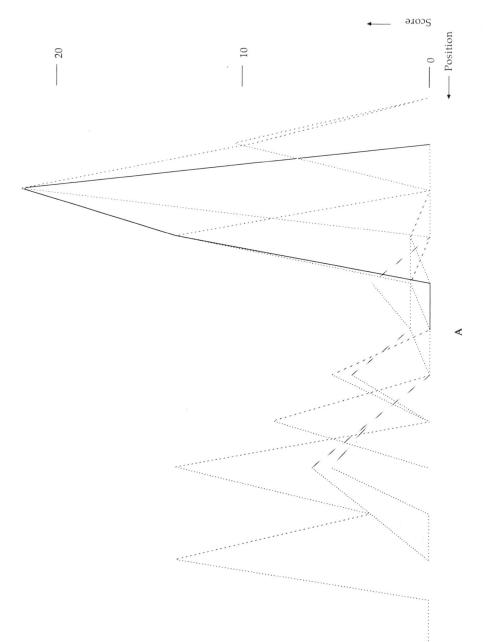

FIGURE 12.   Analysis between the left $k = 7$ pattern and the anticodon stem. Here $W = 5$, $k = 4$, and mm = 0. The dark graph of A is for separation 7. The peak has the pattern shown in B which with 1 mm is given in C. C is the consensus secondary structure of these tRNA sequences.

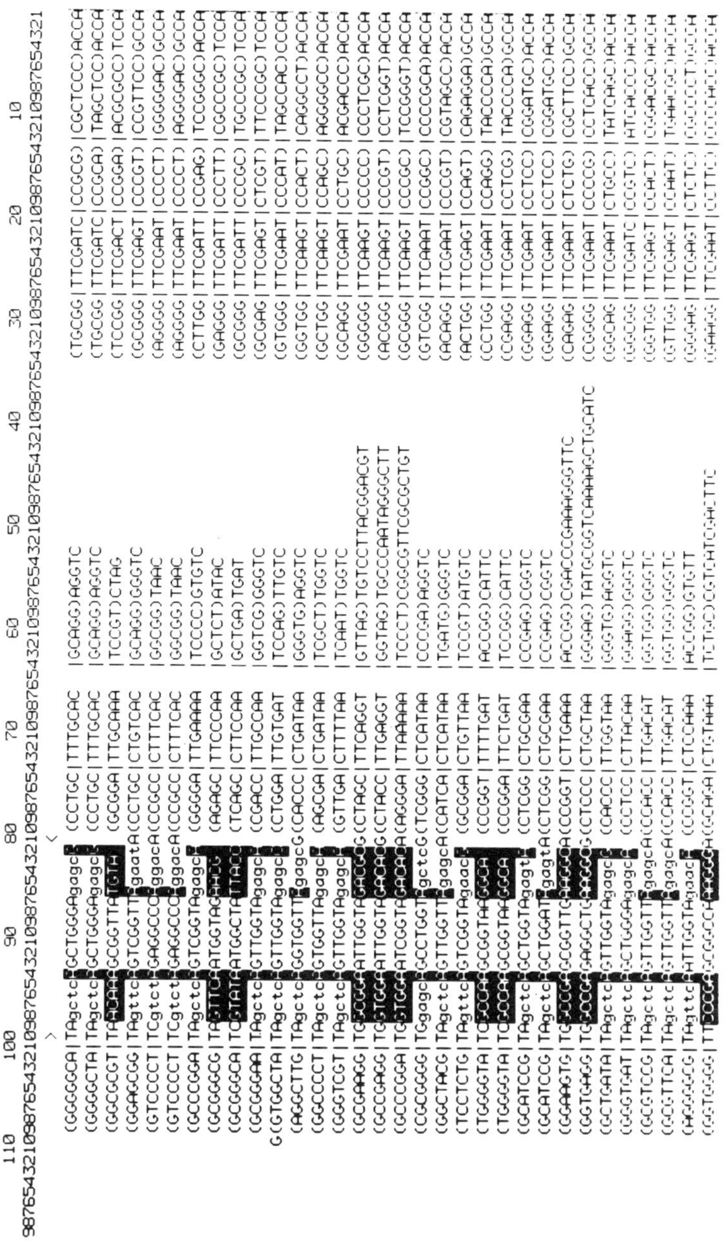

FIGURE 12B.

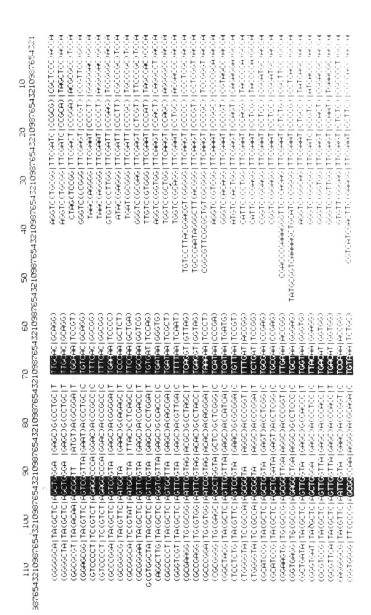

FIGURE 12C.

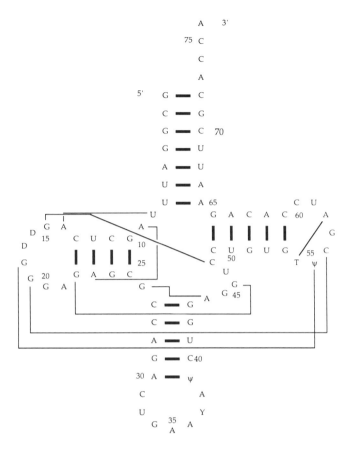

FIGURE 13.   Secondary and tertiary structure of yeast phe tRNA.[13]

VI. CONCLUSIONS

It would seem from the experiences reported in this chapter that the prospects for consensus folding are good, although tertiary interactions might be much more difficult to determine than secondary interactions. Since Levitt's 1969 paper[12] laid the basis that allows this chapter's methods to succeed, it might be asked why the computer development lagged 15 years behind. The reasons relate, it seems to us, to the type of computing previously available: centralized, batch-oriented computer centers. With that resource, it is almost inevitable that the dynamic programming methods be developed first. Dynamic programming is computationally intensive and does not require any human intervention with its recursive calculations. On the other hand, the consensus methods only make sense when some meaningful visual display is provided. Few of us would examine tables of output to recognize where in each sequence a signal was located. Since both reasonable and unreasonable possibilities are produced by consensus, the human is an important part of analysis. Methods such as these are needed to make computational methods into a useful tool for biology.

In the work of Noller and Woese there is the concept of ''proven helixes''.[20] A helix is said to be proven if there is some base pair of the helix that is distinct from the others in the other sequences. Since these authors are studying distinct organisms, they use the double mutation required to maintain the base pair as evidence for the helix as a real structure. While we have not used this device in the program described here, it is quite easy to include this or other modifications in helix definition or scoring.

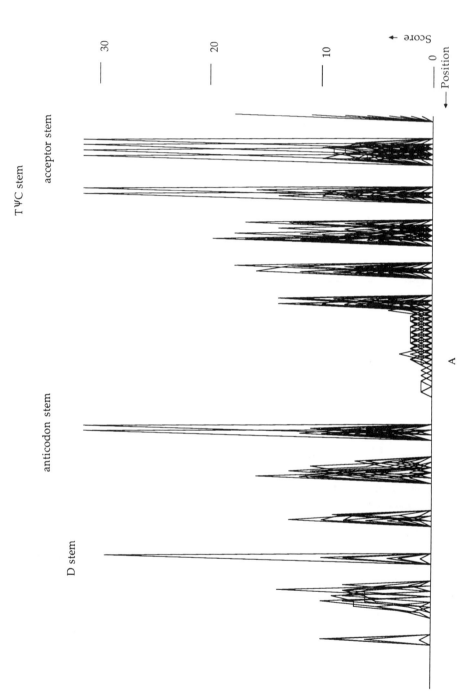

FIGURE 14.   Consensus folding analysis of Figure 12C with W = k = 4 and mm = 1. A shows all separations with the four secondary structure helices indicated. B is the graph for a separation of 9 bases. C shows the potential interaction between the left half of the TΨC stem and the anticodon loop.

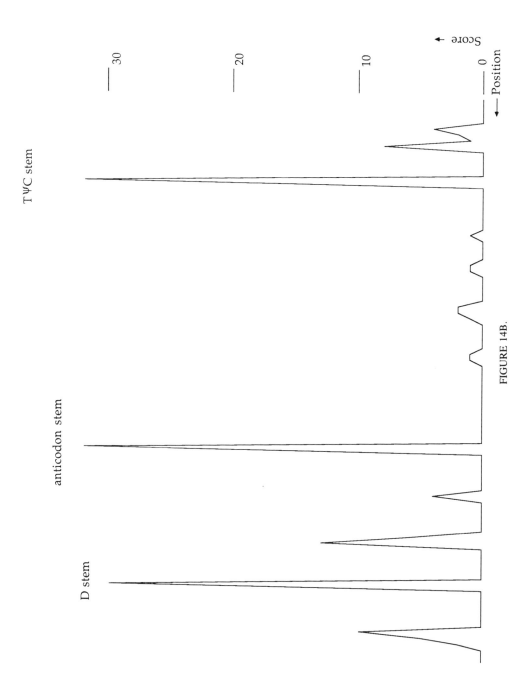

FIGURE 14B.

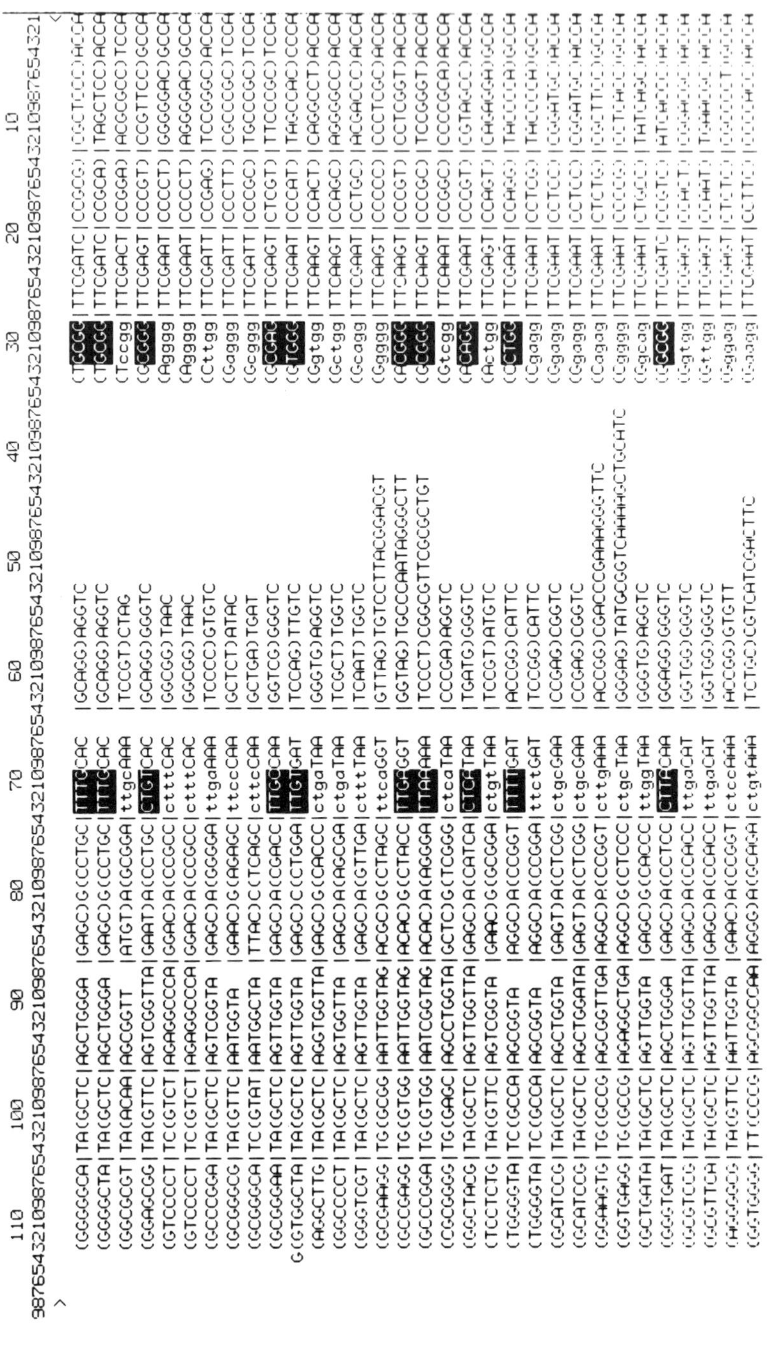

FIGURE 14C.

221

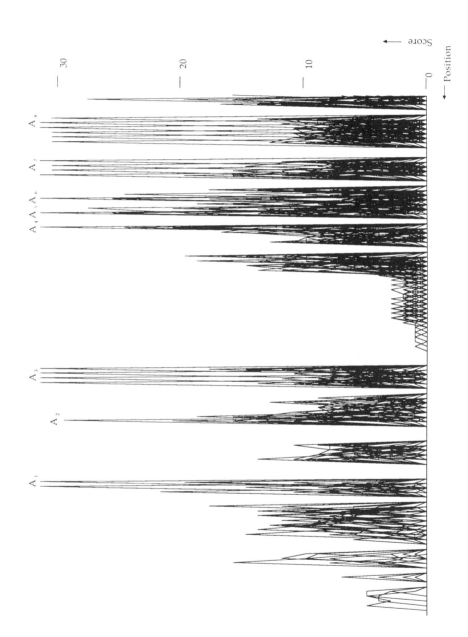

A

FIGURE 15. Consensus folding analysis of Figure 12C with W = k = 2 in A and W = k = 1 in B.

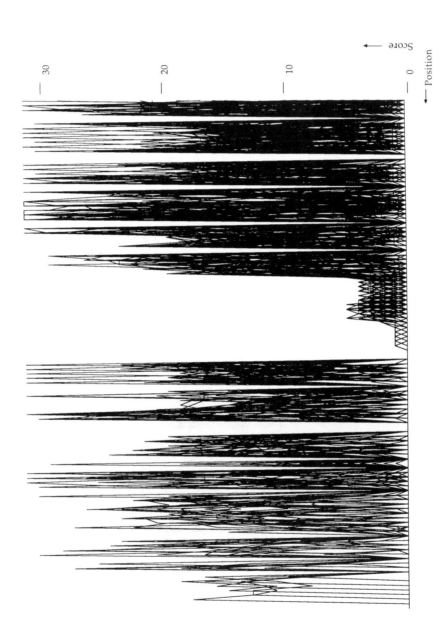

FIGURE 15B.

In closing, we mention that many data sets remain to be examined. The rRNA sequences, 5S, 16S, and 23S, are well analyzed, but it will be instructive and, we hope, revealing to analyze them by these methods. Deeper mathematical and biological questions of inferring rRNA phylogeny via these consensus alignments remain for further study. See Pace et al.[32] for a recent overview of these and related questions.

ACKNOWLEDGMENT

This work was supported by grants from the System Development Foundation and the National Institutes of Health.

REFERENCES

1. **Zuker, M. S.,** The use of dynamic programming algorithms in RNA secondary structure prediction, in *Mathematical Methods for DNA Sequences,* Waterman, M. S., Ed., CRC Press, Boca Raton, Fla., 1988.
2. **White, J.,** An introduction to the geometry and topology of DNA structure, in *Mathematical Methods for DNA Sequences,* Waterman, M. S., Ed., CRC Press, Boca Raton, Fla., 1988.
3. **Benham, C.,** Mechanics and equilibria of supercoiled DNA, in *Mathematical Methods for DNA Sequences,* Waterman, M. S., Ed., CRC Press, Boca Raton, Fla., 1988.
4. **Holley, R. W., Apgar, J., Everett, G. A., Madison, J. T., Marquisee, M., Merrill, S. H., Penswich, J. R., and Zamer, A.,** Structure of a ribonucleic acid, *Science,* 147, 1462, 1965.
5. **Kim, S. H., Suddath, F. L., Quigley, G. J., McPherson, A., Sussman, J. L., Wang, A. H. J., Seeman, N. C., and Rich, A.,** Three-dimensional tertiary structure of yeast phenylalanine transfer RNA, *Science,* 185, 435, 1974.
6. **Tinoco, I., Uhlenbeck, O. C., and Levine, M. D.,** Estimation of secondary structure in ribonucleic acids, *Nature (London),* 230, 362, 1971.
7. **Stein, P. R. and Waterman, M. S.,** On some new sequences generalizing the Catalan and Motzkin numbers, *Discrete Math.,* 26, 261, 1978.
8. **Waterman, M. S.,** Secondary structure of single-stranded nucleic acids, *Stud. Found. Combinatorics Adv. Math. Suppl. Stud.,* 1, 167, 1978.
9. **Waterman, M. S. and Smith, T. F.,** RNA secondary structure: a complete mathematical analysis, *Math. Biosci.,* 42, 257, 1978.
10. **Nussinov, R., Pieczenik, G., Griggs, J. R., and Kleitman, D. J.,** Algorithms for loop matchings, *SIAM J. Appl. Math.,* 35, 68, 1978.
11. **Sankoff, D.,** Simultaneous solution to the RNA folding, alignment and protosequence problem, *SIAM J. Appl. Math.,*
12. **Levitt, M.,** Detailed molecular model for transfer ribonucleic acid, *Nature (London),* 224, 759, 1969.
13. **Lewin, B.,** *Genes,* 2nd ed., John Wiley & Sons, Toronto, 1985.
14. **Sprinzl, M., Moll, J., Meissner, F., and Hartmann, T.,** Compilation of tRNA sequences, *Nucl. Acids Res.,* 132, r1, 1985.
15. **Fox, G. E. and Woese, C. R.,** 5S RNA secondary structure, *Nature (London),* 256, 505, 1975.
16. **Nishikawa, K. and Takemura, S.,** Structure and function of 5S ribosomal ribonucleic acid from *Torulopsis utlis, J. Biochem.,* 76, 935, 1974.
17. **Waterman, M. S.,** Computer analysis of nucleic acid sequences, *Methods of Enzymology,* in press.
18. **Trifonov, E. N. and Bolshoi, G.,** Open and closed 5S ribosomal RNA, the only two universal structures encoded in the nucleotide sequences, *J. Mol. Biol.,* 169, 1, 1983.
19. **Woese, C. R., Magrum, L. J., Gupta, R., Siegel, R. B., Stahl, D. A., Kop, J., Crawford, N., Brosius, J., Gutell, R. R., Hogan, J. J., and Noller, H. F.,** Secondary structure model for bacterial 16S ribosomal RNA: phylogenetic, enzymatic and chemical evidence, *Nucl. Acids. Res.,* 8, 2275, 1980.
20. **Noller, H. F. and Woese, C. R.,** Secondary structure of 16S ribosomal RNA, *Science,* 212, 403, 1981.

21. **Stiegler, P., Carbon, P., Zuker, M., Ebel, J. P., and Ehresmann, C.,** Structural organization of the 16S ribosomal RNA from *E. coli* topography and secondary structure, *Nucl. Acids Res.,* 9, 2153, 1981.

22. **Zwieb, C., Glotz, C., and Brimacombe, R.,** Secondary structure comparisons between small unit ribosomal RNA molecules from six different species, *Nucl. Acids Res.,* 9, 3621, 1981.

23. **Glotz, C., Zwieb, C., Brimacombe, R., Edwards, K., and Kossel, H.,** Secondary structure of the large subunit ribosomal RNA from *Escherichia coli, Zea mays* chloroplast, and human and mouse mitochondrial ribosomes, *Nucl. Acids Res.,* 9, 3287, 1981.

24. **Moazed, D., Stern, S., and Noller, H.,** Rapid chemical probing of confirmation in 16S ribosomal RNA and 30S ribosomal subunits using primer extension, *J. Mol. Biol.,* 187, 399, 1986.

25. **Noller, H. F., Kop, J., Wheaton, V., Brosius, J., Gutell, R. R., Kopylov, A. M., Dohme, F., Herr, W., Stahl, D. A., Gupta, R., and Woese, C.,** Secondary structure model for 23S ribosomal RNA, *Nucl. Acids Res.,* 9, 6167, 1980.

26. **Karlin, S., Ost, F., and Blaisdell, B. E.,** Patterns in DNA and amino acid sequences and their statistical significance, in *Mathematical Methods for DNA Sequences,* Waterman, M. S., Ed., CRC Press, Boca Raton, Fla., 1988.

27. **Waterman, M. S.,** Sequence alignments, in *Mathematical Methods for DNA Sequences,* Waterman, M. S., Ed., CRC Press, Boca Raton, Fla., 1988.

28. **Martinez, H. M.,** An efficient method for finding repeats in molecular sequences, *Nucl. Acids Res.,* 11, 4629, 1983.

29. **Galas, D., Eggert, M., and Waterman, M. S.,** Rigorous pattern recognition methods for DNA sequences, *J. Mol. Biol.,* 186, 117, 1985.

30. **Badadur, R. R.,** *Some Limit Theorems in Statistics,* Society for Industrial and Applied Mathematics, Philadelphia, 1971.

31. **Ellis, R. S.,** *Entropy, Large Deviations, and Statistical Mechanics,* Springer-Verlag, New York, 1985.

32. **Pace, N., Olsen, G., and Woese, C.,** Ribosomal RNA phylogeny and primary lines of evolutionary descent, *Cell,* 45, 325, 1986.

Chapter 9

AN INTRODUCTION TO THE GEOMETRY AND TOPOLOGY OF DNA STRUCTURE

James H. White

TABLE OF CONTENTS

I. INTRODUCTION

The application of topology and geometry to the study of closed circular DNA has developed into an important area of investigation in the past decade and a half.[1-9] The major reason for this is that closed circular DNA exhibits physical and chemical properties that differ in fundamental ways from those of DNAs with a break in one or both strands. These properties, until recently, have been explained in terms of the fact that such DNA have their strands linked[10] with linking number Lk and in terms of two basic characteristics of Lk: (1) that Lk is invariant or unchanged under continuous deformation of the DNA structure and (2) the Lk is the sum of two geometric quantities, twist, Tw, and writhing, Wr.[7]

$$Lk = Tw + Wr$$

These two characteristics have been applied in many ways. Among these are the analysis of supercoiling and linking deficiency,[1] the analysis of enzymatic properties of various types of topoisomerases,[3,4,6] the estimation of the winding of DNA in nucleosomes,[11] the determination of free energy associated with supercoiling,[12-14] and the quantitative analysis of the binding of proteins and small ligands to DNA. From a purely mathematical point of view, there has been the work of Fuller on the decomposition of Lk into biologically meaningful components[15] and the work of Benham surveyed elsewhere in this volume on the mechanics and equilibria of super helical DNA.[16-22]

The purpose of this chapter is to give a detailed introduction to these three concepts, Lk, Tw, and Wr, and to indicate how they are used in some of the applications mentioned above. Sections II through V are devoted to an exposition of the mathematical ideas involved. Section II defines the linking number in three different ways: (1) in terms of crossing numbers, (2) in terms of surface intersections, and (3) in terms of the Gauss map and its associated integral. The three ways are related and examples are given. Section III is devoted to a discussion of the writhing number from both a crossing number and the Gauss map and integral points of view. Examples are given showing the relationship of writhing to coiling in space curves. Section IV defines the twist of one curve about another and discusses several examples of particular importance in the modeling of DNA. Section V presents the fundamental result relating the three quantities, i.e., $Lk = Tw + Wr$, and gives examples of particular importance to DNA. Section VI applies the mathematics of Sections II to V to structural problems in DNA. The half and full ribbon models of DNA are defined, and the twist and writhing of DNA are discussed in detail. The winding in a nucleosome is analyzed, and linking deficiency is explained. Finally, the action of topoisomerases of type 1 and type 2 in reducing linking deficiency is explained using in particular the fundamental relationship of Section V.

This chapter in no way is exhaustive of all of the geometrical and topological methods in examining DNA structure. Instead, it is meant to be an introduction to the kinds of geometric analysis useful in studying DNA. Thus, the applications presented in Section VI give one only a small indication of the types of analysis possible with geometric methods. In particular, these methods are not sufficient to analyze the additional interwinding in catenated or knotted DNA. To do this, one needs the methods of knot theory and oriented link theory. However, the applications given in Section VI are, indeed, the fundamental ones which explain the physical and chemical properties exhibited by supercoiling in DNA. For a much longer and more thorough analysis of the topology of DNA, the reader should address himself to the excellent survey articles in the field.[1,4,5,23] The first and most important mathematical concept to understand concerning closed DNA is that of the linking number.

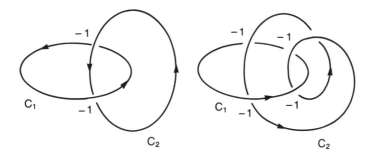

FIGURE 1. Linking numbers of pairs of curves using the index approach.

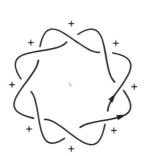

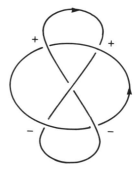

FIGURE 2. Linking of helically intertwined curves with a circular axis.

FIGURE 3. The trapped figure 8: a pair of curves with $Lk = 0$.

II. THE LINKING NUMBER OF TWO CLOSED SPACE CURVES

A. The Index Approach

Let C_1 and C_2 be two closed continuous oriented curves in space. In a projection of these curves into a plane, one of the curves will perhaps cross over the other at a number of points. For example, in Figure 1 there are two examples, one with two such crossings and one with four such crossings. To each of these crossings is associated an index number of $+1$ or -1, according to the direction in which the tangent vector to the top curve must be rotated to coincide with the tangent vector to the bottom curve. If the rotation is clockwise, the number is -1, and if it is counterclockwise, the number is $+1$. Adding all the indices associated to all the crossings and dividing by 2 gives the linking number of the two curves denoted by $Lk(C_2,C_1)$ or simply Lk. Thus, for the first curve in Figure 1 the linking number, Lk, of C_1 and C_2, is $-1 + (-1)$ divided by 2 equals -1, and for the second curve, Lk is $-1 + (-1) + (-1) + (-1)$ divided by 2 equals -2.

An interesting example can be seen in Figure 2. All crossings have sign $+1$. Therefore, $Lk = +4$. This example pictures the case where two closed curves of helical type wind around one another in a right-handed sense, an excellent model for DNA.

In Figure 3, there is pictured a most curious case. There are two $+1$ crossings and two -1 crossings. Hence, $Lk = 0$. The crossing in the middle is not counted since it is a crossing, not of one curve with the other, but of one of the curves with itself. Even though $Lk = 0$, the curves cannot be separated. This example is often called the trapped figure eight.

The linking number has four major properties. First, this number is independent of the planar projection used to calculate it. This is especially important, for the number Lk should

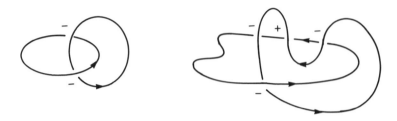

FIGURE 4.   The invariance of Lk under deformation.

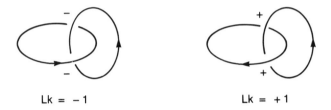

FIGURE 5.   The reversal of the sign of Lk when one of the curves is reversed in orientation.

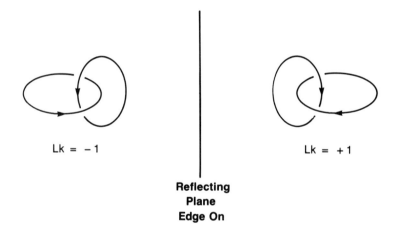

FIGURE 6.   The reversal of the sign of Lk of two curves when reflected in a plane.

be a property of the curves in space and not of any projection. The second major property is that Lk is unchanged if either of the curves is deformed continuously, provided no breaks are made in either curve. Thus, the two curves in Figure 4 have the same linking number. The curves on the left-hand side of Figure 4 have been stretched and deformed to give the curves on the right-hand side, but Lk is the same, since no breaks were made. The third property is that Lk changes sign if the direction of one of the curves is reversed as is illustrated in Figure 5. The final major property is that if a pair of curves is reflected in a plane, then Lk also changes sign. This is illustrated in Figure 6.

B. The Surface Intersection Approach

Another way to compute the linking number of two curves is to use the notion of intersections of one of the curves with a surface spanning the other. Given a piece of a surface bounded by an oriented curve, an orientation may be chosen for the surface in the usual

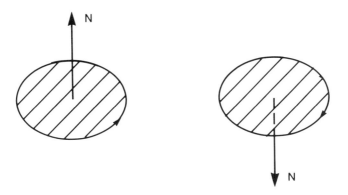

FIGURE 7. The two orientations for a surface.

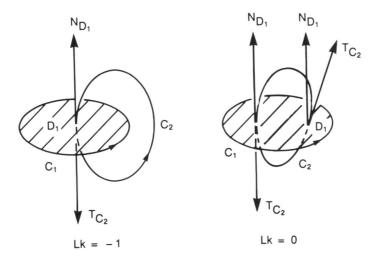

Lk = −1

Lk = 0

FIGURE 8. Linking numbers of pairs of curves using the surface intersection approach.

sense of the classical Stokes' theorem. For example, in the left-hand side of Figure 7 the orientation is given by choosing the upward pointing normal, whereas in the right-hand side the orientation is given by choosing the downward pointing normal.

Let D_1 be an oriented surface whose boundary is one of the closed curves, say C_1. Let C_2 intersect D_1 a number of times. To each such intersection is associated an index number $+1$ or -1, depending on whether the tangent vector to C_2 at the point of intersection points to the same side of the surface as the orienting normal or to the opposite side. Then the linking number Lk is defined as the sum of all these index numbers. In Figure 8 are shown two examples, the one on the left having $Lk = -1$ and the one on the right having $Lk = 0$. An important fact about this definition of Lk is that it does not depend on the choice of spanning surface, a fact proven by elementary methods of algebraic topology.

An interesting example can be found in Figure 9. Here all intersections have index -1, since the tangent vector of C_2 points to the opposite side of the surface from that of the oriented normal. Thus, $Lk = -4$. This is a helical type curve winding in a left-handed fashion about a circular closed curve.

C. The Gauss Integral Approach

A final more mathematically difficult approach to the linking number of two closed space

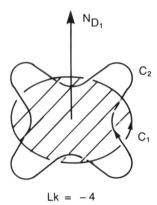

$$Lk = -4$$

FIGURE 9.   The linking number of a helical type curve with its axis using the surface intersection approach.

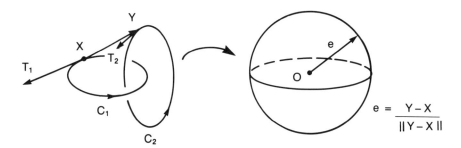

$$e = \frac{Y - X}{\| Y - X \|}$$

FIGURE 10.   The Gauss map.

curves is given by the formula of Gauss. Figure 10 pictures the terms used in the Gauss integral. Let x be an arbitrary point on the curve C_1 and let y be an arbitrary point on C_2. Let T_1 be the unit tangent vector to C_1 at x and let T_2 be the unit tangent vector to C_2 at y. Let $r = \| y - x \|$ be the length of the vector $y - x$, i.e., the vector joining x to y, directed from x to y. Let e be a unit vector along $y - x$, that is, let

$$e = \frac{y - x}{\| y - x \|} = \frac{(y - x)}{r}$$

Finally, let ds_1 and ds_2 be the arc length elements on C_1 at x and on C_2 at y, respectively. Then, it was shown by Gauss that the linking number of C_1 and C_2 is given by the expression:

$$Lk = \frac{1}{4\pi} \iint\limits_{C_1 \times C_2} \frac{e \cdot (T_2 \times T_1)}{r^2} ds_1 \, ds_2 \tag{1}$$

where the integral is taken over pairs of points, and $e \cdot (T_2 \times T_1)$ is the usual triple vector product of e, T_2, and T_1. this integral is difficult in general to compute directly. More often than not, it involves elliptic integrals; nevertheless, it is useful for applications.

Geometrically, this integral can be interpreted in the following way. As was shown above, for each x in C_1 and y in C_2 there is a unique vector e. If this vector is translated in a parallel way to the origin, its endpoint becomes a point on the sphere of radius 1, centered at the origin. Thus, to each pair of points (x, y), x in C_1, y in C_2, there is associated a unique point

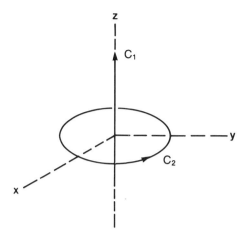

FIGURE 11. The infinite straight line and the circle.

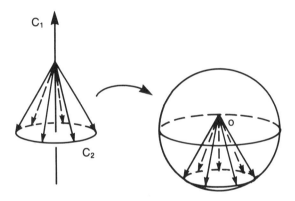

FIGURE 12. The Gauss map for the infinite straight line and
the circle.

on the unit sphere, denoted S^2. The map which makes this association is called the Gauss
map. What the integral expression for Lk measures is how many times the Gauss map sweeps
across the whole unit sphere in a positive or negative manner. The factor of $(4\pi)^{-1}$ in front
of the integral sign is a normalizing factor, for 4π is the surface area of the unit sphere.
Whether a contribution of the Gauss map is positive or negative depends on the sign of the
expression $e \cdot (T_2 \times T_1)$. The following examples illustrate these ideas.

1. The Infinite Straight Line and the Unit Circle

In this case C_1 is the infinitely extending z-axis and C_2 is the unit circle $x^2 + y^2 = 1$ in
the xy-plane. The two curves are oriented in the manner shown in Figure 11. The Gauss
map for one point on the z-axis and all points on the circle is pictured in Figure 12. If the
point on the z-axis is fixed and the point on the circle is allowed to vary over the whole
circle, the Gauss map traces out a circle on the unit sphere. When the point z is above the
xy-plane, the Gauss map traces out a circle in the southern hemisphere. When z is at the
origin, the Gauss map traces out the equator. Finally, when z is below the xy-plane, the
Gauss map traces out a circle in the northern hemisphere. In summary, as z goes from $-\infty$
to $+\infty$, the Gauss map covers the entire sphere exactly once so that Lk is $+1$ or -1
depending on the orientations. In this case $Lk = +1$, as one can see easily using the surface
intersection approach.

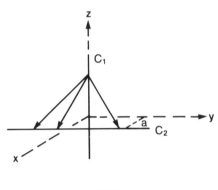

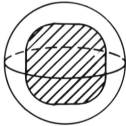

FIGURE 13.   The Gauss map for two straight line segments.

That Equation 1 also gives $Lk = +1$ can be seen as follows. In coordinate expressions, the line C_1 may be written $(0,0,z)$, $-\infty < z < \infty$ and the circle C_2 may be written $(\cos\theta,\sin\theta,0)$, $0 \leq \theta \leq 2\pi$. Hence, x on C_1 may be written as $(0,0,z)$, and y on C_2 as $(\cos\theta,\sin\theta,0)$. In this case, therefore, $y - x = (\cos\theta,\sin\theta,-z)$ and

$$e = \frac{(\cos\theta,\ \sin\theta,\ -z)}{\sqrt{1 + z^2}}$$

$T_1 = (0,0,1)$ and $T_2 = (-\sin\theta,\cos\theta,0)$. Therefore, $T_2 \times T_1 = (\cos\theta,\sin\theta,0)$. Thus,

$$e \cdot T_2 \times T_1 = \frac{1}{\sqrt{1 + z^2}}$$

For C_1, $ds_1 = dz$ and for C_2, $ds_2 = d\theta$ and $r = \sqrt{1 + z^2}$. Putting these expressions into Equation 1 one obtains

$$Lk = \frac{1}{4\pi} \int_{-\infty}^{\infty} \int_{0}^{2\pi} \frac{1}{(1 + z^2)^{3/2}}\, d\theta\, dz$$

$$= \frac{1}{2} \int_{-\infty}^{\infty} \frac{1}{(1 + z^2)^{3/2}}\, dz$$

$$= \frac{1}{2} \int_{-\pi/2}^{\pi/2} \cos\varphi\, d\varphi = 1$$

2. Two Perpendicular Straight Line Segments

In Figure 13 are pictured two perpendicular straight line segments C_1 and C_2, one along the z-axis, and one parallel to the y-axis in the xy-plane displaced slightly from the y-axis a small distance a. Thus, in rectangular coordinates, C_1 may be written as $(0,0,z)$, $-\epsilon \leqslant z \leqslant +\epsilon$ and C_2 may be written as $(a,y,0)$, $-\delta \leqslant y \leqslant +\delta$. In Figure 13 the Gauss map is shown for this pair. It is simply a patch on the face of the unit sphere. The larger the displacement a, the smaller the size of the patch. As a gets very small and approaches zero, the patch covers approximately one half the sphere. Thus, the Gauss integral is approximately $\pm 1/2$, depending on the choice of sign for a. This can be shown directly from formula as follows: C_1 has representation $(0,0,z)$, hence $T_1 = (0,0,1)$ and $ds_1 = dz$. C_2 has representation $(a,y,0)$; hence, $T_2 = (0,1,0)$ and $ds_2 = dy$. Thus, $T_2 \times T_1 = (1,0,0)$. Now

$$e = \frac{(a,\ y,\ -z)}{\sqrt{a^2 + y^2 + z^2}}$$

so that

$$e \cdot T_2 \times T_1 = \frac{a}{\sqrt{a^2 + y^2 + z^2}}$$

the Gauss integral becomes

$$\frac{1}{4\pi} \int_{-\delta}^{+\delta} \int_{-\epsilon}^{+\epsilon} \frac{a}{(a^2 + y^2 + z^2)^{3/2}} dz dy$$

Note that if a is positive, the integral is positive and the crossing is positive, and if a is negative, the integral is negative and the crossing is negative.

To show the integral is $+1/2$ when a goes to zero from the positive side, one need only make the substitutions $y' = a^{-1}y$, $z' = a^{-1}z$ then the integral becomes

$$\frac{1}{4\pi} \int_{-\delta/a}^{+\delta/a} \int_{-\epsilon/a}^{+\epsilon/a} \frac{1}{(1 + y'^2 + z'^2)^{3/2}} dz' dy'$$

In the limit this integral becomes

$$\frac{1}{4\pi} \int_{-\infty}^{\infty} \int_{-\infty}^{\infty} \frac{1}{(1 + y'^2 + z'^2)^{3/2}} dz' dy'$$

which, in polar coordinates, becomes

$$\frac{1}{4\pi} \int_0^{2\pi} \int_0^{\infty} \frac{1}{(1 + r^2)^{3/2}} r\, dr\, d\theta$$

$$= \frac{1}{2} \int_0 \frac{1}{(1 + r^2)^{3/2}} r\, dr = \frac{1}{2}$$

In a similar manner, one can show that if a approaches zero from the negative side, the integral becomes $-1/2$.

D. Relationship Between the Index Approach and the Gauss Integral Approach

Recall that in measuring Lk using the integral approach one attaches a number $\pm 1/2$ to each crossing in a planar projection. The sum of these is, then Lk. To see the connection directly between these numbers and the Gauss integral approach, one need only refer to the

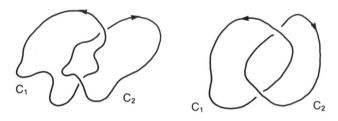

FIGURE 14.   Deformation of a pair of curves to measure *Lk* via the two straight line segments technique.

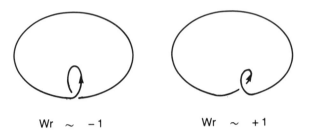

FIGURE 15.   The writhing number of curves with one coil.

second example in Section C in which the Gauss integral yielded $\pm \frac{1}{2}$ depending on the sign of the crossing.

The approach is exemplified in Figure 14. To compute *Lk* for C_1 and C_2 one adds the two numbers $-\frac{1}{2}$ and $-\frac{1}{2}$ to get -1. However, *Lk* remains the same under any continuous deformation of either curve C_1 or C_2. Thus, one may deform the curves on the left-hand side of Figure 14 to the ones on the right-hand side without changing *Lk*. On the right-hand side the two curves lie in the same plane except near the crossings where they appear as line segments perpendicular to one another, both crossings being negative. The Gauss integral for the portions of the curves near the crossings is $-\frac{1}{2}$ for each crossing. The Gauss integral for the remainder is zero because all three vectors T_1, T_2, and e lie in the same plane, and hence, $e \cdot T_2 \times T_1 = 0$. Thus, the total Gauss integral becomes the sum of the integrals near crossings and so equals -1.

III. THE WRITHING NUMBER OF A CLOSED SPACE CURVE

A. The Index Approach

Let C be a continuous closed oriented curve in space. In a projection of this curve into a plane, this curve will perhaps cross over itself a number of times. To each of these crossings is associated an index number of $+1$ or -1 as in the linking number section. Adding all of these indices gives the directed writhing number of the curve C, the direction being that of the projection. The actual writhing number, denoted $Wr(C)$ or simply Wr, of a curve C is defined as the average overall possible projections of the directed writhing numbers. Thus the curves in Figure 15 will have respectively one crossing with index -1 and $+1$ in almost all projections, except for a few from the side, so $Wr = -1$ and $+1$.

An easy way to understand the idea of averaging the directed writhing number is as follows. Make a wire model of the curve C and suspend it in space by a string. Then look at it from the sides, from under it, from above it, etc. In all the views, the curve will appear to cross itself a number of times or perhaps, will not cross itself at all. Compute the directed writhing number for all views and average them. The result will give Wr for the curve.

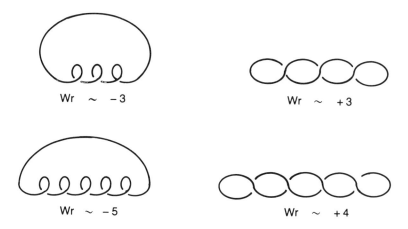

FIGURE 16. The writhing number of curves with multiple coils.

Thus, in Figure 1 Wr is not exactly ± 1 since there are side views where no crossings are observed. Thus, Wr is slightly larger than -1 in one case and slightly less than $+1$ in the other.

It is also clear from this analysis that if a curve C ever passes very close to itself, the passing will give a contribution of $+1$ or -1 because in almost all views the passing will appear to be a crossing.

Now, unlike Lk, if the orientation of C is reversed, the directed writhing number is unchanged, since both crossing segments reverse, and hence, Wr is unchanged. Furthermore, unlike Lk, Wr does indeed change under deformation of the curve C. For example, any unknotted curve such as those in Figure 15 can be deformed into a circle. The former has Wr close to ± 1, whereas the latter has $Wr = 0$. In Figure 16 there are additional examples of space curves with different Wr. Note that the more the coiling, the greater Wr in absolute value.

If a curve is passed through itself, then the writhing number of the curve just before the self-passage differs by 2 from the writhing number of the curve just after the self-passage. This is due to the fact that the segments have the same orientation, but are reversed as to which one is on the top and which one is on the bottom. Thus, the two curves in Figure 15 really differ only by a self-passage.

B. The Gauss Integral Approach

There are an integral expression and Gauss map for Wr which are exact counterparts to the ones for Lk in Section II.C. Let x and y be two points of the curve C. Let T_1 be the unit tangent vector to C at x and T_2 the unit tangent vector to C at y. Let $r = \|y - x\|$ and $e = \frac{1}{r}(y - x)$. Finally, let ds_1 and ds_2 be the arc length elements at x and y, respectively. Then,

$$Wr = \frac{1}{4\pi} \iint\limits_{C \times C} \frac{e \cdot T_2 \times T_1}{r^2} ds_1 ds_2$$

This is the Gauss integral for a single curve.

For most curves this integral is too complex to compute. However, there are two important observations that should be made. First, if C is a plane curve with no self-intersections, then $Wr = 0$. This is due to the fact that e, T_1, and T_2 all lie in the same plane, and hence $e \cdot T_2 \times T_1 = 0$. Thus, $Wr = 0$. Second, if C is deformed into a plane curve except for

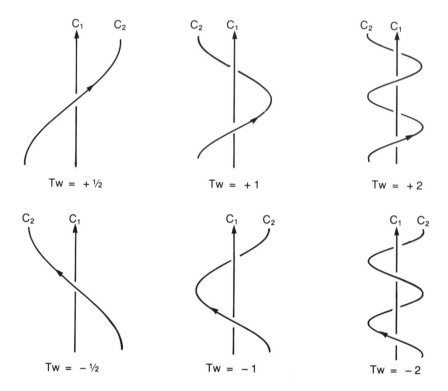

FIGURE 17.   The twist of helices about a linear axis.

a finite number of crossings at which the curve crosses itself in a perpendicular fashion, then one can use an analysis exactly similar to that in Section II.D to determine that the Gauss integral is the sum of numbers ± 1 attached to these crossings.

A few remarks about the existence of the integral are in order here. As the point y approaches the point x, r approaches zero. Thus, there is some question about the finiteness of the integral. Suffice it to say that this integral indeed is finite, but the proof[7] is beyond the intent of this chapter.

Fortunately, one need hardly ever compute the writhing number of a curve directly, for this number and the linking number of the curve with another curve are related to the twist of the two curves. This last quantity is much easier to compute. The next section defines the twist and gives the procedure to compute it.

IV. THE TWIST OF ONE CURVE ABOUT ANOTHER

A. The Ribbon-Like Correspondence Surface Approach

Basically, the twist of one curve C_2 about another curve C_1, denoted $Tw(C_2,C_1)$ or simply Tw, measures the magnitude of the spinning of C_2 around C_1. In the simplest case, that of a helix spinning around its axis, Tw is just the number of times the helix revolves about the axis. This number is positive if the helix is right-handed and negative if left-handed. Examples are given in Figure 17.

The twist can also be measured by means of the spinning of a vector pointing from the curve C_1 to the curve C_2. In Figure 18 the vector spins through an angle of 2π, and in this case, the twist is the total angle turned divided by 2π. For the case of a helical type curve winding about a closed circle for its axis, the twist may be defined in an analogous way by means of a spinning vector (see Figure 19).

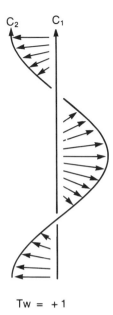

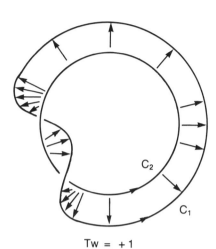

$$Tw = +1$$

$$Tw = +1$$

FIGURE 18. The spinning arrow approach to the twist of a helix with linear axis.

FIGURE 19. The spinning arrow approach to the twist of a helical curve with circular axis.

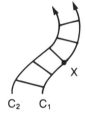

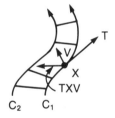

FIGURE 20. A is a graphical representation of a correspondence surface. B pictures the spanning vectors T and V to the correspondence surface at a point x of C_1.

For the more general cases in which C_1 is not linear or planar, the definition of the twist is much more complex for the concept is no longer geometrically obvious. To define the twist in general one needs not just the two curves C_1 and C_2, but the ribbon-like surface joining and bounded by the two curves called the correspondence surface.[11] In the examples in Figure 18 and 19, this surface is the one generated by a line along the spinning vector field joining a point on C_1 to a corresponding point on C_2. In all cases, the correspondence surface is assumed to be differentiable (or smooth) near the curve C_1. This insures that there is a tangent plane to the surface at every point of C_1. In Figure 20 a portion of a correspondence surface between two curves is drawn. Let T be the unit tangent vector to the curve C_1 at a point x. Let V be a unit vector perpendicular to T at x, but tangent to the surface at x pointing in the direction of C_2. Thus, T and V are two perpendicular unit vectors which span the tangent plane to the correspondence surface at x on C_1. Then, their cross-product $T \times V$ is a unit vector perpendicular to the surface at x. As the point x is allowed to vary along the curve C_1, T, and V and $T \times V$ also vary. How V varies is measured by its derivative. The twist, Tw, is defined to be the measure of the total change of V in the direction of $T \times V$ as x moves along the entire curve. It is given by the line integral over the curve C_1:

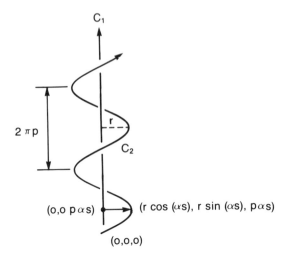

FIGURE 21.   A circular helix of radius r and pitch $2\pi p$ about a linear axis.

$$Tw = Tw(C_2, C_1) = \frac{1}{2\pi} \int_{C_1} (T \times V) \cdot dV \qquad (2)$$

The factor of $\frac{1}{2\pi}$ is in front of the integral so that twist is normalized in turns rather than radians.

In general, twist is not an integer and most definitely changes under deformations of either the curve C_1 or the correspondence surface. Furthermore, the twist depends on the ordering of the curves, i.e., the twist of C_2 about C_1 is not necessarily the twist of C_1 about C_2. These concepts are illustrated in the following examples.

1. The Solenoidal Helix with Straight Line Axis

Let C_2 be a right-handed helix of constant radius r whose axis C_1 is a straight line segment of length L. A diagrammatic illustration of this example is pictured in Figure 21. Then without loss of generality one may assume the axis is the z-axis in space and write the vector equation for C_2 as:

$$y(s) = (r \cos(\alpha s),\ r \sin(\alpha s),\ p\alpha s)$$

where $y(s)$ is the vector pointing from the origin to a point on the curve, $\alpha = \dfrac{2\pi n}{L}$, and s is the length measured along the axis, $0 \leq s \leq L$. Thus, as s goes from 0 to L, the helix winds about the axis C_1 n times with pitch $2\pi p$, so that $2\pi p n = L$.

To compute $Tw(C_2, C_1)$, one needs to establish the correspondence surface. This is formed by vectors connecting a point $(0,0,p\alpha s)$ on the axis C_1 to its corresponding point $(r\cos(\alpha s), r\sin(\alpha s), p\alpha s)$ on the helix C_2. The difference of these two vectors, $(r\cos(\alpha s), r\sin(\alpha s), 0)$, directed from C_1 to C_2 is called the correspondence vector, and the correspondence vectors generate the correspondence surface.

Next to use Formula 2 to compute the twist, one needs to find T and V. T is clearly the unit vector to the z-axis so that $T = (0,0,1)$. To find V, one need only observe that since the correspondence vector generates the surface, it is also tangent to the surface. Furthermore it is perpendicular to T, since the dot product

$$(r \cos(\alpha s),\ r \sin(\alpha s),\ 0) \cdot (0,\ 0,\ 1)\ =\ 0$$

Thus, one may choose V to be a unit vector along the correspondence vector,

$$V\ =\ (\cos(\alpha s),\ \sin(\alpha s),\ 0)$$

Then $T \times V = (-\sin(\alpha s), \cos(\alpha s), 0)$. Finally,

$$\frac{dV}{ds}\ =\ (-\alpha \sin(\alpha s),\ \alpha \cos(\alpha s),\ 0)$$

and therefore,

$$(T \times V) \cdot \frac{dV}{ds}\ =\ \alpha$$

Using Formula 2 to compute $Tw(C_2, C_1)$, one obtains

$$
\begin{aligned}
Tw(C_2,\ C_1)\ &=\ \frac{1}{2\pi} \int_{C_1} (T \times V) \cdot dV \\
&=\ \frac{1}{2\pi} \int_0^L (T \times V) \cdot \frac{dV}{ds} ds \\
&=\ \frac{1}{2\pi} \int_0^L \alpha ds\ =\ \frac{n}{L} \int_0^L ds\ =\ n
\end{aligned}
\tag{3}
$$

where the arc length s of C_1 is used as the parameter of the straight line axis. Thus, the integral expression for twist yields the expected result that $Tw(C_2, C_1) = n$.

It is of special interest to reverse the roles of C_2 and C_1 and compute $Tw(C_1, C_2)$ of C_1 about C_2. The correspondence surface is the same as the one above, and indeed, the correspondence vector is the same except that it is the negative of the one above, for it connects the point $(r\cos(\alpha s), r\sin(\alpha s), p\alpha s)$ on C_2 to $(0, 0, p\alpha s)$ on C_1, and hence, is $(-r\cos(\alpha s), -r\sin(\alpha s), 0)$.

To use Formula 2 one needs again to find T and V. In this case T is the unit vector to the curve C_2 and may be computed from the equation

$$T\ =\ \frac{dy/ds}{\|dy/ds\|}\ =\ \frac{(-r \sin(\alpha s),\ r \cos(\alpha s),\ p)}{(r^2 + p^2)^{1/2}}$$

The correspondence vector $(-r\cos(\alpha s), -r\sin(\alpha s), 0)$ is perpendicular to T and tangent to the surface. Therefore, V may be chosen to be a unit vector along this vector, i.e.,

$$V\ =\ (-\cos(\alpha s),\ -\sin(\alpha s),\ 0)$$

Then

$$T \times V\ =\ \frac{(p \sin(\alpha s),\ -p \cos(\alpha s),\ r)}{(r^2 + p^2)^{1/2}}$$

Finally,

$$\frac{dV}{ds} = (\alpha \sin(\alpha s),\ \alpha \cos(\alpha s),\ 0)$$

and, therefore,

$$(T \times V) \cdot \frac{dV}{ds} = \frac{p\alpha}{(r^2 + p^2)^{1/2}}$$

Using Equation 2 to compute $Tw(C_1, C_2)$ one obtains

$$Tw(C_1,\ C_2) = \frac{1}{2\pi} \int_{C_2} (T \times V) \cdot dV$$

$$= \frac{1}{2\pi} \int_0^L (T \times V) \cdot \frac{dV}{ds} ds$$

$$= \frac{1}{2\pi} \int_0^L \frac{p\alpha}{(r^2 + p^2)^{1/2}} ds = \frac{np}{(r^2 + p^2)^{1/2}}$$

Recalling that $Tw(C_2, C_1) = n$, one sees that Tw definitely depends on the choice of ordering of the curves C_1 and C_2.

The above computations have been made for the right-handed helical case. However, the same analyses work for left-handed helixes winding about a linear axis. If one denotes by C_2^* the left-handed helix corresponding to C_2, the corresponding results are

$$Tw(C_2^*,\ C_1) = -Tw(C_2,\ C_1) = -n$$

and

$$Tw(C_1,\ C_2^*) = Tw(C_1,\ C_2) = \frac{-np}{(r^2 + p^2)^{1/2}}$$

2. Symmetric Solenoidal Helixes

The results obtained in the first example are for what has been termed the half ribbon model. However, they may be used to obtain the twist of a full ribbon model, i.e., the twist of symmetric solenoidal helixes about one another. This is the case where the helix C_2 is reflected through the axis C_1 to obtain a new helix C_2'. The twist of C_2' about C_2, $Tw(C_2', C_2)$ is exactly the same as $Tw(C_1, C_2)$ because the unit vector V along the correspondence vector is the same in both cases (Figure 22). Thus, the result obtained is

$$Tw(C_2',\ C_2) = \frac{np}{(r^2 + p^2)^{1/2}} \qquad (4)$$

i.e., the twist of a helix winding about its symmetrical counterpart n times is not n, the twist of one of the helixes about the axis, but depends strongly on the geometry of the configuration. For helixes of low pitch (p approaching zero) $Tw(C_2', C_2)$ is very small. Conversely, for helixes of very large pitch p compared to r, $Tw(C_2', C)$ approaches n.

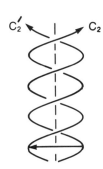 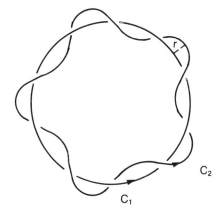

FIGURE 22.   Symmetric solenoidal or circular he-   FIGURE 23.   A helical curve wrapping around a to-
lixes about a linear axis.   rus of radius r whose axis is a circle.

3. The Helical Curve with a Closed Circular Axis

Let C_2 be a helical type curve winding in a right-handed uniform sense about a closed circular axis C_1 (Figure 23). This case can best be described in the following manner. C_1 is as a circle of radius R and hence, curvature $\kappa = \dfrac{1}{R}$. Its length is therefore $L = 2\pi R$. Imagine an inner tube or torus of radius $r < R$ with C_1 as its central axis. The curve C_2 is a helical type curve of uniform pitch lying on the surface of the torus winding in a right-handed sense about the curve C_1. Suppose that C_2 winds about C_1 n times. Then it is clear that $Lk(C_2,C_1) = n$. Furthermore, a straightforward calculation of the twist,[11] $Tw(C_2,C_1)$, shows that

$$Tw(C_2, C_1) = n \tag{5}$$

In this case the correspondence vector generating the correspondence surface is directed from a point on the circle C_1 to the corresponding point on the curve C_2. This case can be thought of as the case in which the model in the first example is bent so that the linear axis becomes a circle.

Reversing the roles of C_1 and C_2 leads to a much more difficult computation. In this case the twist of C_1 about C_2 is given by the integral[11]

$$Tw(C_1, C_2) = \frac{1}{2\pi} \int_0^{2\pi n} \{(1 - r\kappa \cos \theta)^2 + (rn\kappa)^2\}^{-1/2} d\theta \tag{6}$$

This is a difficult elliptical integral in general. However, in the special case that $r\kappa \ll 1$, i.e., the radius of the torus is very very small compared to the radius of the circle C_1, the term $r\kappa\cos\theta$ can be ignored, and

$$Tw(C_1, C_2) \cong \frac{1}{2\pi} \int_0^{2\pi n} (1 + (rn\kappa)^2)^{-1/2} d\theta$$

$$= n(1 + (rn\kappa)^2)^{-1/2}$$

This answer contrasts sharply to $Tw(C_2,C_1) = n$. If one arbitrarily defines a "pitch" by $2\pi p$, so that $2\pi pn = L = 2\pi R = \dfrac{2\pi}{\kappa}$, then

$$Tw(C_1, C_2) = \frac{np}{(r^2 + p^2)^{1/2}} \tag{7}$$

which is exactly analogous to the expression in Subsection 1.

In the case that $r\kappa < 1$, but is not very very small, then one must use the full solution to the elliptical integral. In this case

$$Tw(C_1, C_2) = \left(\frac{2ng}{\pi\mu}\right) K(\epsilon) \tag{8}$$

where

$$\frac{g}{\mu} = ((r^2\kappa^2(n^2 + 1) + 1)^2 - 4r^2\kappa^2)^{-1/2}$$

and

$$\epsilon^2 = \frac{1}{2}(1 - ((n^2 - 1)r^2\kappa^2 + 1) \times ((n^2 + 1)r^2\kappa^2 + 1)^2 - 4r^2\kappa^2)^{-1/2}$$

where $K(\epsilon)$ is the well-known complete elliptical integral. This is a formidable expression, but is very useful in applications.

As in the linear case these results can be adapted to deal with the case of a helical type curve C_2^* winding in a left-handed fashion about the axis C_1. In this case, $Lk(C_2^*, C_1) = -n$, and

$$Tw(C_2^*, C_1) = -Tw(C_2, C_1)$$
$$Tw,(C_1, C_2^*) = -Tw(C_1, C_2)$$

4. The Superhelix Whose Axis Is the Solenoidal Helix with Straight Line Axis

Let C_2 be the solenoidal helix with straight line axis C_1 described in 1. Let C_3 be a superhelical type curve winding in a right-handed manner about the helix C_2. This case is pictured in Figure 24 and can be described in the following manner.

Imagine a thin piece of rubber tubing of radius ρ which is bent into helical type surface, i.e., its central axis traces out the curve C_2. Then C_3 can be drawn on the surface of this tubing winding in a right-handed manner and in a uniform way (i.e., pitch uniform) about the axis C_2. Thus, C_2 is a helix which lies on a cylinder of radius r, and C_3 is a superhelix lying on a helical type surface with radius ρ. Suppose further that C_3 actually winds about C_2 m times. Then, the twist $Tw(C_3, C_2)$ can be computed[11] and found to be

$$Tw(C_3, C_2) = m + \frac{np}{(r^2 + p^2)^{1/2}} \tag{9}$$

In this case the correspondence surface is generated by the vectors joining a point of C_2 to the corresponding point of C_3.

The twist of a curve C_3^* winding m times about the curve C_2 in a left-handed fashion is given by the formula

$$Tw(C_3^*, C_2) = -m + \frac{np}{(r^2 + p^2)^{1/2}}$$

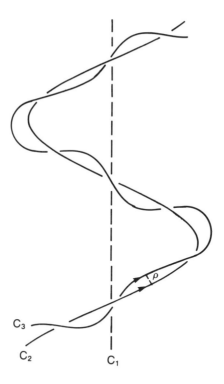

FIGURE 24. A superhelical curve wrapping around a
torus of radius ρ whose axis is a helix.

Finally, the twist of a curve C_3 winding m times in a right-handed manner about a left-handed helix C_2^* is given by the formula

$$Tw(C_3, C_2^*) = m - \frac{np}{(r^2 + p^2)^{1/2}} \tag{10}$$

It is well worth noting that these last three expressions for the twist involving not only the winding of C_3 (or C_3^*) about C_2 (or C_2^*), but also the geometry of the helix C_2 (or C_2^*) itself. Indeed, the term $\frac{np}{(r^2+p^2)^{1/2}}$ (or $\frac{-np}{(r^2+p^2)^{1/2}}$) is nothing other than $Tw(C_1,C_2)$ [or $Tw(C_1,C_2^*)$].

The twist of C_2 about C_3 is also computable[11] and strongly involves the geometry of both helixes.

5. The Superhelix Whose Axis Is the Helical Curve with a Closed Circular Axis

Let C_2 be the helical type curve winding in a uniform manner about a closed circular axis. Let C_3 be a superhelical type curve winding in a right-handed manner about the helix C_2. Basically this is the case where the example in the previous subsection is closed up. The result for the twist is entirely analogous to that in subsection 4, namely,

$$Tw(C_3, C_2) = m + Tw(C_1, C_2)$$

where m is the number of times C_3 winds about C_2.

If C_3^* is a superhelical curve winding in a left-handed fashion m times about C_2, then

$$Tw(C_3^*, C_2) = -m + Tw(C_1, C_2)$$

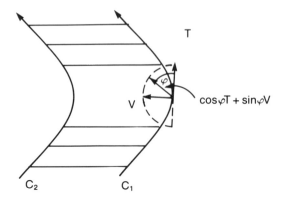

FIGURE 25.   The half circle of vectors in the tangent plane
to the correspondence surface at a point of the boundary curve.

B. The Gauss Integral Approach

In Sections II and III, integral expressions were given for the linking number and the
writhing number. These integrals give a measure of how many times and in what manner
the unit sphere is covered by vectors joining points of either the two curves in the case of
the linking number or points of the same curve in the case of writhing. The integral expression

$$Tw(C_2, C_1) = \frac{1}{2\pi} \int_{C_1} T \times V \cdot dV$$

also derives from a similar kind of Gauss map integral.

The Gauss map for the twist is defined as follows. At each point x on C_1 one considers
the half-tangent plane spanned by the vectors T and positive vectors along V, i.e., the portion
of the tangent plane to the correspondence surface at x that lies on the positive V side of T
(see Figure 25). In this half-plane there are unit vectors starting at x and lying in the half-
plane. Any such vector can be written in the form $\cos\varphi T + \sin\varphi V$ where $0 \leq \varphi \leq \pi$. Thus,
the endpoints of these vectors trace out a half-circle in the tangent plane at x. If each of
these vectors is translated to the origin, its endpoint becomes a point on the sphere of radius
1, centered at the origin. Indeed, if the entire half-circle of vectors is translated to the origin,
an entire half-great circle on the sphere is traced out. Finally, if this procedure is carried
out for all points x on C_1, one obtains the Gauss map for the twist. As in the case of linking,
the twist measures how many times and with what sign the Gauss map just defined sweeps
across the unit sphere. Once again this integral is normalized by a factor of $(4\pi)^{-1}$. Each
half-circle contributing to the Gauss map will be positive or negative depending on the sign
of the twist term $T \times V \cdot dV$ at the point in question.

The simplest illustration of this map is for the circular helix winding about the linear axis
(see Figure 26). In this case C_1 is the straight line axis and C_2 is the circular helix. T is the
unit vector along the axis, i.e., (0,0,1) and V is the unit vector pointing from the axis to
the helix, perpendicular to T, i.e., $V = (\cos(\alpha s), \sin(\alpha s), 0)$. The half-circles have their
centers on the axis and spin around the axis as the point on the axis moves up. Thus, the
Gauss map sweeps across the sphere in a counterclockwise fashion, covering the whole
sphere exactly once for each turn of the helix. When normalized by the factor of $(4\pi)^{-1}$,
the twist is one for each turn of the helix.

V. THE FUNDAMENTAL FORMULA $Lk = Tw + Wr$

The three quantities Lk, Wr, and Tw are related by a fundamental equation in special
cases, and it is this equation which proves to be so useful in applications to DNA. The case

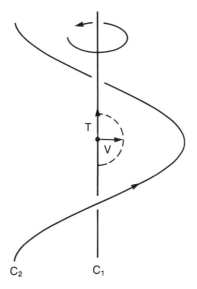

FIGURE 26. The spinning half circle which generates the Gauss map for the twist of a helix about a linear axis.

of primary interest is the case in which C_1 and C_2 are two oriented curves which bound a ribbon-like correspondence surface. The surface is also assumed to be differentiable at C_1 and not to intersect C_1 (other than having C_1 as its boundary). In this case, the three quantities $Lk(C_2,C_1)$, $Tw(C_2,C_1)$, and $Wr(C_1)$ are related by the fundamental formula

$$Lk(C_2, C_1) = Tw(C_2, C_1) + Wr(C_1) \qquad (11)$$

Examples are given in Figure 27. In Figure 27a and b, $Lk = Tw = Wr = 0$. In Figure 27c, $Lk = Tw = +1$, $Wr(C_1) = 0$.

There is one major consequence of this equation that should be immediately noted. Although the left-hand side, $Lk(C_2,C_1)$, is a topological invariant, the two terms on the right-hand side, $Tw(C_2,C_1)$ and $Wr(C_1)$ are not, and in fact, vary under deformations. Therefore, as long as the boundary curves C_1 and C_2 are not broken, any change in Tw must be compensated by an equal in magnitude but opposite in sign change in Wr. For example, if one lifts the top branch of the ribbon in Figure 28, $Wr(C_1)$ begins to decrease and $Tw(C_2,C_1)$ begins to increase. Then with an appropriate deformation, one can eventually deform the ribbon into that of Figure 27c. In this whole process $Lk(C_2,C_1) = +1$; $Wr(C_1)$ changes from approximately $+1$ to 0, and $Tw(C_2,C_1)$ changes from approximately 0 to $+1$.

A second application of formula illustrates how to use twist to decrease or increase linking. Suppose that in Figure 27a there is a break in one of the boundary curves C_2 of the ribbon surface. If this break is filled in, $Lk = Tw = Wr = 0$. However, if one side of the broken section is rotated about the curve C_1 in a right-handed manner exactly once and then reannealed, then Tw has been changed from 0 to $+1$ and so has Lk. Since C_1 remains unchanged, $Wr(C_1)$ remains equal to 0. Thus, Equation 11 is verified. The end product will be the ribbon surface in Figure 27c. Clearly, the direction of rotation determines the sign of the twist. Further, if the broken part is rotated n times in the same direction about C_1 and then reannealed, then twist and linking will be changed in magnitude by n.

A third application of the formula illustrates how to use a change in writhing to decrease or increase linking. If the ribbon in Figure 28 has a break in the entire ribbon surface on

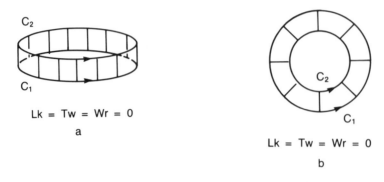

$Lk = Tw = Wr = 0$

a

$Lk = Tw = Wr = 0$

b

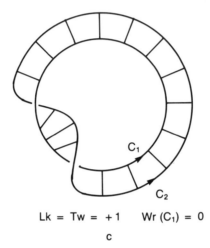

$Lk = Tw = +1 \qquad Wr(C_1) = 0$

c

FIGURE 27.   Pictorial examples demonstrating $Lk = Tw + Wr$ for ribbon models.

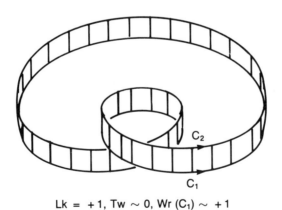

$Lk = +1, Tw \sim 0, Wr(C_1) \sim +1$

FIGURE 28.   A ribbon model with $Lk = +1$, $Tw \sim 0$ Wr
$\sim +1$.

the top loop and if the bottom loop is passed through this break to become the top loop and then if the original break is resealed, then, in this process, $Wr(C_1)$ has changed from approximately $+1$ to approximately -1, Tw is basically unchanged, and Lk has decreased by 2. Thus, the formula is once again verified. Of course, this process can be reversed to increase Lk by 2.

Equation 11 may also be used directly to compute the writing number of some of the special curves from Section IV. For example, if C_2 is a helical curve winding n times in a right-handed manner about a circular axis C_1, then $Lk(C_1,C_2) = n$, and by Equation 7,

$Tw(C_1,C_2) = \dfrac{np}{(r^2+p^2)^{1/2}}$. Therefore, by Equation 11

$$Wr(C_2) = n\left(1 - \frac{p}{(r^2 + p^2)^{1/2}}\right)$$

Thus, the contribution per turn of the helix to the twist is $\dfrac{p}{(r^2+p^2)^{1/2}}$ and to the writing is

$1 - \dfrac{p}{(r^2+p^2)^{1/2}}$. If C_2^* is a helical curve winding n times in a left-handed manner about C_1, then $Lk(C_1,C_2^*) = -n$, $Tw(C_1,C_2) = -Tw(C_1,C_2^*)$, and $Wr(C_2^*) = -Wr(C_2)$.

The proof[7] of Equation 11 is beyond the scope of this chapter. However, the idea is as follows. One shows that the Gauss maps and integrals are so related that $Lk(C_2,C_1) = Tw(C_2,C_1) + Wr(C_1)$. What this means is that if the Gauss map for Lk sweeps across a point, say p_0, on the unit sphere m times, if the Gauss map for Wr sweeps across p_0, r times, and if the Gauss map for Tw sweeps across p_0, s times, then one can show by mathematical analysis that $m = r + s$. However, a detailed understanding of the proof is not necessary for applications. The three applications listed above all verified the theorem, and it is these that will be used mostly in molecular biology.

VI. APPLICATIONS TO DNA

In the application of the concepts Lk, Tw, and Wr, two models will be used: (1) the so-called full ribbon model[8] and (2) the so-called half ribbon model.[9] Although not necessary for the general theory, the DNA double helix model used will be the classical Crick-Watson model which completes one turn of the helix about every 10.5 bp. The full ribbon model will be one in which the two curves C_1 and C_2 described in Sections II, III, IV, and V will be chosen to pass along the phosphodiester-sugar backbone chains. Hereafter, these curves will be denoted C and W. Twist, Tw, will denote $Tw(W,C)$. Writhing, Wr, will denote $Wr(C)$, and in case the DNA is closed circular, linking number, Lk, will denote $Lk(W,C)$. The correspondence surface which enables one to define Tw will be the ribbon-like surface generated by lines which join a base on C to its complementary base on W. Essentially, this is the model pictured in Figure 22.

The half ribbon model is defined as follows. The entire double helical structure of the Crick-Watson model has an axis, to be denoted A. In the simple linear model, A is a straight line about which C turns as a helix. In the simplest closed circular model, A is a circle about which C turns as a helix. The half ribbon model will be one in which the two curves C_1 and C_2 described in Sections II to V will be chosen to be the curves A and C (or W), respectively. Tw will denote $Tw(C,A)$, Wr will denote $Wr(A)$, and in the case the DNA is closed circular, Lk will denote $Lk(C,A)$. The correspondence surface which enables one to define Tw will be the ribbon-like surface generated by lines which join a base on C to its corresponding point on the axis A (see Figures 21 and 23).

Both the full and half ribbon models are useful in studying DNA. The model most often used is the half ribbon one because the axis A is an easy curve to analyze in most cases. However, there are complex structures in DNA such as cruciforms or denatured zones which make the axis A undefinable. In these cases, the full ribbon model is useful since the curves C and W are always defined. In most simple cases of closed circular DNA there is an interesting relationship between the two models. Since the curve W can be deformed into the axis A in a continuous manner, $Lk(C,A) = Lk(C,W)$. However, $Lk(C,W) = Lk(W,C)$. Therefore, Lk for either model is the same, and thus one can speak of the *linking number of DNA* without concern about the model. It must be emphasized that this is not the case with either Tw or Wr. However, because of formula and the fact that $Lk(C,A) = Lk(W,C)$, one can state $Tw(W,C) + Wr(C) = Tw(C,A) + Wr(A)$ or $Wr(C) - Wr(A) = Tw(C,A) - Tw(W,C)$. These two formulas relate the twists and writhing numbers of the two models.

A. Twist and Writhing of DNA

The first application will be to use the results of the first four sections to compute twist and writhing numbers for representative models of DNA.[11]

1. Linear DNA

For the case of linear Crick-Watson DNA, one may use Equation 3 to compute that if C coils about A, n times, $Tw(C,A) = n$. Thus, if the DNA is B bp in length, its twist, Tw, is equal to $\dfrac{B}{10.5}$, since it takes 10.5 bp to make one revolution of the helix. To compute the twist of one strand W about the other C, $Tw(W,C)$ we may use Equation 4 to find that $Tw(W,C) = \dfrac{np}{(r^2+p^2)^{1/2}}$ where r is the radius of the double helical structure, i.e., the radius of the cylinder on which C and W lie, $2\pi p$ is the pitch of the helix, and n is the number of times the helix winds about the axis A. For the classical structure $2\pi p = 3.36nm$ and $r = 1.0nm$. Hence, $p = 0.54nm$. Thus, $Tw(W,C) = \dfrac{.54n}{(1+(.54)^2)^{1/2}} = 0.47n$. Thus, if the DNA is B bp long, $Tw(W,C) = \dfrac{0.47B}{10.5}$. It is of interest to note that the twist of one strand about the other is approximately one half of the twist of a strand about the axis. In the literature,[9] this quantity $\dfrac{p}{(r^2+p^2)^{1/2}}$ is often denoted $\sin \alpha$ where α is the helical pitch angle. In this case $\sin \alpha = 0.47$ so that α is approximately $28°$.

2. Closed Circular DNA in which the Axis Is a Circle

If the axis A of the DNA is a closed circle and the DNA strand C winds about A, n times, then one may use Equation 5 to obtain that $Tw(C,A) = n$. Furthermore, since A is a plane circle, one may use the results of Section III to obtain $Wr(A) = 0$ and then use Equation 11 to find that $Lk(C,A) = n$. Thus, in this simple case, $Lk(C,A) = Tw(C,A)$.

In this case when $Wr(A) = 0$, $Lk(C,A)$ is usually denoted Lk_0. Lk_0 is the linking number of the relaxed state of the closed circular DNA. The number of base pairs being approximately 10.5 per turn of the helical structure, one finds that if a closed circular DNA of B bp length is in its relaxed state, then $Lk_0 = \dfrac{B}{10.5}$. For example, if a DNA is 2100 bp in length, $Lk_0 = 200$.

To compute the twist of W about C, one may use Equation 6 and divide into two subcases. If R is the radius of the circle A, if r is the radius of the DNA, and if $r \ll R$, i.e., r is very small compared to R, then, by Equation 7, $Tw(W,C) = \dfrac{np}{(r^2+p^2)^{1/2}}$, where $p = R/n$. For most DNA, $r \ll R$, since most DNA are quite long. This case essentially reduces to the linear case, and one can show that $Tw(W,C) = 0.47n$. Since $Lk(C,A) = Lk(W,C) = n$, one can use the equation to show that $Wr(C) = n - 0.47n = 0.53n$. Thus, for each segment of the DNA strand which revolves once about the axis, the contribution to Tw is 0.47 and that to Wr is 0.53.

The other subcase to be discussed is the case where R is closer to r, i.e., $r < R$ but not necessarily $\ll R$. In this case, one must use the complicated expression in Equation 8 to compute Tw. Once Tw is found, then since $Lk = n$, one may use the formula to compute Wr, i.e., $Wr = n - Tw$. Since most DNA are fairly long, this expression is rarely used. It does however have more applications in computing the writhing number of catenated DNA.

3. Superhelical DNA and Winding in a Nucleosome

If the axis A of a DNA is itself a helix winding about a linear axis, the DNA is said to be supercoiled (see Figure 24). In this case, the DNA strand C is a superhelix, i.e., a helix winding about a helix. If the axis A winds about its axis n times in a right-handed sense, and the superhelix C winds about A m times in a right-handed sense, then one may use Equation 9 to compute the twist $Tw(C,A) = m + \dfrac{np}{(r^2+p^2)^{1/2}}$ where $2\pi p$ is the pitch of the helix A and r is the radius of the cylinder on which the helix A lies. If the axis A winds about its axis n times in a left-handed sense and C winds m times about A in a right-handed sense, then by Equation 10 $Tw(C,A) = m - \dfrac{np}{(r^2+p^2)^{1/2}}$.[11]

This last expression can be applied to the winding of DNA in a nucleosome as follows. DNA does not exist simply as a double helical structure by itself, but has a great deal of associated structure. In particular, DNA is known to wrap in a left-handed sense around nucleosomes. These entities can be thought of in simple terms as cylinders on which the axis of the DNA sits as a left-handed helix. Thus, the double helical structure becomes a superhelical structure. When the axis of the DNA is on the nucleosome, the number of base pairs per turn is no longer 10.5. According to the most recent X-ray data,[24,25] when DNA is wrapped about the nucleosome in a left-handed sense, there is approximately one duplex turn for each 10 bp. Thus, if there are B bp on the nucleosome, there are $\dfrac{B}{10}$ duplex turns, so that $m = \dfrac{B}{10}$. Furthermore, the same data gives information about the radius r of the nucleosomal cylinder and the pitch $2\pi p$ of the left-handed helix. In fact, $r = 4.3nm$ and $2\pi p = 2.8nm$, so that the quantity $\dfrac{p}{(r^2+p^2)^{1/2}} \cong \dfrac{1}{10}$. Hence, if the helix wraps around n times, $Tw(C,A) = \dfrac{1}{10}(B-n)$. If the same DNA of B base pairs were extended linearly, where the latest data gives the number of base pairs per turn as 10.54, then $Tw(C,A) = \dfrac{B}{10.54}$. Thus by wrapping the DNA left-handedly on the nucleosome, $Tw(C,A)$ changes from $\dfrac{B}{10.54}$ to $\dfrac{B-n}{10}$. Usually[25] the number of base pairs is approximately 146 and n is approximately 1.85. Thus, $Tw(C,A)$ changes from 13.85 to 14.41 and hence, increases by 0.56. If one compares the writhing number of the axis A of the linearly extended DNA in which case A is straight line with $Wr(A) = 0$ and the writhing number of the left-handedly wrapped axis in which case by the results at the end of Section V $Wr(A)$ is approximately -1.65, the net change in $Wr(A)$ is -1.65. Thus the total change in $Tw(C,A)$ plus that of $Wr(A)$ is -1.09. This can be interpreted by Equation 11 as the net change in linking. This change of approximately -1 is called the linking deficiency due to nucleosomal wrapping. Of course, these numbers are only a close approximation, but they give a reasonable analysis of the linking deficiency problem.

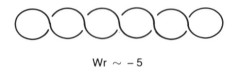

Wr ~ −5

FIGURE 29. An interwound helix with multiple negative coils.

B. Analysis of Enzymatic Action

The second application will be to use the results of Sections II to V to analyze two different types of enzymatic activity. As was observed earlier, if a closed circular DNA is in its so-called relaxed state, its linking number is Lk_0. However, since DNA has associated nucleosomal winding, its actual linking number is *decreased* by approximately 1 for each nucleosome. When these DNAs are isolated from nature, they therefore appear to be *underwound* relative to the relaxed state, and indeed, in the electron microscope they appear to be contorted or coiled up rings with many crossings. Such behavior is called *supercoiling*. The actual linking number Lk is therefore less than Lk_0, and the quantity $Lk - Lk_0 = \Delta Lk$ is called the *linking number difference*. The reason for the supercoiling can be described in the following manner. Any change from Lk_0 to Lk can be divided into a change in Tw and a change in Wr. Apparently the DNA prefers the change in Wr to the change in Tw, i.e., the DNA is conformationally more stable if its change in Tw is minimized (kept as close as possible to 10.5 bp per turn). Therefore, change in Lk is compensated mostly by change in Wr. In the relaxed state $Wr = 0$; in the state of reduced linking $Wr < 0$. The more negative Lk, the more negative coiling that arises from the negative Wr. It appears that more often than not, this negative supercoiling takes the form of an interwound helix as shown in Figure 29. In this special case there are five negative crossings.

Some years after the discovery of the fact that closed circular DNA is underwound,[10] it was discovered that there are enzymes which can actually change the linking number. These enzymes fall into two main categories: Type 1 topoisomerases form a transient single stranded break, allow a DNA chain to pass through the break, and then reseal the break and Type 2 topoisomerases create a transient double-stranded break, allow a DNA chain passage, and then reseal the break without a rotation of the broken ends.

1. Type 1 Topoisomerases: Enzymes which Change Lk by 1

Type 1 topoisomerases are thought to "relax" the supercoiling due to the large negative linking number difference. The larger the difference, the quicker the reaction, or the closer Lk is to Lk_0, the slower the reaction. To show how one can use the ideas of Sections II to V to model the reaction, one proceeds as follows. Figure 30A is shown a ribbon-like surface with boundaries C and A. $Lk(C,A) = -1$, $Wr(A) \cong -1$, and $Tw(C,A) \cong 0$. The first step in a Type 1 topoisomerase reaction will break the curve C at the point p. The second step will be to rotate the curve C about A once in right-handed fashion. The third step will be to reseal the broken curve C at p. The endproduct is shown in Figure 30B. Speaking geometrically, what has transpired in this process is that $Tw(C,A)$ has increased by $+1$ (second step) and that $Wr(A)$ has remained unchanged. Therefore, by the fundamental Equation 11, Lk has increased by $+1$ and therefore changes from -1 to 0.

Energetically, the increase in twist will be used to eliminate the negativity of the writhing of A to yield a completely relaxed ribbon such as the one shown in Figure 27a.

This analysis can apply in an obvious way to underwound DNA. If a DNA, say for example SV-40, has $Lk_0 = 500$, but is underwound so that $Lk = 475$ with 25 negative supercoils, then, with some simplification, one can say that $Lk(C,A) = 475$, $Tw(C,A) \cong 500$, and $Wr(A) \cong -25$, where C is one of the backbones and A is the axis. A reaction such as the one outlined above will increase $Tw(C,A)$ by $+1$, which increase will be absorbed

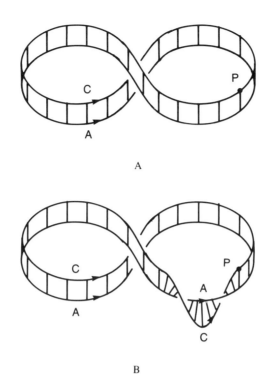

A

B

FIGURE 30.   A represents an interwound ribbon model.
The break is made at p and the ribbon rotated so that C
revolves about A in a right-handed manner to give the
model in B.

to eliminate one of the supercoils. Thus, after the reaction, $Lk(C,A) = 476$, $Tw(C,A) \cong$
500, and $Wr(A) \cong -24$. Naturally, reiteration of this reaction will increase $Lk(C,A)$ and
then $Wr(A)$ by 1 each time. Eventually, one will arrive at the case where $Lk = Lk_0$ and
$Wr(A) = 0$.

2. Type 2 Topoisomerases: Enzymes which Change Lk by 2

One of the actions of Type 2 topoisomerases is also the relaxation of negative supercoiling.
In the reaction of topoisomerases of Type 1, the change in the linking number was due to
an increase in the twist and a subsequent modification. In the case of topoisomerases of
Type 2, the change in linking is due to an increase in writhing. To model the reaction, one
may proceed as follows. One starts with the ribbon-like surface shown in Figure 31A,
bounded by curves C and A. In this case $Lk(C,A) = -2$, $Wr(A) \cong -2$, and $Tw(C,A) \cong$
0. The first step in a Type 2 topoisomerase reaction will be a complete break of the ribbon
at the point p and q. The second step will be to pass the top part of the ribbon through the
break. The third step will be to reseal the break in the ribbon, without any rotation of either
edge C or A. The end product is displayed in Figure 31B. Geometrically, what has transpired
in this process is that $Wr(A)$ has increased by 2, since A has passed through itself, and
$Tw(C,A)$ has remained unchanged. Therefore, Lk has increased by $+2$ and therefore changes
from -2 to 0. The increase in writhing by 2 will completely compensate for the $Wr(A)$ ($=$
-2), so that $Wr(A) = 0$ and the result will be a completely relaxed ribbon.

This analysis may be applied to DNA in the following manner. If the SV-40 molecule is
underwound as before with 25 negative supercoils, then once again $Lk(C,A) = 475$, $Tw(C,A)$
$\cong 500$, and $Wr(A) \cong -25$. A reaction of a Type 2 topoisomerase breaks the entire duplex
structure at one region, passes another region through the break, and then reseals the original

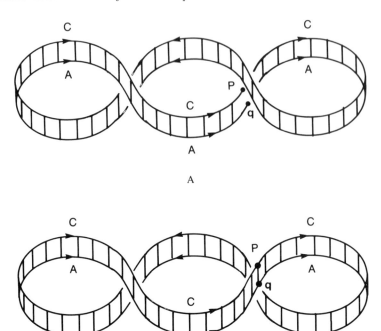

FIGURE 31.   A represents an interwound ribbon model. A full break is made at *p*
and *q*, and the top branch is passed through to give the model in B.

break. In this process, the axis A of the DNA is passed through itself so that $Wr(A)$ increases
by 2. $Tw(C,A)$ is left unchanged, and therefore $Lk(C,A)$ increases by 2. Thus, after the
reaction $Lk(C,A) = Lk = 477$, $Tw(C,A) \cong 500$, and $Wr(A) \cong -23$. Naturally, reiteration
of this reaction changes Lk by $+2$ and $Wr(A)$ by $+2$. This, therefore, is a method to reduce
the underwound DNA to its reduced state.

REFERENCES

1. **Bauer, W. R.,** Structure and reactions of closed duplex DNA, *Annu. Rev. Biophys. Bioeng.*, 7, 287, 1978.
2. **Bauer, W. R., Crick, F. H. C., and White, J. H.,** Supercoiled DNA, *Sci. Am.*, 243, 100, 1980.
3. **Gellert, M.,** DNA topoisomerases, *Annu. Rev. Biochem.*, 50, 879, 1981.
4. **Wang, J. C.,** DNA topoisomerases, *Annu. Rev. Biochem.*, 54, 655, 1985.
5. **Wasserman, S. A. and Cozzarelli, N. R.,** Biochemical topology, *Science*, 232, 951, 1986.
6. **Cozzarelli, N. R.,** DNA gyrase and the supercoiling of DNA, *Science*, 207, 953, 1980.
7. **White, J. H.,** Self-linking and the Gauss integral in higher dimensions, *Am. J. Math.*, 91, 693, 1969.
8. **Crick, F. H. C.,** Linking numbers and nucleosomes, *Proc. Natl. Acad. Sci. U.S.A.*, 73, 285, 1976.
9. **Fuller, F. B.,** The writhing number of a space curve, *Proc. Natl. Acad. Sci. U.S.A.*, 68, 815, 1971.
10. **Vinograd, J. and Lebowitz, J.,** Physical and topological properties of circular DNA, *J. Gen. Physiol.*, 49, 103, 1965.
11. **White, J. H. and Bauer, W. R.,** Calculation of the twist and writhe for representative models of DNA, *J. Mol. Biol.*, 189, 329, 1986.
12. **Bauer, W. R. and Vinograd, J.,** *Progress in Molecular and Subcellular Biology*, Springer-Verlag, New York, 1985.

13. **Pulleybank, D. E., Shure, M., Tang, D., Vinograd, J., and Vosberg, H.-P.,** Action of nicking-closing enzymes on supercoiled and non-supercoiled closed circular DNA, *Proc. Natl. Acad. Sci. U.S.A.,* 72, 4280, 1975.

14. **Depew, R. E. and Wang, J. C.,** Conformational fluctuations of DNA helix, *Proc. Natl. Acad. Sci. U.S.A.,* 72, 4275, 1975.

15. **Fuller, F. B.,** Decomposition of the linking number of a closed ribbon, *Proc. Natl. Acad. Sci. U.S.A.,* 75, 3557, 1978.

16. **Benham, C. J.,** Torsional stress and local denaturation in supercoiled DNA, *Proc. Natl. Acad. Sci. U.S.A.,* 76, 3870, 1979.

17. **Benham, C. J.,** The equilibrium statistical mechanics of the helix-coil transition in torsionally stressed DNA, *J. Chem. Phys.,* 72, 3633, 1980.

18. **Benham, C. J.,** Theoretical analysis of conformational equilibria in superhelical DNA, *Annu. Rev. Biophys. Biophys. Chem.,* 14, 23, 1985.

19. **Benham, C. J.,** An elastic model of the large-scale structure of duplex DNA, *Biopolymers,* 18, 609, 1979.

20. **Benham, C. J.,** Elastic model of supercoiling, *Proc. Natl. Acad. Sci. U.S.A.,* 74, 2397, 1977.

21. **Benham, C. J.,** Geometry and mechanics of DNA superhelicity, *Biopolymers,* 22, 2477, 1983.

22. **Benham, C. J.,** Cruciform formation at inverted repeat sequences in supercoiled DNA, *Biopolymers,* 21, 679, 1982.

23. **Walba, D. M.,** Topological stereochemistry, *Tetrahedron,* 41, 3161, 1985.

24. **Klug, A. and Lutter, L. C.,** The helical periodicity of DNA on the nucleosome, *Nucleic Acids Res.,* 9, 4267, 1981.

25. **Uberbacher, E. C., Ramakrishnav, V., Olins, D. E., and Bunick, G. J.,** Neutron Scattering studies of nucleosome structure at low ionic strength, *Biochemistry,* 22, 4916, 1983.

Chapter 10

MECHANICS AND EQUILIBRIA OF SUPERHELICAL DNA

Craig J. Benham

TABLE OF CONTENTS

I. DNA SUPERHELICITY IN BIOLOGICAL SYSTEMS

DNA within living systems is constrained so that the stresses imposed upon it can be regulated. The constraint that is most amenable to in vitro experimental investigation involves the covalent bonding together of the two ends of each duplex strand to form a ring molecule in which each strand is a continuous circle.[1] This restricts the molecule to conformations having a fixed value of the linking number Lk, which in turn has the effect of topologically coupling its secondary and tertiary structures through White's formula[2,3]

$$Lk = Tw + Wr \tag{1}$$

as described elsewhere in this volume. If the covalent continuity of one strand is disrupted at a single site, the molecule is said to be nicked. Local rotation of the ends temporarily created by transient nicking permits the linking number to be changed. The relaxed state of a circular molecule is phenomenologically defined to have the twist and writhe characteristic of the singly nicked species under the given environmental conditions.[4]

The stress experienced by a closed circular molecule depends upon its linking difference $\alpha = \Delta Lk = Lk - Lk_0$, the amount by which the molecular linking number differs from its relaxed value. In principle, the linking difference α can be modulated in two ways. First, Lk itself may be altered, which requires the introduction of transient strand breaks. Both eukaryotic and prokaryotic organisms produce topoisomerase enzymes which perform this function.[5,6] Type I topoisomerases act, usually without need of a source of free energy, to relax the DNA. Type II enzymes, using ATP as an energy source, generally act to decrease Lk below Lk_0. The dynamic balance between these activities maintains prokaryotic DNA in a negatively superhelical, underlinked state (i.e., $\alpha < 0$).[7] Alternatively, α can be modulated without disrupting strand continuity by changing the value of the relaxed linking number Lk_0. This can occur through any alteration of the local environment that changes either the unstressed twist or the relaxed tertiary structure of the molecule.

Closed circular molecules have become the paradigm examples of stressed DNA for in vitro investigation, largely because they are amenable to the manipulation of and sorting by their linking numbers.[8] Experimental results have shown that several physiologically important regulatory events are highly sensitive to the degree of superhelical stress imposed on the molecule in vitro. These include the initiation of transcription[9,10] and replication,[11] transposition,[12] integrative recombination and the uptake of homologous single strands,[13] and the recognition of and binding to several classes of regulatory enzymes.[14,15] There is also important (but necessarily more circumstantial) evidence that these physiological functions of DNA are also regulated by the degree of superhelical stress imposed on the molecule in vivo.[16,17] In particular, DNA within malignantly transformed cells is maintained at more extreme negative superhelicities than the corresponding DNA in normal cells.[18,19]

Many types of DNAs occur as closed circles, including plasmids, episomes, mitochondrial DNA, and the genomic DNAs of prokaryotes and many viruses.[20] Although much of the DNA within living systems is not circular, it still may have stresses imposed upon it that are analogous to those present in closed ring molecules.[21] The DNA within eukaryotic chromosomes is intricately associated with basic histone and nonhistone proteins to form a chromatin fiber. Within this fiber the DNA duplex is wound around a histone core to form a nucleosome.[22] The fiber consisting of a string of nucleosomes in turn is wound into higher order structures that associate with a protein scaffolding.[23] The DNA within the chromatin fiber is attached to this scaffolding so as to preclude local rotations at the attachment site.[24] Thus the portion of the DNA between adjacent attachment sites is constrained as a topological domain analogous to a closed circle, upon which superhelical stresses may be imposed.[25] Because the relaxed state of the domain has twist and writhe characteristic of the nicked species under identical conditions, it will depend sensitively on the chromatin structure and in particular on the degree of nucleosomal winding present. As the tertiary structure of the DNA within the domain is determined by its interactions with histones and the other molecules comprising chromatin, any stresses imposed upon DNA under these circumstances will be primarily torsional in character.

The highly structured environment of DNA within chromatin provides several additional methods by which stresses may be regulated. A change in the association with nucleosomes, such as the fiber taking up additional nucleosomes or being stripped of some, will alter the effective relaxed state of the domain, hence its imposed superhelical stresses. Differences in nucleosomal association have been observed between transcriptionally active and inactive chromatin.[26,27] The binding to or disassociation of this fiber with histone H1, which serves to bridge the gap between nucleosomes, will influence both the effective superhelicity of a domain and the susceptibility of the DNA at the sites involved to other influences, such as bending deformations or interactions with other molecules. Relative motions of or conformational transitions within nucleosomes can also alter the stresses upon local regions of the DNA.[28,29]

The genomic DNAs of many bacteria and other prokaryotes are both circular and attached to the cell wall.[11,20,21] Thus its molecular linking number can be regulated by events similar to those experienced by other, smaller closed circles. However, experimental evidence suggests that the prokaryotic genome is subdivided into topological domains similar to those found in eukaryotic chromatin.[30] Torsional stress can be imposed upon domains within the molecule independent of the state of neighboring sites.[31] The nature of these periodic constraints is not understood at present.

The linking difference imposed upon a superhelical domain of DNA must be accommodated by changes in the total twist and/or by writhing. In addition to smooth flexural and torsional deformations away from the relaxed secondary structure, local conformational transitions may occur within susceptible sequences to alternative secondary structures.[32-35] Because physiologically supercoiled DNA is negatively superhelical (i.e., $\alpha < 0$), local transitions to conformations that are less twisted in the right-handed sense than the B-form can be energetically favored. Although the transition itself requires free energy, it produces a net decrease of the local twist which acts to relieve strain elsewhere in the molecule. When the imposed superhelicity becomes sufficiently large that the strain energy relieved elsewhere exceeds the cost of transition, the transition becomes energetically favored to occur. (Similar considerations apply to transitions to overtwisted secondary structures in positively supercoiled domains, although this is not a physiologically important case.) Which particular torsional, flexural, and transconformational alternatives are feasible for a particular molecule and how their competition determines the superhelical conformational equilibria is the subject of this chapter.

First we consider the conformations and energetics of the DNA secondary structures which are important in negatively superhelical molecules.

II. DNA CONFORMATIONS AND ENERGETICS

DNA is a highly polymorphic molecule. In addition to the familiar Watson-Crick B-form there are numerous other secondary structures which it can assume under specific circumstances. These include alternative helical duplex conformations, both right- and left-handed, as well as triple helixes, and structures involving disruption of the interstrand base pairing, such as the denatured and cruciform conformations.[36-39] Each of these structures has its own sequence specificity and conditions for stability. Each has an unstressed conformation, characterized by the number A of base pairs per right-handed turn of the helix. (Left-handed helixes have $A < 0$, while untwisted forms have $A^{-1} = 0$.) Deformation of a secondary

Table 1
CONFORMATIONAL AND ENERGETIC PROPERTIES OF DNA SECONDARY STRUCTURES[a]

Sequence	B-DNA All	Z-DNA Alternate purine-pyrimidine[41]	A-DNA Prefers G + C-rich[36]	Denatured All	Cruciform Inverted repeat
A (bp/turn)	10.4 (42)	−12	11	Untwisted	Untwisted
B (erg-cm $\times$ 10^{-19})	2.2 (39,43)	6 (44)	?	0.1 (39)	—[b]
C (erg-cm $\times$ 10^{-19})	2.4 (45,46)	?	?	0.12 (47)	—[b]
a (kcal/mol)[c]	—	5.0 (48,49)	3.6 (50)	7 (51)	variable[d]
b (kcal/mol)[c]	—	0.3—0.4 (48,49)	1.0 (50)	1 for AT, 2 for GC	0.0

[a]   Values given are for physiological conditions of solvent, temperature, pressure, and ionic strength.

[b]   Torsional and bending deformations in the cruciform arms do not affect the rest of the domain. The mechanical properties of the region joining the cruciform to the rest of the duplex are not known.

[c]   The values for the cooperativity free energy a and the free energy per base pair b are for transitions from the B-form to the alternate conformation under physiological conditions.

[d]   This value depends upon the length and composition of the DNA sequence intervening between the repeat copies.

structure away from its unstressed shape, either by twisting or bending, requires free energy. Experiments have shown that DNA secondary structures have the effective mechanical properties of symmetric, linearly elastic rods.[40] If a segment of length L of a given secondary structure is torsionally deformed away from its unstressed helicity by an amount $\tau(s)$ radians per unit length at each position s and if its local curvature differs from its unstressed value by $\kappa(s)$, then the free energy required for these deformations is given by

$$G = \frac{1}{2} \int_0^L B\kappa^2(s) + C\tau^2(s) \, ds \qquad (2)$$

Here B and C are the molecular bending and torsional stiffnesses, respectively. Both B and C, as well as the unstressed shape of each conformation, may vary with base sequence. The values of these and other important parameters relating to superhelical equilibria, where known, are given in Table 1.

The familiar B-form is the energetically most favored duplex DNA conformation under physiological conditions of temperature, pressure, ionic strength, and solvent in vitro (and presumably also in vivo). In this structure the molecule remains approximately straight, with an average helical twist of 34° per base pair, so A_B = 10.4 base pairs per turn. The B-form of DNA is deformable both by flexure and by twisting, with (sequence average) values of its bending stiffness B and its torsional stiffness C given in Table 1. Both B and C are known to vary slightly with base sequence, with GC pairs being stiffer than AT pairs.[52] The magnitude of the torsional stiffness suggests that the B-form is actually quite flexible to twisting. The root-mean-square fluctuation in the interbase pair twist angle that will occur at room temperature due to random thermal motion for a molecule having torsional stiffness in this range is approximately 5° in either direction out of an average value of 34°.

In addition to the B-form, there are numerous other secondary structures which DNA can assume under specific circumstances.[36,37] These include several other helical duplexes, such as the right-handed A-form and the left-handed Z-form. These alternative secondary structures usually are not equally accessible to all sequences of base pairs, but instead occur preferentially or exclusively at specific sites. For example, the right-handed A-form appears to prefer G + C-rich sequences, while the left-handed Z-form seems to require alternating purine-pyrimidine sequences. These alternative secondary structures do not occur in unstressed DNA under physiological conditions, but can be induced by chemical or thermo-dynamic modification of the environment.[37,41] The A-form can be induced in fibers by lowering the humidity[53] or in solutions by choosing a solvent that contains a large component of methanol or ethanol.[50] Like the B-form, these alternative helical structures are mechanically deformable. However, not all the mechanical stiffnesses of these helixes have been measured to date. It is known that the Z-form is about three times stiffer to bending than the B-form.[44]

In addition to duplex helical secondary structures, several other DNA conformations occur which involve some degree of disruption of interstrand base pairing. In the locally denatured (also called melted) state the hydrogen bonding between the strands is disrupted at a site, leaving two disordered single strands. The two strands may still twist around each other, although they are not base paired. Free energy is required for this interstrand rotation, arising primarily as entropy resulting from the conformational restrictions involved.[51] Also, this conformation has a small but positive bending stiffness, which arises from the known resistance of the individual single strands to flexure.[39] The magnitude of this stiffness depends upon the degree of base stacking that is retained by the individual strands. The value given in Table 1 for the denatured bending stiffness is derived from that measured for single strands. The denatured state may be induced in DNA by elevation of temperature beyond the physiological range. Experiments have shown that thermal motion at room temperature transiently separates base pairs enough to permit hydrogen exchange.[54] This happens to approximately 2% of base pairs at any time at room temperature. Also, an effectively denatured local state may occur at the junction between two other helical states, such as B- and Z-forms.

Another type of disruption of the duplex may occur at sites having inverted repeat homology. The bases that occur on the same strand at the sites of the two repeat copies may base pair together to form an intrastrand helical structure called a hairpin.[33,38] As this commonly happens to both strands simultaneously, a cruciform structure results. As the two strands of the duplex are physically separated at the cruciform site, they do not twist around each other there. The only way that the extent of the local interstrand twist may vary is for the cruciform either to be further extended or to partially revert back to the interstrand B-form. Because the junction between B-form and the cruciform has unknown flexibility, it is possible that the presence of this type of altered secondary structure may have dramatic effects on the amounts or dispositions of local flexural deformations.

In addition to the B-form, each base pair in a DNA sequence will have one or more alternative structures that it can assume. Every base pair can denature, while those in alternating purine-pyrimidine sequences can also assume the Z-form. Base pairs that occur in inverted repeat sequences may participate in cruciform formation. Cooperative conformational transitions between alternative secondary structures can occur at local sites along a molecule. To analyze these transconformation reactions, a conformational reference state is chosen as the unstressed form of that secondary structure which is most stable under the given environmental conditions. This conformational reference state may depend upon base sequence, and hence vary along the molecule. Under physiological environmental conditions the B-form is the standard reference state.

The transition of a base pair to an alternative conformation has an energetic cost comprised of two components. First, there is a cooperativity free energy a, which is the cost of producing a pair of junctions between states. Its value will depend upon the identities of the states involved. Also, transforming each base pair will cost an amount b of free energy. A homopolymeric transition is one in which b has the same value for all base pairs involved.[55] The B-Z transition within a simple alternating copolymeric sequence and denaturation of a poly-A sequence are examples of homopolymeric transitions. The free energy cost of a homopolymeric transition of n sequential base pairs to a single run of the alternative conformation in an unconstrained molecule is

$$G_{\text{trans}} = a + bn \tag{3a}$$

A transition in which the value of b depends upon the identity of the base pair and also perhaps upon the identities of its neighbors is heteropolymeric in character. The energetic cost of a heteropolymeric transition of n contiguous base pairs to the alternative conformation in an unconstrained molecule is

$$G_{\text{trans}} = a + \sum_{i=1}^{i=n} b_i \tag{3b}$$

where b_i is the free energy of transforming the ith base pair in the run. Values of a and b for the conformational transitions that are important in supercoiled molecules are given in Table 1.

Because each alternative conformation has a distinct secondary structure, the local unstressed helical twist of a site depends upon which conformation it is in. The transition of n base pairs from a conformation having A_0 base pairs per turn to one having A_n base pairs per turn changes the helicity by an amount

$$\frac{1}{\bar{A}} = \frac{1}{A_n} - \frac{1}{A_0} \tag{4}$$

Some DNA conformations, including the Z-form, have fundamental structural unit that is a multiple of a base pair.[41] Transitions involving such a conformation must extend over an integer number of structural units.

III. CONFORMATIONAL EQUILIBRIA OF SUPERHELICAL DNA

A. Superhelical Deformations and Their Free Energies

The states accessible to a superhelically constrained DNA molecule must be torsionally and/or flexurally deformed away from their relaxed conformation so as to accommodate the imposed linking difference α. This deformation may be partitioned between local conformational transitions and residual deformations:

$$\alpha = \alpha_{\text{trans}} + \alpha_{\text{res}} \tag{5}$$

That portion of the linking difference which is expressed as conformational transitions is given by:

$$\alpha_{\text{trans}} = \sum_i \left(\frac{n_i}{\bar{A}_i} + \psi_i \right) \tag{6}$$

where n_i is the number of transformed base pairs at the ith site of transition, $\bar{A}_i^{-1}$ is the change of helicity characteristic of that transition and ψ_i is the change of local twist (measured in turns) at the junctions between the ith site of transition and the rest of the domain. The portion α_{res} of the linking difference that is not accommodated by transitions must be manifested as smooth torsional and/or flexural deformations of the secondary structures away from their relaxed conformations:

$$\alpha_{\text{res}} = \Delta Tw + \Delta Wr \tag{7}$$

There are several degrees of specificity with which the deformations comprising α_{res} may be treated, as described below.

The complete specification of the state of a superhelical molecule involves both discrete and continuously varying parameters. There are a finite number of distinct local transitions to alternate secondary structures, each of which determines a value of α_{trans}. The residual linking difference is accommodated by continuously varying smooth torsional and flexural deformations of the secondary structures away from their unstressed conformations.

The free energy associated to each state of a superhelical molecule has the form:

$$G = G_{trans} + G_{res} \tag{8}$$

For a particular state of secondary structure the free energy G_{trans} associated to the regions of altered conformation is given by

$$G_{trans} = \sum_{j} \left(a_j + \sum_{i=1}^{n_j} b_i \right) \tag{9}$$

Here j enumerates the regions of altered secondary structure, each of which is of length n_j.

The free energy G_{res} that is associated to the residual deformation α_{res} may be specified in different ways depending upon the level of detail that is desired. The least specific way involves ascribing to the residual linking difference a quadratic free energy deduced from experiment. There the introduction of transient single strand breaks in a population of identical circular DNA molecules has been shown to result in a Boltzmann distribution of linking numbers around the relaxed state.[56,57] This allows a quadratic phenomenological free energy to be associated to α for states near the relaxed state. Using this experimental expression, a free energy is ascribed to α_{res} as follows:

$$G_{res} = \frac{K \, \alpha_{res}^2}{2} \tag{10}$$

where $K = 2200RT/N$ for a DNA sequence of N base pairs.[56] It must be cautioned that this experiment only measures the phenomenological free energy near the relaxed state. Little is known at present regarding the free energy associated to α when the molecule is substantially supercoiled. To assume that the same law pertains at all superhelicities that have been verified only near the relaxed state involves considerable extrapolation. Theoretical evidence suggests that this assumption may not be valid, but unambiguous experimental information addressing this question is lacking. This technique is of limited utility both because the free energy associated to α_{res} is not known with confidence and because the means of accommodating the residual deformation are not specified. Whether torsional or flexural deformations predominate and under what circumstances they may do so are important questions that cannot be addressed using this approach. On the other hand, computations based on this approach are relatively tractable because there are a discrete, indeed finite, collection of accessible states determined by the set of all possible transitions available to the domain. There is no continuous component to the specification of these states.

A slightly more detailed analysis accounts explicitly for the torsional deformations of the alternative secondary structure. This approach is required in cases where the alternative conformation has a small torsional stiffness relative to that of the relaxed secondary structure. In this situation a large amount of the imposed linking difference can be accommodated by smooth torsional deformations of the alternative secondary structure, which profoundly influences the competitive advantage of the transition. This is the situation for the locally denatured conformation, whose torsional stiffness is between one and two orders of magnitude smaller than that of the B-form.[47] To analyze this case one specifies the torsional deformation τ_j, measured in radians per unit length, of the n_j base pairs that are transformed at the jth site. (At mechanical equilibrium τ_j is a constant throughout a region where the torsional stiffness C is fixed — see Section V below.) Then the residual linking difference α_{res} is partitioned between the τ_js and $\bar{\alpha}$, the latter being accommodated by presently unspecified torsional and flexural deformations throughout the domain:

$$\alpha_{res} = \bar{\alpha} + \sum_j \frac{n_j \tau_j}{2\pi} \tag{11}$$

This partitioning may be accomplished in a continuum of ways, so the τ_js are continuous parameters. Now the free energy associated with residual deformations has the form:

$$G_{res} = \frac{K\,\bar{\alpha}^2}{2} + \sum_j \frac{C_j n_j \tau_j^2}{2} \tag{12a}$$

where C_j is the torsional stiffness of the secondary structure at the jth site of transition. If all transition is to a single type of alternative secondary structure, then

$$G_{res} = \frac{K\,\bar{\alpha}^2}{2} + \frac{Cn\tau^2}{2} \tag{12b}$$

where n is the total number of transformed base pairs at all sites. If $n = 0$, then $\bar{\alpha} = \alpha_{res} = \alpha$, which is the actual linking difference imposed on the domain.

A slight modification of this approach treats the torsional part of the superhelical deformation in detail and the flexural part in a nonspecific manner, usually by assuming that Wr is invariant. Now the superhelical parameter is ΔTw, which is partitioned between smooth deformations throughout the domain and conformational transitions. This method is easy to implement as an analytic technique because the total twist, which is the imposed constraint, is extensive.[58,59] It will be exactly correct in situations where the tertiary structure is held invariant, as may occur in physiologically important cases through the constraining action of nucleosomes on eukaryotic DNA.

The most specific but least tractable method of accounting for the residual linking difference treats explicitly the torsional and flexural deformations by which α_{res} may be accommodated. Once α_{trans} is fixed, the collection of possible deformations of this type is constrained by the constancy of α_{res} (see Section V). Because there are infinitely many ways in which a particular value of α_{res} may be accommodated by smooth deformations, there is a high dimensional continuum of possible states which must be considered. Each one has free energy G_{res} associated to its smooth torsional and flexural deformations of the form given by Equation 2. This approach, although more general than the nonspecific association of a quadratic free energy to α_{res}, is considerably more complicated to implement in practice.

There may be other contributions to the free energy of a state that are not included at present. In particular, the entropy resulting from the restrictions imposed by the coupling of twisting and bending through White's formula is not well understood at present. Modifications may be made to it to account for any new sources of free energy as they become known.

B. Equilibrium Statistical Mechanics

At thermodynamic equilibrium a population of identical superhelical DNA molecules will be distributed among its accessible states according to Boltzmann's law.[60] This central tenet of statistical mechanics states that the equilibrium properties of a system derive from its governing partition function Z, which is constructed from an enumeration of the states accessible to that system. If these states are discrete in nature, indexed by i, and if the free energy of state i is G_i, then the partition function of this system is given by

$$Z = \sum_i \exp(-G_i/kT) \tag{13a}$$

where k is Boltzmann's constant and T is the absolute temperature. If the states of the system vary continuously they may be enumerated by some continuous parameter μ over an interval $\mu_0 < \mu < \mu_1$. Then the partition function is given by

$$Z = \int_{\mu_0}^{\mu_1} exp(-G(\mu)/kT)d\mu \tag{13b}$$

If the states of the system include both discrete and continuous parameters, the partition function has a mixed form:[59]

$$Z = \sum_i [exp(-G_i/kT)]\int_{\mu_0}^{\mu_1} exp(-G(\mu)/kT)d\mu \tag{13c}$$

The equilibrium properties of a system can be determined from its governing partition function. The probability of the system being in state i, also equal to the fractional occupancy of this state for a population at equilibrium, is given by

$$p_i = \frac{exp(-G_i/kT)}{Z} \tag{14}$$

The fractional occupancy of each state will vary according to the relative contribution of its Boltzmann factor to the overall partition function. States whose free energy exceeds the minimum value will be occupied at equilibrium, but they will be less populated the higher their free energy is above that minimum. If the value of parameter ξ in state i is ξ_i, then its expected value at equilibrium in a discrete transition is

$$\bar{\xi} = \frac{\sum_i \xi_i exp(-G_i/kT)}{Z} \tag{15}$$

Equations corresponding to 14 and 15 also may be found when the states of the system are continuous or of mixed type.

Although this formalism is conceptually simple, its application to the rigorous analysis of superhelical equilibria is greatly complicated by the number and complexity of the states involved. For example, because every base pair is susceptible to denaturation, a molecule of N base pairs has 2^N states of local denaturation. Even for short molecules (i.e., $N = 1000$) this is a forbiddingly large number. Most DNAs also have a large number of sites whose sequences permit transitions to other conformations in addition to melting, which renders the number of states of secondary structure even larger. Moreover, for each state of secondary structure there is a continuum of ways of partitioning α_{res} between smooth torsional deformations and writhing. Further, there are many tertiary structures having a given value of Wr. Any fixed amount of smooth torsional deformation also can be partitioned along the molecule in an infinite number of ways. Thus the specification of all conformational states of a superhelical DNA molecule is so complex as to preclude a complete statistical mechanical analysis at present.

To make progress in understanding superhelical equilibria, one must analyze simpler problems than the most general one. Several types of simplifications that are computationally tractable still provide useful results. One could, for example, not consider the partitioning of the residual linking number in complete detail, provided that one can assign a reasonably accurate value to $G(\alpha_{res})$ or to $G(\overline{\alpha})$. The competition among secondary structures may be limited to a small number of the energetically least expensive alternatives. For example, one could analyze the relative competition between two types of transitions, such as denaturation at the A + T-richest site vs. extrusion of a single cruciform. The second basic simplification technique involves finding those states which are local minima of the free energy (or of the action in the cases of tertiary structure — see Section V) in the space of all accessible conformations. If more than one such state is found, the competition among them may be analyzed using Boltzmann's theory. In the following sections analyses of these types are developed and their important results are described.

In the next two sections we examine the equilibria of secondary and tertiary structure, respectively.

IV. SECONDARY STRUCTURAL EQUILIBRIA

The imposition of negative superhelicity on a domain of DNA provides a means of influencing the local secondary structure at specific sites throughout the domain. The practical importance of this phenomenon may be inferred from the observation that many types of regulatory regions within genomic DNA have sequences that suggest susceptibility to specific types of conformational transitions. These include alternating purine-pyrimidine sequences, susceptible to the B-Z transition, at enhancer sites[41] and A + T-rich regions within initiation sites for DNA transcription and replication.[61-63] Inverted repeats susceptible to cruciform extrusion occur at other regulatory sites, including origins of transcription and replication.[64] There is also strong evidence that the activity of certain of these regulatory sites is influenced by changes in superhelicity, suggesting that the conformational transition to which they are susceptible may play a role in their regulatory action.[64]

A. Statistical Mechanics of Paradigm Transitions

Homopolymeric and heteropolymeric transitions and cruciform extrusion are the three formally distinct types of cooperative conformational transitions that are important in superhelical DNA molecules. We derive first the partition function governing transition at a single site in each of these three cases. Then we consider the analysis of competing transitions at multiple sites within a domain of DNA.[65-67]

The free energy of a homopolymeric transition depends only on two quantities, the number n of fundamental repeat units (usually base pairs) that are transformed and the number r of runs in which the transformation occurs. In general there will be a large number of states having the same free energy. A computationally simpler partition function results when the degree of degeneracy of the energy levels is high. For a domain containing N base pairs, of which N_s sequential base pairs are susceptible to this homopolymeric transition, the number of ways of choosing n base pairs for transformation in r runs is

$$M(n,r) = \binom{n - 1}{r - 1}\binom{N_s - n + 1}{r} \tag{16a}$$

For fixed values of N_s and n there is a maximum number of runs that are possible, given by

$$r_{max} = \begin{cases} N_s - n + 1, & \text{if } n > [N_s + 1]/2 \\ n, & \text{otherwise} \end{cases} \tag{16b}$$

where the square brackets denote the greatest integer function. The residual linking difference α_{res} is partitioned between smooth deformations of the alternative secondary structure, of τ radians per unit length, and other deformations $\bar{\alpha}$ throughout the domain:

$$\alpha_{res} = \alpha - \frac{n}{A} - r\,\psi = \bar{\alpha} + \frac{n\tau}{2\pi} \qquad (17)$$

There are a continuum of ways in which this partitioning may be accomplished, which may be enumerated using the parameter τ. In this paradigm case we assume quadratic free energy laws for τ and for $\bar{\alpha}$, so G_{res} is given by Equation 12b above. The transitional free energy is

$$G_{trans}(n,r) = \begin{cases} ar + bn, & \text{if } n > 0 \\ 0, & \text{if } n = r = 0 \end{cases} \qquad (18)$$

Then the governing partion function for this transition at a particular value of the linking difference α is[66]

$$Z = e^{-G(0,0)/kT} + \sum_{n=1}^{NS}\left(\sum_{r=1}^{r_{max}} M(n,r)e^{-G_{trans}(n,r)/kT}\int_{-\infty}^{\infty} e^{-G_{res}(n,r)/kT}\,d\tau\right) \qquad (19a)$$

If more than one region is susceptible to this homopolymeric transition, the limits of summation and the degeneracy factor $M(n,r)$ must be modified accordingly.

The analysis of a heteropolymeric transition is considerably more complex in practice, because conformational degeneracy cannot be used to simplify the calculation of the partition function. Instead, an exact calculation requires that every state be accounted for individually.[59] If there is a single run of susceptible fundamental repeat units of length N, then there are 2^N possible states of transition. Each such state has transitional free energy given by Equation 9 above. The residual linking difference α_{res} may be partitioned between torsional deformations of the alternate conformations and unspecified deformations $\bar{\alpha}$ elsewhere, so the free energy G_{res} again has the form given in Equation 12b above. The partition function governing this transition is

$$Z = e^{(-G(0,0)/kT)} + \sum_{n=1}^{N}\left[\left(\sum_{w_n} e^{-G_{trans}/kT}\right)\int_{-\infty}^{\infty} e^{-G_{res}/kT}\,d\tau\right] \qquad (19b)$$

where w_n enumerates all states with n transformed base pairs, and G_{trans} is the transition free energy of such a state, as given in Equation 9 above.

The heteropolymeric transition of greatest practical importance in superhelical DNA is local denaturation, for which the free energies of transition under physiological conditions are $b = 1$ kcal for an AT base pair, and $b = 2$ kcal for a GC pair. Because every base pair is susceptible to this transition, the number of possible states of secondary structure grows extremely rapidly with DNA segment length. In practice it is only tractable to perform a complete analysis on extremely short DNA lengths, at most about 100 bp.[59] To treat longer segments, one must approximate by considering only those states whose free energy does not exceed that of the most favorable state by more than a specified amount.

The cruciform transition requires a rather different analysis because of its unusual energetics and its torsionally undeformable character.[65] Consider a superhelical domain of length N and linking difference α, which contains a single perfect inverted repeat sequence. Suppose that each copy of this repeat contains N_{IR} base pairs, the copies being separated by N_L

intervening base pairs that lack inverted repeat homology. The states of this cruciform may be indexed by i, the number of intrastrand base pairs in a single arm of the cruciform. Then $i = 0$ corresponds to the unextruded state, where the domain is entirely interstrand duplex B-form, while $1 \leq i \leq N_{IR}$ are the states where the cruciform is partially or entirely extruded. In each state the number N_C of interstrand pairs that are disrupted in the formation of the cruciform is

$$N_C(i) = \begin{cases} N_L + 2i + N_D, & \text{if } i > 0 \\ 0, & \text{if } i = 0 \end{cases} \tag{20}$$

where N_D is the number of base pairs that are disrupted in the junction region joining the base of the cruciform to the interstrand duplex. The free energy G_{trans} associated with each state of extrusion of the cruciform is

$$G_{trans} = \begin{cases} 0, & \text{if } i = 0, \\ a_D + a_L + bN_L + 2\gamma kT \ln N_L, & \text{if } i > 0 \end{cases} \tag{21}$$

Here a_D is the free energy associated with the formation of the junction region, while $a_L + bN_L$ is the free energy needed to denature the sequence between the inverted repeat copies. The logarithmic contribution results from the loop entropy of the single-stranded loops at the ends of the cruciform arms. Note that the free energy of formation of each cruciform does not vary with the arm length i, provided that $i > 0$. This is because the extension of the partially extruded cruciform disrupts a number of interstrand base pairs equal to the number of intrastrand pairs that are formed in the two arms. To a first approximation this is an isoenergetic process, so all extruded states of a perfect inverted repeat have the same transition free energy. The slight variations that can occur due to sequence effects (viz., interstrand AT base pairs disrupting as intrastrand GC pairs form of vice versa) do not have a significant effect on the equilibrium.

Because the two strands comprising the cruciform are physically separated in space, they do not twist around each other. Thus the change of helicity consequent on the cruciform transition is $\bar{A}^{-1} = -A_B^{-1}$, where A_B is the number of base pairs per turn of the relaxed duplex conformation. Because the cruciform structure is torsionally undeformable, the continuous partitioning of the residual linking difference does not arise in this case, so

$$\alpha_{res} = \alpha + \frac{N_C(i)}{A_B} \tag{22}$$

and the free energy associated to state i is

$$G(i) = \frac{K \alpha_{res}^2}{2} + G_{trans} \tag{23}$$

The partition function governing the extrusion of a perfect inverted repeat then is[65]

$$Z = e^{-G(0)/kT} + \sum_{i=1}^{N_{IR}} e^{-G(i)/kT} \tag{24}$$

Two complications arise when this analysis is applied to actual DNA sequences. First, most DNAs of interest contain numerous sequences possessing some degree of inverted repeat homology. These cannot all form cruciforms together. If there are two interleaved inverted repeats with one copy of the first sequence lying in the region intervening between the copies of the second repeat, then both cruciforms cannot extrude simultaneously. Second, many DNA molecules contain sequences which possess partial inverted repeat homology. Often the two copies match closely, but not exactly. If such a sequence were to extrude a cruciform, its arms would have sites where the intrastrand base pairing cannot occur. It is not clear at present what effect these disruptions will have on the free energy of transition.

An average DNA molecule commonly has several sites that are particularly susceptible to transition. These may include A + T-rich regions, alternating purine-pyrimidine sequences susceptible to the B-Z transition, and sites possessing a high degree of inverted repeat homology. To understand the effects of superhelicity on DNA secondary structure, it is important to consider how multiple transitions of these sorts compete at equilibrium. The analysis involved in treating this question may be constructed from the pieces described earlier.[67]

To illustrate this procedure, we consider a DNA molecule of N base pairs which contains a single perfect inverted repeat and a single Z-susceptible site of length N_Z.[66] The states of this system now are indexed by four parameters — the number of Z-form base pairs n_Z and the number r_Z of runs in which they occur, the number i of intrastrand base pairs in each cruciform arm, all of which are discrete, and the part τ of the residual linking difference that is partitioned to torsional deformation of the Z-form site. The residual linking difference α_{res} is

$$\alpha_{res} = \alpha - \frac{N_C(i)}{\overline{A}_C} - \frac{n_Z}{\overline{A}_Z} \tag{25}$$

where $\overline{A}_Z^{-1}$ and $\overline{A}_C^{-1}$ are the changes of helicity associated to the B-Z transition and to cruciform extrusion, respectively. The free energy of a given state is comprised of three contributions,

$$G(n_Z, r_Z, i, \alpha_{res}) = G_Z + G_C + G(\alpha_{res}) \tag{26}$$

where G_Z is given by Equation 18, G_C by Equation 21, and $G(\alpha_{res})$ by Equation 12b. The partition function governing this system is

$$Z = \sum_{i=0}^{N_{IR}} e^{(-G_C/kT)} \left\{ I_0 + \sum_{n_Z=1}^{N_Z} \left[I_0 + \sum_{r_Z=1}^{r_{Z(max)}} M(n_Z, r_Z) e^{(-G_Z/kT)} \right] \right\} \tag{27a}$$

where

$$I_0 = exp\left(-K \left[\alpha + \frac{N_C(i)}{A_B} \right]^2 /2kT \right) \tag{27b}$$

$$I_{N_Z} = \int_{-\infty}^{\infty} e^{-G(\alpha_{res})/kT} \, d\tau \tag{27c}$$

The complexity of this type of analysis clearly increases rapidly with the number of competing transitions being considered.

B. Approximate Transition Analysis — Minimum Energy States

The statistical-mechanical formalism described above provides an exact methodology for analyzing conformational equilibria. Unfortunately, its use in superhelical problems is constrained by the intrinsic complexity of the phenomena being described. The computations involved in using these techniques, unless they address a simple problem involving transitions at a small number of short sites, are intractably complex to perform unless simplifications are introduced. Fortunately, in many circumstances the molecular transition behavior can be analyzed effectively by the simpler approximation methods described here.[58,68] These suffice, for example, to determine which transition will be the first to occur as α is decreased from zero, when this transition occurs and how its extent changes with α. As α is decreased further, one can determine whether another transition somewhere else on the domain also becomes favored and if so how it competes with the first one.

This analysis finds those states whose free energies are local minima in the space of all configurations consistent with constraints. The competition among these states then is analyzed using Boltzmann statistics. To illustrate this method in its simplest form, we consider a homopolymeric transition at a single site whose cooperativity free energy exceeds its transition free energy sufficiently that all transition will occur effectively in a single run. Both B-Z transitions at an alternating copolymeric sequence and local denaturation at the A + T-richest site satisfy these criteria reasonably well at physiological temperatures and ionic strengths. The states of this system are specified by two parameters, the number n of sequential base pairs that are transformed and the amount τ (in radians per unit length) by which this alternative secondary structure is twisted away from its unstressed conformation. It is known that τ will be constant, throughout the transformed site at mechanical equilibrium, provided the effective torsional stiffness does not vary[69] (see Section V). This assumption will be accurate for the types of transitions being considered here. We suppose the domain of DNA consists of N bp and is superhelically constrained by a linking difference α. This approach slightly generalizes a previous presentation, where the superhelical constraint was ΔTw.[58,68]

That portion $\overline{\alpha}$ of the imposed linking difference that is not expressed either as the conformational transition or as the smooth torsional deformation of the alternative secondary structure must occur as smooth torsional or flexural deformations throughout the domain. It is given by

$$\overline{\alpha} = \alpha - \frac{n}{\overline{A}} - \left(\frac{n\tau}{2\pi}\right) \tag{28}$$

where $\overline{A}$ is the change of helicity of the transition, and the unwinding of the junctions is neglected. If a quadratic free energy is associated to $\overline{\alpha}$ with coefficient $K = c/N$, then the free energy of the state determined by τ and n is

$$G(n,\pi) = \begin{cases} c\alpha^2/2N, & \text{if } n = 0 \\ a + bn + \dfrac{Cn\tau^2}{2} + \dfrac{c\overline{\alpha}}{2N}, & \text{if } n > 0 \end{cases} \tag{29}$$

Stable locally transformed states do not exist for all values of α. There is an extremum of $G(n,\tau)$ having $n > 0$ only for linking differences satisfying the following quadratic inequality:

$$c^2\alpha^2 + 8\pi^2CN\left(\frac{c\alpha}{\overline{A}} - Nb\right) > 0 \tag{30}$$

That is, a stable state with $n > 0$ exists only for values of α satisfying $\alpha < \alpha_1$ or $\alpha > \alpha_2$, where the α_is are the roots of the quadratic expression in Equation 30 above. It follows that $\alpha_2 > 0$, while α_1 has the opposite sign as b. For linking differences satisfying this criterion, the extremum of $G(n,\tau)$ is a minimum which occurs at the values

$$n = \frac{2\pi\alpha}{\varsigma} + \frac{4\pi^2 CN}{c\varsigma}\left[\frac{2\pi}{\overline{A}} - \varsigma\right] \tag{31a}$$

and

$$\tau = -\frac{2\pi}{\overline{A}} + \varsigma \tag{31b}$$

where

$$\varsigma = \pm \left[\frac{4\pi^2}{\overline{A}^2} + \frac{2b}{C}\right]^{1/2} \tag{31c}$$

Here the positive sign is chosen for ζ when $\alpha > \alpha_2$, the negative sign when $\alpha < \alpha_1$. At this minimum $\overline{\alpha}$, that portion of the linking difference not absorbed either in the transition to or the smooth torsional deformation of the alternative secondary structure has a constant value independent of changes in α given by:

$$\overline{\alpha} = 2\pi CN\tau/c \tag{31d}$$

These results show that, for any value of α, there is at most a single minimum energy state in which local transition to the alternate conformation occurs. In this state the value τ of the torsional deformation of the alternative secondary structure is a constant, as is $\overline{\alpha}$. All changes in $|\alpha|$ act entirely to alter length n of the region of transition, without changing either the residual linking difference or the torsional deformation density τ of the alternate secondary structure, up to the point where the entire susceptible site has been transformed. It follows from Equation 29 that the free energy associated to this transformed state increases linearly with the magnitude of the imposed linking difference. In contrast, the free energy of the untransformed state increases quadratically with α. As the linking difference is decreased from zero, a point will come where the transformed and the untransformed states have the same values of free energy. Beyond this point the transformed state is energetically favored at equilibrium.

The competition between these two states at equilibrium is analyzed by applying Boltzmann's theorem to them. The two state partition function governing this transition should include the degeneracy of the states of transformation. If the stable locally transformed state has n sequential base pairs in the alternative conformation, and the susceptible site is of length N_s, then there are $N_s - n + 1$ choices of which n base pairs transform. Although the quantitative results found by applying Boltzmann's theorem in this context will not be precisely accurate because states near that of local minimum free energy have been ignored, comparison calculations show that the effect of this approximation is slight.

The analysis described above applies to transitions to torsionally deformable alternative conformations. When the transition involves cruciform extrusion, a slightly different and somewhat simpler analysis results.[65] The only variable now is i, the number of intrastrand base pairs in each cruciform arm. The free energy associated to a state is

$$G(i) = \begin{cases} K\alpha^2/2, & \text{if } i = 0 \\ G_{\text{trans}} + K(\alpha + [N_C(i)])^2/2, & \text{if } i > 0 \end{cases} \tag{32}$$

where $N_C(i)$ is the linear function of i given in Equation 20, and G_{trans} is shown by Equation 21. When the value of i at which $G(i)$ is a local minimum is computed, one finds that such a state exists for $i > 0$ only if $\alpha < 0$. In this state the entire linking difference is absorbed by the cruciform extrusion, so the residual linking difference is $\alpha_{res} = 0$. Thus, as α is decreased from zero in a molecule whose only available transition is cruciform extrusion at a single inverted repeat, a competition occurs between the extruded and the unextruded states. The equilibrium distribution between these states may be found from Boltzmann's theorem. The number of base pairs participating in the cruciform increases with $|\alpha|$, up to the point where the entire inverted repeat is involved. For intermediate states of extrusion, the rest of the duplex is entirely relaxed. Superhelical stresses only occur in the unextruded or in the completely extruded states.

One may extend this analytic technique to encompass the competition among transitions at multiple sites.[68] However, each additional site requires the introduction of two new variables, the number of transformed base pairs there and the torsional deformation of the alternate conformation involved. (Only one additional variable is needed if cruciform extrusion is involved.) The treatment of large numbers of competing sites in this way becomes computationally complex.

The inclusion of the variable τ describing the torsional deformation of the transformed site is especially important when the alternative secondary structure has a small torsional stiffness relative to the untransformed (usually B-form) state. A large amount of the linking difference can be absorbed as torsional deformation in such cases, which profoundly influences the competitive advantage of transition. For transitions to conformations whose torsional stiffness roughly equals that of B-DNA, these torsional deformations of the local secondary structure become less important. In such cases this analysis may be amended to ignore τ. Now the inclusion of more competing sites introduces one new variable per site, resulting in a simpler analysis. However, under physiological environmental conditions, local denaturation at A + T-rich sites is an important and energetically feasible alternative whose analysis requires the inclusion of τ.

C. Competing Transitions in Superhelical DNA — Results

DNA has many types of secondary structures that are stable in specific sequences under particular environmental conditions.[36,37,40] Many of these, although of considerable physicochemical interest, do not appear to be physiologically important in living systems. Although the methods described above may be applied to the analysis of superhelically stressed transitions in general, the results of greatest practical interest pertain to the behavior of molecules within physiological ranges of pressure, temperature, ionic strength, solvent conditions, and imposed superhelicities. Here the DNAs unstressed secondary structure is entirely B-form, and the imposed linking differences are negative, $\alpha < 0$. Of all the alternative secondary structures that the DNA could possibly assume, only those having a smaller right-handed unstressed twist than the B-form will be candidates for local transitions under these conditions. As described in the previous section, a given transconformation reaction will be energetically favored to occur when the strain relief it provides by localizing some of the negative linking difference as undertwist at the transition site exceeds the energetic cost of performing it.

Specific transitions that have been suggested to be important in superhelical molecules under physiological environmental conditions include local denaturation at A + T-rich regions,[32,58] cruciform extrusion at inverted repeats,[33,34,65] and B-Z transitions at susceptible alternating purine-pyrimidine sequences.[35] An average DNA molecule will contain numerous sites that are susceptible to transitions of these types. For example, the pBR322 molecule contains approximately 200 sites having a significant degree of inverted repeat homology, of which about a dozen have the repeat copies sufficiently close together so that cruciform extrusion is energetically competitive there. It also contains several dozen short sites whose sequence suggests susceptibility to the B-Z transition, as well as numerous A + T-rich regions of various lengths. In order to understand the superhelical equilibria in a molecule such as this, it is important to determine how the energetically most favored alternative transitions compete. Although molecules of this complexity have not been analyzed rigorously to date, calculations made on several prototype competitions provide information regarding the general principles governing competing transitions. Because the values of some of the free energy parameters involved in this analysis are not known to good accuracy at present, quantitatively accurate predictions from theory are not currently possible. However, the qualitative conclusions that are found regarding the transition behavior have been shown to be robust when these parameters are altered.

The basic principle behind this work is to analyze competitions in a pairwise manner. The molecule is regarded as having exactly two sites, each of which is susceptible to a single transition. The analysis is performed either with the more rigorous statistical mechanical techniques of Section IV.A or with the approximate methods of Section IV.B.[67] The general results are found not to depend significantly on which method is chosen, although more information may be gleaned from the more powerful statistical techniques. Here we will summarize the most important qualitative conclusions regarding superhelical transitions. Additional details may be found in the references provided.

First, a transconformation reaction will be energetically favored to occur in a sufficiently negatively supercoiled molecule containing a single site susceptible to either cruciform extrusion,[65] denaturation,[58,59] or transition to Z-form.[35] When considered separately, each type of transition will occur at a value of α determined by details of sequence and environmental conditions. The numbers of base pairs participating in a transition at the point where it becomes energetically favored also depends upon the length of the domain and the sequence of the susceptible site. In contrast to these cases, transition to A-form is not energetically favorable under physiological environmental conditions because it only relieves about three degrees of twist per base pair, not enough to offset its cost.[68]

The B-Z transition provides the most torsional relaxation per transformed base pair (about 65°), while its costs in free energy are comparable to those of other transitions. For this reason it will occur at less extreme superhelicities than the alternatives under physiologically reasonable in vitro conditions.[66,68] Because the sites susceptible to transition to Z-form are usually short (i.e., generally less than 20 bp, sometimes only 6 or 8 pairs), the extent of transition at the point where it is favored to occur often encompasses the entire site. That is, the transition acts effectively as a switch from entirely B-form to entirely Z-form. If there are several sites susceptible to this transition, it will occur first only at one location. This can be any site whose length exceeds the number of transformed base pairs at the onset of transition. If there is no site that long, transition will occur at the longest susceptible location and will have the character of a switch. As α is decreased further below the point of onset of this first transition, the equilibrium behavior becomes quite complex, determined by the competition among all the available alternatives, not just among the Z-susceptible sites.

The free energy needed to extrude a cruciform at a perfect inverted repeat depends primarily on the size N_L and composition of the sequence intervening between the repeat copies (see Equation 21). In a domain containing a single inverted repeat, the cruciform will extrude at less extreme negative linking differences when N_L is smaller, other things being equal.[65] Similarly, in a domain containing multiple inverted repeats (but no sites susceptible to other transitions), that cruciform will extrude first whose free energy of formation is smallest. If N_C, the maximum size of this first cruciform, satisfies $N_C/A_B > -\alpha$, then partial extrusion suffices to absorb the entire imposed linking difference. At more extreme negative superhelicities a coordinated transition may occur in which the extrusion of a longer but energetically more costly cruciform having a larger value of N_C is coupled to the reabsorption of the original cruciform.[65] In a DNA molecule containing numerous inverted repeats, the set of cruciforms that extrude at equilibrium may vary in an intricate manner as α is decreased, with coordinated extrusions and reversions happening at numerous thresholds.

Local denaturation under physiological conditions is largely confined to the A + T-richest portions of the molecule.[59] If this is the only transition available to a domain, as α is decreased from zero, denaturation will occur at the most A + T-rich single site available. Only if the A + T-rich region is surrounded by G + C-rich sites will a point arrive where it becomes energetically cheaper to start another transition elsewhere than to extend a region of denaturation that already exists.

Certain principles of transition apply to all three types considered here. First, under physiological environmental conditions, each of these transconformation reactions has a high initiation free energy relative to the cost of extending a preexisting region of transition. This means that the opening of a second transition site is generally more expensive than extending a preexisting region of altered secondary structure, if that is sequentially permitted. Only when the entire susceptible site has been transformed will transition elsewhere become energetically favored to occur. These additional transitions need not be simply transformations at other sites. Depending upon the sequences at the site involved, they may be coupled to coordinated reversions of existing regions of alternate secondary structure back to the B-form. Second, as α is decreased from zero, the first transition will occur at less extreme specific linking differences $\sigma = \alpha/Lk_0$ in longer molecules, other factors remaining fixed.[66,68] Although the exact calculations on denaturation could only be carried out on short segments of DNA to date,[59] where the melting was shown to occur at extreme values of σ, this scaling implies that denaturation can occur at physiological linking differences in longer domains (i.e., $N > 500$ base pairs).

The analysis of superhelical transitions in domains containing regions susceptible to all three types of alternative secondary structures is quite complex. Only partial information is available at present. Which of the three types of transitions will occur first as $|\alpha|$ is decreased from zero in a molecule containing regions susceptible to each type will depend upon the details of the sequences involved as well as on the values of the temperature and other thermodynamic variables. Specifically, the determining parameters for this question are the relative cost of each transition vs. the amount of torsional relief they afford. The Z-form in transition relieves about 65° of twist per base pair participating, whereas the cruciform extrustion relieves only 34°/bp. Local denaturation relieves about between 34 and 55°, depending upon the magnitude of the linking difference and the length N of the DNA involved. This variability results from the torsional flexibility of the denatured form, which allows it to absorb large amounts of the residual deformation at small incremental energetic costs. Because the B-Z transition affords the greatest superhelical relief, this will be the first transition to occur under physiological conditions. As α is decreased beyond the point where the entire susceptible site of the first transition is in the Z-form, a complex competition ensues. Depending on details of the system involved, either denaturation or cruciform extrusion can be the second transition to occur. In either case this transition can be a simple opening of a second site, or it can involve the coupled reversion of the Z-form site back to the B-form.[66] How cruciforms compete with denaturations depends upon the amount of superhelicity imposed and on the sequences at the sites involved. If the molecule is substantially supercoiled and the inverted repeat is short, then denaturation may be the preferred transition. If the inverted repeat is long enough to absorb the entire linking difference while the intervening region is short so the energetic cost of extrusion is small, then cruciform extrusion will be the preferred transition.

V. TERTIARY STRUCTURAL EQUILIBRIA

The analyses of superhelical tertiary structure that have been developed to date find the stable equilibrium conformations of an elastic DNA molecule subject to the constraint imposed by the constancy of the linking number.[69-71] The secondary structure is regarded as fixed, and the conformational energy arises from smooth elastic deformations of these secondary structures away from their unstressed shapes, either by bending or by twisting. In its simplest form this approach may be used to treat the conformational tertiary equilibria in a domain that is entirely in the B-form, hence only slightly supercoiled.

The nature of the equilibrium found here is qualitatively different from that found in the statistical mechanical analysis of secondary structure given in Section IV.A. There the equilibrium is dynamic in nature, consisting of a distribution of a population among the accessible states. The lowest energy state is relatively the most populated, but other states nearby also are occupied, even though they do not have a local minimum free energy. In the present analysis the equilibrium is mechanical and static in nature. Only conformations that are local minima of the analogous action (defined below) in the configuration space are found, not distributions among all accessible states. In this regard the present analysis is similar to the treatment of local minimum energy secondary structures in the approximate analysis presented in Section IV.B.

The various secondary structures of DNA are regarded as having the mechanical properties of symmetric, linearly elastic rods. A piece of DNA which is torsionally and flexurally smoothly deformed away from its lowest energy shape will experience elastic restoring stresses across each cross section. These stresses are mechanically resolvable into a force $N(s)$ and a torque $M(s)$ acting at the center of each cross section, which may vary with position s along the rod.[69,70] In a constrained mechanical equilibrium conformation these forces and torques are balanced. This implies that the force vector N must be constant everywhere. The equilibrium condition on the torque is equivalent to an extremal condition on a quantity called the analogous action S. The stable equilibria are given by those extremals which are local minima of S. This is a consequence of the formal identity between the equations governing equilibria in symmetric, linearly elastic rods and those determining the motion of symmetric tops about a fixed point.[72] First noted by Kirchhoff, this identity is called the Kirchhoff kinetic analogy. The analogous action S is the difference between the elastic deformation strain energy K (analogous to the kinetic energy of a top) and the analogous potential energy V:

$$S = K - V = \int_0^L \frac{B\kappa^2(s)}{2} + \frac{C\tau^2(s)}{2} \, ds - \int_0^L N \cos \theta(s) \, ds \qquad (33)$$

where $N = |N|$, L is the length of the rod and $\theta(s)$ is the angle between the local tangent vector to the rod at position s and the force vector N.

The computations involved in this analysis are facilitated if the shape of the molecule is expressed using the Euler angles $\theta(s)$, $\phi(s)$, and $\psi(s)$.[69,71] These three angles describe the orientation of the unit tangent vector to the center of the molecule at each position s with respect to the fixed lab axes. The coordinates of a point along the rod may be recovered from these Euler angles as

$$x(s) = \int_0^s \sin \theta(s) \sin \phi(s) \, ds \qquad (34a)$$

$$y(s) = -\int_0^s \sin \theta(s) \cos \phi(s) \, ds \qquad (34b)$$

$$z(s) = \int_0^s \cos\theta(s)\,ds \tag{34c}$$

In terms of these Euler angles the analogous action is given by:[69]

$$S = \int_0^L \frac{B}{2}(\dot\phi^2 \sin^2\phi + \dot\theta^2) + \frac{C}{2}(\dot\phi\cos\theta + \dot\psi)^2 - N\cos\theta\,ds \tag{35}$$

The constraint imposed by the constancy of the linking number may also be expressed as an integral using the Euler angles as generalized coordinates:[71]

$$\Delta Lk = \frac{1}{2\pi}\int_0^L \dot\psi + \frac{\left(\dot\phi - \dfrac{2\pi}{L}\right)\cos\theta - \dot\theta\sin\left(\dfrac{2\pi s}{L} - \phi\right)}{1 - \sin\theta\cos\left(\dfrac{2\pi s}{L} - \phi\right)}ds \tag{36}$$

The superhelically constrained equilibrium tertiary structures are found by solving an iso-perimetric variational problem: to determine the extremals of the action integral subject to the constancy of the linking integral and the condition of smooth ring closure. One can show that the equilibrium Euler angles satisfy the following differential equations:[71]

$$\dot\theta^2 = 2\beta_3 - \eta\cos\theta - \frac{(\beta_2 - \gamma\beta_1\cos\theta)^2}{\sin^2\theta} \tag{37a}$$

$$\dot\phi = \frac{\beta_2 - \gamma\beta_1\cos\theta}{\sin^2\theta} \tag{37b}$$

$$\dot\psi = \beta_1 - \frac{\beta_2 - \gamma\beta_1\cos\theta}{\sin^2\theta}\cos\theta \tag{37c}$$

Here the β_is are constants of integration, $\gamma = C/B$, and $\eta = 2N/B$. The first of these equations may be solved in terms of the Jacobi elliptic function Sn to be[71]

$$\cos\theta(s) = u_1 + (u_2 - u_1)Sn^2(qs) \tag{38}$$

Here $-1 \leq u_1 \leq u_2 \leq 1$ are the limits of motion of $\cos\theta$. From this result the differential equations for ϕ and ψ may be solved by quadratures involving elliptic integrals.[69] In the equilibrium conformations the Euler angle θ oscillates between extrema θ_1 and θ_2. The number of oscillations of θ along the domain is an integer whose value depends upon q. When the torsional and bending stiffnesses have constant values at every point along the molecule, the equilibrium structure will be torsionally deformed a constant amount everywhere.[69]

The condition of smooth ring closure requires that the domain itself and its tangent indicatrix curve both be closed. These restrictions impose several conditions on the admissible solutions involving the allowed values of the constants of integration and the limits u_1 and u_2 of motion of θ. When this problem is solved, the equilibria are found to have the structure of toroidal helixes. The number of oscillations of θ as this structure is traversed is at least two.[71]

Interwound structures and others that involve points of molecular self-contact do not appear in this analysis because it assumes that no external forces are imposed. A completely satisfactory treatment of tertiary structure that encompasses cases having forces of self-contact has not been presented to date. However, interwound structures are expected to be equilibrium configurations which may compete effectively with toroidal conformations.

Another factor that is not included in this mechanical equilibrium analysis as presently formulated is configurational entropy. The global constraint imposed by the constancy of Lk severely restricts the accessible states of the system. This produces an entropic effect that will alter the effective free energy of configurations. At present there is little information regarding configurational entropy associated with superhelical tertiary structures. In particular, the entropy associated to toroidal vs. interwound structures is not understood. It has been claimed that this configurational entropy will not dominate over other sources of free energy.[73]

Small angle X-ray scattering experiments confirm that the superhelical equilibria of closed circular molecules usually have the structure of toroidal helixes,[74] although in one instance an interwound configuration was found.[75] The factors that determine which equilibrium is preferred are not known at present. It is possible that entropy is the factor favoring the toroidal configurations because there are so many more low energy toroidal configurations with a given writhing than there are interwound ones.

VI. GENERAL FORMULATIONS AND OTHER PROBLEMS

The analysis of conformational equilibria described in this chapter provides important information regarding superhelical DNA structure. It has resulted in numerous predictions regarding superhelical molecules. Although most of these predictions are beyond present experimental techniques to test, those that have been tested have all been verified.[34,41,49,64,74] In certain cases the application of these theoretical techniques to experimental results has permitted the evaluation of free energy parameters that were not previously known.[49]

One may amalgamate the analyses of secondary and tertiary structures described above to develop a unified treatment of superhelical equilibria. Although the calculations involved in carrying out such an analysis would be forbiddingly complex, in principle the construction of such a theory is a straightforward extension of the previous work involving the construction of a partition function encompassing all the available states of the system.

The enumeration of the accessible states first requires specifying all possible secondary structures available to the domain. For a fixed value of α each state of secondary structure has a specific amount of residual linking difference that must be accommodated by smooth deformations. Next, one must find those smoothly deformed configurations having this value of the residual linking difference. For static equilibria this is done by solving an isoperimetric problem as described in the previous section. If one wishes to consider dynamic equilibria involving tertiary structure, one must include all such smoothly deformed structures, not just those having minimum energy. In this case the space of all possible tertiary structures becomes a subvariety of an infinite dimensional manifold. An analysis of this type must be performed for each possible state of secondary structure. Next, a free energy is assigned to each state of transition and smooth deformation according to the principles described above. Finally, a partition function Z is constructed having mixed form of the type shown in Equation 13c. This Z may then be analyzed to determine the equilibrium properties of the system, at least in principle.

In addition to its extreme complexity, this program is impractical to pursue at present because several attributes of superhelical molecules are not sufficiently understood. Most importantly, the configurational entropy associated with tertiary structures will contribute to overall free energies in a manner that has not been completely analyzed. Also, the structural implications of the constancy of Lk have not been fully examined. It is clear that this constraint couples the torsional and flexural states of the molecule, because when Lk is fixed changes in Wr must be compensated by corresponding changes in Tw. However, it is not known precisely how tight this coupling is. For instance, in the configuration space of all possible tertiary structures of a smoothly closed molecule, does that subset consisting of structures having a particular value of Wr form a connected set? If so, one can sample all configurations having that value of Wr without altering Tw, suggesting a relatively loose coupling between these parameters. If not, then the transition between certain pairs of tertiary structures would require transient changes of Tw. In the most extreme case this subset might be an entirely disconnected collection of isolated points, so then transitions between any pair of configurations in this set would always require transient changes of Tw.

The complete treatment of DNA superhelicity requires an understanding of kinetics as well as of equilibria. Although knowledge of the conformational equilibria is useful, it is also important to know whether these equilibria are achieved in practice and if so how fast they are approached. The theoretical analysis of the kinetics of superhelical DNA configurations is subject in its infancy. However, experimental evidence suggests that kinetic phenomena may be quite complex. For example, it is known that the introduction of transient strand breaks results in the rapid approach to an equilibrium distribution around the relaxed state.[56,57] In contrast, there is some preliminary evidence suggesting that cruciform extrusion may sometimes, but not always, proceed rapidly to equilibrium. If the sequence intervening between the repeat copies is either G + C-rich or long, then the strand separation that is a necessary preliminary to cruciform extrusion may constitute a large free energy barrier to transition.[76,77] A reasonably complete treatment of the kinetics of superhelical structural transitions has yet to be developed.

ACKNOWLEDGMENTS

This work was supported in part by grants DMB 84-03523 and DMB 86-13371 from the National Science Foundation.

REFERENCES

1. **Vinograd, J. and Lebowitz, J.,** Physical and topological properties of circular DNA, *J. Gen. Physiol.,* 49, 103, 1965.
2. **White, J. H.,** Self-linking and the Gauss integral in higher dimensions, *Am. J. Math.,* 91, 693, 1969.
3. **Fuller, F. B.,** The writhing number of a space curve, *Proc. Natl. Acad. Sci. U.S.A.,* 68, 815, 1971.
4. **Bauer, W. R.,** Structure and reactions of closed duplex DNA, *Annu. Rev. Biophys. Bioeng.,* 7, 287, 1978.
5. **Gellert, M.,** DNA topoisomerases, *Annu. Rev. Biochem.,* 50, 879, 1981.
6. **Cozzarelli, N. R.,** DNA gyrase and the supercoiling of DNA, *Science,* 207, 953, 1980.
7. **Richardson, S. M. H., Higgins, C. F., and Lilley, D. M. J.,** The genetic control of DNA supercoiling in *Salmonella typhimurium, EMBO J.,* 3, 1745, 1984.
8. **Keller, W.,** Determination of the number of superhelical turns in simian virus 40 DNA by gel electrophoresis, *Proc. Natl. Acad. Sci. U.S.A.,* 72, 4876, 1975.
9. **Wells, R. D., Goodman, T., Hillen, W., Horn, G., Klein, R., Larson, J., Mueller, U., Neuendorf, S., Panayotatos, N., and Stirdivant, S.,** DNA structure and gene regulation, *Prog. Nucl. Acids Res. Mol. Biol.,* 24, 167, 1980.
10. **Smith, G. R.,** DNA supercoiling: another level for regulating gene expression, *Cell,* 24, 599, 1981.
11. **Kornberg, A.,** *DNA Replication,* W. H. Freeman, San Francisco, 1980.
12. **Sternglanz, R., DiNardo, S., Voelkel, K., Nishimura, Y., Hirota, Y., Becherer, K., Zumstein, L., and Wang, J. C.,** Mutations in the gene coding for *Escherichia coli* DNA topoisomerase I affect transcription and transposition, *Proc. Natl. Acad. Sci. U.S.A.,* 78, 2747, 1981.
13. **Radding, C. M.,** Genetic recombination: strand transfer and mismatch repair, *Annu. Rev. Biochem.,* 47, 847, 1978.
14. **Wang, J. C.,** Interactions between twisted DNAs and enzymes: the effects of superhelical turns, *J. Mol. Biol.,* 87, 797, 1974.

15. **Salemme, F. R.,** A model for catabolite activator protein binding to supercoiled DNA, *Proc. Natl. Acad. Sci. U.S.A.,* 79, 5263, 1982.

16. **Mattern, M. R. and Painter, R. B.,** Dependence of mammalian DNA replication on DNA supercoiling, *Biochim. Biophys. Acta,* 563, 293, 1979.

17. **Larson, A. and Weintraub, H.,** An altered DNA conformation detected by S1 nuclease occurs at specific regions in active chick globin chromatin, *Cell,* 29, 609, 1982.

18. **Luchnik, A. N. and Glaser, V. M.,** DNA topological linking numbers in malignantly transformed Syrian hamster cells, *Mol. Gen. Genet.,* 183, 553, 1981.

19. **Hartwig, M., Matthes, E., and Arnold, W.,** Extremely underwound chromosomal DNA in nucleoids of mouse sarcoma cells, *Cancer Lett.,* 13, 153, 1981.

20. **Helinski, D. R. and Clewell, D. B.,** Circular DNA, *Annu. Rev. Biochem.,* 40, 899, 1971.

21. **Alberts, B., Bray, D., Lewis, J., Raff, M., Roberts, R., and Watson, J. D.,** *The Molecular Biology of the Cell,* Garland Press, New York, 1983.

22. **McGhee, J. D. and Felsenfeld, G.,** Nucleosome structure, *Annu. Rev. Biochem.,* 49, 1115, 1980.

23. **Igo-Kemenes, T., Hoerz, W., and Zachau, H. G.,** Chromatin, *Annu. Rev. Biochem.,* 51, 89, 1982.

24. **Vogelstein, B., Pardoll, D. M., and Coffey, D. S.,** Supercoiled loops and eucaryotic DNA replication, *Cell,* 22, 79, 1980.

25. **Lilley, D. M. J.,** Eukaryotic genes — are they under torsional stress? *Nature (London),* 305, 276, 1983.

26. **Johnson, E. M., Campbell, G. R., and Allfrey, V. G.,** Different nucleosome structures on transcribing and non-transcribing ribosomal gene sequences, *Science,* 206, 1192, 1979.

27. **Smith, R. D., Seale, R. J., and Yu, J.,** Transcribed chromatin exhibits an altered nucleosomal spacing, *Proc. Natl. Acad. Sci. U.S.A.,* 80, 5505, 1983.

28. **Gordon, V. C., Knobler, C. M., Olins, D. E., and Schumaker, V. N.,** Conformational changes of the chromatin subunit, *Proc. Natl. Acad. Sci. U.S.A.,* 75, 660, 1978.

29. **Prior, C. P., Cantor, C. R., Johnson, E. M., Littau, V. C., and Allfrey, V. G.,** Reversible changes in nucleosome structure and histone H3 accessibility in transcriptionally active and inactive states of rDNA chromatin, *Cell,* 34, 1033, 1983.

30. **Sinden, R. R. and Pettijohn, D. E.,** Chromosomes in living *Escherichia coli* cells are segregated into domains of supercoiling, *Proc. Natl. Acad. Sci. U.S.A.,* 78, 224, 1981.

31. **Pettijohn, D. E. and Pfenninger, O.,** Supercoils in prokaryotic DNA restrained *in vivo, Proc. Natl. Acad. Sci. U.S.A.,* 77, 1331, 1980.

32. **Vinograd, J., Lebowitz, J., and Watson, R.,** Early and late helix-coil transitions in closed circular DNA, *J. Mol. Biol.,* 33, 173, 1968.

33. **Woodworth-Gutai, M. and Lebowitz, J.,** Introduction of interrupted secondary structure in supercoiled DNA as a function of superhelix density: consideration of hairpin structures in superhelical DNA, *J. Virol.,* 18, 195, 1976.

34. **Lilley, D. M. J.,** The inverted repeat as a recognizable structural feature in supercoiled DNA molecules, *Proc. Natl. Acad. Sci. U.S.A.,* 77, 6468, 1980.

35. **Benham, C. J.,** Theoretical analysis of transitions between B- and Z-conformations in torsionally stressed DNA, *Nature (London),* 286, 637, 1980.

36. **Bram, S. and Tougard, P.,** Polymorphism of natural DNA, *Nature (London),* 239, 128, 1972.

37. **Zimmerman, S. B.,** The three-dimensional structure of DNA, *Annu. Rev. Biochem.,* 51, 395, 1982.

38. **Gierer, A.,** Model for DNA and protein interactions and the function of the operator, *Nature (London),* 212, 1480, 1966.

39. **Bloomfield, V. A., Crothers, D. M., and Tinoco, I.,** *Physical Chemistry of Nucleic Acids,* Harper & Row, New York, 1974.

40. **Record, M. T., Mazur, S. J., Melancon, P., Roe, J. H., Shaner, S. L., and Unger, L.,** Double helical DNA: conformations, physical properties, and interactions with ligands, *Annu. Rev. Biochem.,* 50, 997, 1981.

41. **Rich, A., Nordheim, A., and Wang, A. H.-J.,** The chemistry and biology of left-handed Z-DNA, *Annu. Rev. Biochem.,* 53, 791, 1984.

42. **Wang, J. C.,** Helical repeat of DNA in solution, *Proc. Natl. Acad. Sci. U.S.A.,* 76, 200, 1979.

43. **Hagerman, P. J.,** Investigation of the flexibility of DNA using transient electric birefringence, *Biopolymers,* 20, 1503, 1981.

44. **Thomas, T. J. and Bloomfield, V. A.,** Chain flexibility and hydrodynamics of the B- and Z-forms of poly(dG-dC)·poly(dG-dC), *Nucl. Acids Res.,* 11, 1919, 1983.

45. **Barkley, M. D. and Zimm, B. H.,** Theory of twisting and bending of chain molecules: analysis of the fluorescence depolarization of DNA, *J. Chem. Phys.,* 70, 2991, 1979.

46. **Shore, D. and Baldwin, R. L.,** Energetics of DNA twisting, *J. Mol. Biol.,* 170, 957, 1983.

47. **Crothers, D. and Spatz, H.,** Theory of friction-limited DNA unwinding, *Biopolymers,* 10, 1949, 1971.

48. **Klysik, J., Stirdivant, S. M., Singleton, C. K., Zacharias, W., and Wells, R. D.,** Effects of 5 cytosine methylation on the B-Z transition in DNA restriction fragments and recombinant plasmids, *J. Mol. Biol.,* 168, 51, 1983.

49. **Peck, L. and Wang, J. C.,** Energetics of B-to-Z transition in DNA, *Proc. Natl. Acad. Sci. U.S.A.,* 80, 6206, 1983.

50. **Ivanov, I., Minchenkova, L., Minyat, E., Frank-Kamenetskii, M., and Schyolkina, A.,** The B to A transition of DNA in solution, *J. Mol. Biol.,* 87, 817, 1974.

51. **Crothers, D. M. and Zimm, B. H.,** Theory of the melting transition of synthetic polynucleotides: evaluation of the stacking energy, *J. Mol. Biol.,* 9, 1, 1964.

52. **Hogan, M., LeGrange, J., and Austin, B.,** Dependence of DNA helix flexibility on base composition, *Nature (London),* 304, 752, 1983.

53. **Mahendrasingam, A., Pigram, W., Fuller, W., Brahms, J., and Vergne, J.,** Conformational transitions in the synthetic polynucleotide poly[d(G-C)]·poly[d(G-C)] double helix, *J. Mol. Biol.,* 168, 897, 1983.

54. **Mandal, C., Kallenbach, N., and Englander, S. W.,** Base-pair opening and closing reactions in the double helix, *J. Mol. Biol.,* 135, 391, 1980.

55. **Poland, D. and Scheraga, H. A.,** *Theory of Helix-Coil Transitions in Biopolymers,* Academic Press, New York, 1970.

56. **Pulleyblank, D. E., Shure, M., Tang, D., Vinograd, J., and Vosberg, H.-P.,** Action of nicking-closing enzyme on supercoiled and non-supercoiled closed circular DNA: formation of a Boltzmann distribution of topological isomers, *Proc. Natl. Acad. Sci. U.S.A.,* 72, 4280, 1975.

57. **Depew, R. E. and Wang, J. C.,** Conformational fluctuations of DNA helix, *Proc. Natl. Acad. Sci. U.S.A.,* 72, 4275, 1975.

58. **Benham, C. J.,** Torsional stress and local denaturation in supercoiled DNA, *Proc. Natl. Acad. Sci. U.S.A.,* 76, 3870, 1979.

59. **Benham, C. J.,** The equilibrium statistical mechanics of the helix-coil transition in torsionally stressed DNA, *J. Chem. Phys.,* 72, 3633, 1980.

60. **Eisenberg, D. and Crothers, D. M.,** *Physical Chemistry with Applications to the Life Sciences,* Benjamin/ Cummings Publishing, Menlo Park, Calif., 1979, chap. 14.

61. **Vollenweider, H. J., Fiandt, M., and Szybalski, W.,** A relationship between DNA helix stability and recognition sites for RNA polymerase, *Science,* 205, 508, 1979.

62. **van Mansfield, A., Langeveld, S., Baas, P., Jansz, H., van der Marel, G., Veeneman, G., and van Boom, J.,** Recognition sequence of bacteriophage φX174 gene A protein — an initiator of DNA replication, *Nature (London),* 288, 561, 1980.

63. **Gotoh, O. and Tagashira, Y.,** Locations of frequently opening regions on natural DNA and their relationship to functional loci, *Biopolymers,* 20, 1043, 1981.

64. **Sheflin, L. G. and Kowalski, D.,** Altered DNA conformations detected by mung bean nuclease occur in promoter and terminator regions of supercoiled pBR322 DNA, *Nucl. Acids Res.,* 13, 6137, 1985.

65. **Benham, C. J.,** Cruciform formation at inverted repeat sequences in supercoiled DNA, *Biopolymers,* 21, 679, 1982.

66. **Benham, C. J.,** Statistical mechanical analysis of competing conformational transitions in superhelical DNA, *Cold Spring Harbor Symp. Quant. Biol.,* 47, 219, 1982.

67. **Benham, C. J.,** Theoretical analysis of conformational equilibria in superhelical DNA, *Annu. Rev. Biophys. Biophys. Chem.,* 14, 23, 1985.

68. **Benham, C. J.,** Theoretical analysis of competitive conformational transitions in torsionally stressed DNA, *J. Mol. Biol.,* 150, 43, 1981.

69. **Benham, C. J.,** An elastic model of the large-scale structure of duplex DNA, *Biopolymers,* 18, 609, 1979.

70. **Benham, C. J.,** Elastic model of supercoiling, *Proc. Natl. Acad. Sci. U.S.A.,* 74, 2397, 1977.

71. **Benham, C. J.,** Geometry and mechanics of DNA superhelicity, *Biopolymers,* 22, 2477, 1983.

72. **Love, A. E. H.,** *A Treatise on the Mathematical Theory of Elasticity,* Dover Publishing, New York, 1944.

73. **Laiken, N.,** Theoretical model for the equilibrium behavior of DNA superhelices, *Biopolymers,* 12, 11, 1973.

74. **Brady, G., Fein, D., Lambertson, H., Grassian, V., Foos, D., and Benham, C. J.,** X-ray scattering from the superhelix in circular DNA, *Proc. Natl. Acad. Sci. U.S.A.,* 80, 741, 1983.

75. **Brady, G., Foos, D., and Benham, C. J.,** Evidence for an interwound form for the superhelix in circular DNA, *Biopolymers,* 23, 2963, 1984.

76. **Gellert, M., O'Dea, M., and Mizuuchi, K.,** Slow cruciform transitions in palindromic DNA, *Proc. Natl. Acad. Sci. U.S.A.,* 80, 5545, 1983.

77. **Greaves, D. R., Patient, R. K., and Lilley, D. M. J.,** Facile cruciform formation from a *Xenopus* globin gene, *J. Mol. Biol.,* 185, 461, 1985.

INDEX